To Hugh,

Memories of St Mary's

Alasdair Know.

Affectionate memoRIes
to a dear frigend and
colleague.

Dean Craig.

DOCTORS AT WAR

Oscar Craig
Emeritus Consultant, St Mary's Hospital, London W2
Past Director, Clinical Studies, St Mary's Hospital Medical School,
London W2

Alasdair Fraser
Emeritus Consultant, St Mary's Hospital, London W2
Past Director, Clinical Studies, St Mary's Hospital Medical School,
London W2

DOCTORS AT WAR

by

OSCAR CRAIG AND
ALASDAIR FRASER

The Memoir Club

First published in 2007 by
The Memoir Club
Stanhope Old Hall
Stanhope
Weardale
County Durham

British Library Cataloguing in
Publication Data.
A catalogue record for this book
is available from the
British Library

ISBN: 978-1-84104-171-1

Typeset by TW Typesetting, Plymouth, Devon
Printed by Biddles Ltd, King's Lynn

Dedication

This book is dedicated to St Mary's Hospital Medical School and to all the students who have studied there and the teachers who taught them.

Contents

List of Illustrations

Foreword

These letters, written during wars from 1897 until the Peace of 1945, and discovered amongst the archives of the *St Mary's Gazette*, were preserved and prepared for publication by Dr Oscar Craig and Dr Alasdair Fraser, both consultants at St Mary's. This cache of letters presents a unique saga of war as seen by doctors and nurses at the forefront of battle. Their experience of the horrors at close quarters in war have been vividly described in this series of unsolicited letters to the Editor of the *Gazette*. They were not professional journalists but doctors and nurses who were at war and wrote of their immediate experiences. Neither were they politically correct but expressed honest comments on their lives as soldiers. The *Gazette* itself was a boost to morale; a super efficient Royal Engineers' postal service delivered them to widely scattered parts of the world.

The lives of Regimental Medical Officers (RMO) are perceptibly described, and range from the bush warfare of Benin to the campaigns in South Africa, the Western and Eastern fronts of WWI to the worldwide theatres of war in WWII. The RMO is forward at the edge of the battle supervising stretcher-bearers and performing skilled first aid. The Royal Naval Surgeon is equally exposed.

Shown through these letters is the development of surgery dealing with missile injuries, improvement in the evacuation of the wounded, the surgical techniques of primary excision with delayed primary or secondary closure described from each generation of war surgeons. To shorten the distance and time to surgery the Casualty Clearing Stations (CCS) were moved closer to the battle.

Here is told the incredible results that emanated from those pioneers of St Mary's – Almroth Wright and Alexander Fleming. The development of Anti-typhoid (TAB), Tetanus Toxoid, antigas serum and later penicillin can all be traced. Vivid descriptions of the body's reaction to the early vaccines are given.

Tropical medicine and the principles of field hygiene are given their proper recognition; the medical morbidity and death rates were always higher than the surgical cases.

One of the outstanding letters was from one of the medical students who had just returned from the Belsen Concentration Camp describing the horrors they had seen and had dealt with.

There is also a cool, calm, clinical account of the Japanese inhuman conduct in one of the better Far East POW Camps. The Stanley Camp in Hong Kong although awful was not as bad as those in Sumatra or Java. The horror of the death of Dr John Diver in one of these camps is recorded for posterity to remember the sadism of the Japanese conqueror. After liberation POWs were evacuated with diseases, infective and from starvation and with stress effects they would endure for their lifetime.

The Army Medical Services Museum in Aldershot has twenty-three VCs on display; this book shows why.

Drs Oscar Craig and Alasdair Fraser have rendered an invaluable service to the medical history of warfare by discovering and publishing these letters. To make them of more interest they have researched the lives of the letter-writers and often their postwar careers.

This is a book which should be read by doctors, nurses, medical students and historians. It should be compulsory for gung-ho politicians.

Major-General Norman Kirby, OBE, FRCS

Acknowledgements

We wish to thank Kevin Brown. archivist to St Mary's Hospital and the last editor of the *St Mary's Hospital Medical School Gazette* for permission to print the letters from the *Gazette* for without his permission this book could not have been written.

The authors also wish to thank the St Mary's Development Trust for funding the publication of this book.

Preface

In July 1844 a plot of land in Paddington was given by the Lord Bishop of London, to build a hospital originally called the Paddington and Marylebone Hospital, but later St Mary's Hospital because of its close proximity to St Mary's Church. The foundation stone was laid by Prince Albert in 1845. The decision to build an associated medical school was finalised in 1851 and formally opened in 1854. The Medical School *Gazette* was produced and published by the students of the school until the school was joined to the medical schools of Westminster and Charing Cross in the new Imperial College School of Medicine in the latter part of the twentieth century.

Letters written by St Mary's Hospital Medical School graduates were found in the archives of the school by Alasdair Fraser. These letters had been published in the Medical School *Gazette* and each described personal experiences during service in various wars, the Benin Expedition, the Boer War and World Wars I and II. They illustrated the duties and difficulties of medical officers at and behind the front line. From these letters, the changing pattern of human behaviour in battle from the nineteenth to the twentieth century unfolds as does the chivalry and patriotism of the fighting man. They illustrate the horrors of war, suffering, courage and sacrifice and the tragic loss of young lives.

The duties of the medical officers differ in many significant ways from those of the civilian doctor. In civil practice there is a crucial doctor/patient relationship but the military doctor has an officer/soldier relationship. For most doctors this is a difficult transition as he may then have to give priority in treatment to those men most likely to return to the front line of combat. During World Wars I and II civilian doctors recruited into the armed forces made up most of the medical force. In World War I half of the nation's doctors were serving with the forces. They found themselves dealing with issues outside their normal practice, especially those of public health, preventative medicine, epidemics of infectious diseases, body infestations and poor hygiene, venereal disease, malingerers and shell shock. Seldom were they free from danger and they were called upon for the immediacy of front line treatment. They had responsibility for sanitation, water supplies, and the routine physical and psychological care of the fighting force. The nature of war wounds and their contamination were a constant challenge and surgery under enemy fire proved an additional hazard.

The part played by St Mary's Hospital doctors and nurses was considerable, and no doubt equalled by others from sister hospitals and medical schools. However there were two St Mary's doctors whose work had an influence of gigantic proportions on the health of the entire fighting force, namely Sir Almroth Wright and Sir Alexander Fleming. Their contribution is mentioned in some of the letters in this book but the overall influence of their work permeates the accounts of events. It is remarkable that these two very different medical titans, master and pupil, worked in the same laboratory at St Mary's Hospital and played such a major part in the outcome of two world wars, where disease and sickness were as much the enemy as bullets and shells.

The letters in this book are a record of the time when patriotism was foremost in the minds of those engaged in battle for their country and its beliefs. The question is unanswered as to whether or not this strong emotive force still exists or could be called upon for similar conflicts. Chivalry in war was also a respected human quality and is portrayed in these letters. In the Boer War, the Boers apologised to those British medical staff they bombarded thinking they were an ammunition convoy, and ceased as soon as they discovered their mistake.

The role of the non-combatant was respected by both sides; often captured doctors were released to return to their comrades.

The Red Cross, founded in 1864, was to help wounded or captured soldiers and the symbol of the cross was respected on both sides. Is this the same today? We have heard of ships displaying the red cross being bombarded in the recent wars.

The Geneva Convention formed in 1864 was concerned with the protection of wounded soldiers and the control of materials of war such as the dum-dum bullets, whose explosive force caused untold damage and suffering. Today we fear the manufacture of chemical and bacterial weaponry and nuclear explosives. Fortunately the doctors' duty still includes the care of the wounded from whatever side. The letters give examples of this. We have to ask if this duty would still apply and though lacking in evidence we trust it would.

Many St Mary's doctors did distinguished service in the Boer War of 1899–1902, and the Roll of Honour lists six who gave their lives. In World War I many served in the Army, Navy and Air Force and many had high rank and distinction. Sir John Goodwin was appointed Director General of the Army Medical Service in 1918. Sir E.W.C. Bradfield became Director General of the Indian Medical Service. Many consultants served with temporary high ranks, among them Sir Almroth Wright and Sir Alexander Fleming. Of the large number serving in the forces in World War I, forty-four lost their lives. In World War II St Mary's Hospital was in the thick of the bombing of London and the staff and students played crucial roles in dealing with civilian casualties. Six hundred St Mary's graduates served in the forces. Thirty-one received decorations, forty-one were mentioned in dispatches and twenty-one gave their lives.

In these conflicts many students wished to volunteer for active service in fighting units, and some did, but the War Office encouraged students to continue their studies and enlist as medical officers. It was pointed out that their value to the armed forces was greater as qualified doctors. A number of letters written to the *Gazette* from the front supports this advice and reinforces the invaluable service given by medical graduates of many schools to their country and the forces fighting for it.

These letters from the front are a testament to the part played by St Mary's graduates at war.

(The letters have been reproduced exactly as written by the authors. No attempt has been made to edit the variations in spelling, the punctuation or the style of the prose. To have done so might alter the character or tone they convey.)

CHAPTER 1

The Benin Expedition of 1897

Benin was a powerful kingdom in the South Nigerian rainforest. It was founded in the thirteenth century AD, and has been a colony of the Portuguese, a French Protectorate in 1892 and conquered by the British in 1897. The Portuguese used Benin to supply cloth, beads and slaves, and the slave-trade was encouraged by its ruler, the Oba. It was noted for its culture of life-sized bronze heads and ivories and thousands of its art objects and antiquities were brought back to England following the expedition of 1897. Benin embraced Marxism in 1972 and changed its name from Dahomey to The Peoples' Republic of Benin. Marxism was abandoned in 1989 and it became the Republic of Benin. It has a population of 6,517,000 and covers an area of 43,472 square miles.

The Benin Expedition resulted from the ambush and massacre of a party of British officers and traders who travelled to Benin to open advantageous trade relations. Lt. James Phillips, an officer under Ralph Moor, the governor of the Niger Coast Protectorate, sent a message to King Oba announcing an impending 'visit'. The 'visit' was made by a small force of ten British officers and a column of 200 African porters. The group was ambushed and among the dead were Phillips and eight other British officers. The massacre caused a public outcry which compelled Lord Salisbury's government to send a punitive force. In February 1897, 1,200 British soldiers, which included a Naval squadron and Marines, and the local Niger Coast Protectorate Force invaded Benin. A member of the Naval ships was Petty Officer Callaghan, the father of a future Prime Minister, James Callaghan. Dr Felix Roth (1865–1921), a graduate of St Mary's Hospital Medical School, at the age of twenty eight, joined the Niger Coast Force and served in the Benin Expedition. He wrote letters to the St Mary's Hospital Medical School *Gazette* which were published in March 1899 and they covered the period from 7 February to 22 February 1897.

A Diary of a Surgeon with the Benin Punitive Expedition
By Felix N. Roth MRCS, LRCP

Colonel Bruce Hamilton, Major Landon, Captains Carter, Ringer and Searle and Gregory of H.M.S. Theseus, myself and 260 Protectorate troops, one Maxim (automatic machine gun, manufactured by Vickers), two seven-pounders, and carriers arrived at Ceri from the first landing place,

Warriga, at 4.00 p.m. on February 6th, 1897. We are up here before the naval men in order to cut a path for them and clear the ground for their camp, and look after its sanitary arrangements. As soon as we arrived we encamped in the native village; pickets were out for the night, and just at the present moment the officer is going his rounds, the bugle having sounded the last post. It is a strange life, black troops lying about all over the place, laughing and gibbering like a lot of monkeys. A dull cloudy night, and plenty of mosquitoes to keep us all awake, gives a man time to think what the future will bring, when once we have started into the Benin country.

February 7th
Ceri.

I slept last night on the ground in a native hut, it being too late to rig up a bed or couch. This morning I looked after the sanitary arrangements of the camp for the naval column; that means we have to make everything comfortable for the naval brigade, which is expected on the 10th or 11th of February. We are called the advance guard and have plenty of work. We cut roads, build trenches, get up stores from Warriga; in fact we have to do all the nursing, as it were, so that the naval men will not be exposed in the severe climate, and may have as little as possible to do. Searle and Carter are looking after the troops to-day, Landon and Ringer are busy with the carriers, arranging stores, and Gregory of H.M.S. Theseus is taking positions.

February 8th
Ceri.

We are still at this place, getting things (houses, etc.) ready for the naval column. We did a lot of work to-day. I found a spring and have dammed it up so that a large number of men can draw water from it. To-night Major Galwey, our consul, and Executive Commander Bacon have got a canoe and boys and are reconnoitring up the Ologbo Creek to find out if there is any branch connecting with Benin city. We think there must be a branch, as we cannot understand how else the Benin city people can obtain their drinking water. It is rather a risky undertaking for the two men, but they are both cautious, and will no doubt bring back a lot of useful information. They cannot go during the day, as when we tried a little while back one of our officers was fired upon. In so far as I can find out, we shall cut a road from Ceri to a position opposite Ologbo Town, which is a few miles distant from here. We shall then shell Ologbo itself, land some black troops, and build a suspension bridge, which has been prepared by the naval men. The span is about 70 or 80 yards; we are not sure of the length, but shall know in a day or two. We will then most probably form a big base there, land the naval brigade and stores, etc., and make a start to cut the bush path which leads to Benin. The following is to be the order of procedure:-

Captain Turner, of the Protectorate, will scout with about 60 Bini men, the same who did the scouting for the Ashanti Expedition in 1873. These men will work through the bush to find out where the natives may be lurking; they will be supported by our black troops, but how many I do not know. Then come the bush cutters and more black troops, with two doctors, one being myself. We shall do this until we get close to Benin, when a naval column will come up and help to take the city; this is to take place within seven or eight days. There may be a little fighting, but such care will be taken that I think few men will be killed. Urini is the native name for Benin City. So far all the white men are fit; I trust few will go down with fever.

February 9th
Ceri.

It is really quite a sight to see the black troops quartered in this native town of Ceri; there are 250 of them. One is tumbling over them all day, or rather all night, as during the day they are hard at work in the camp which we are making for the white troops here. The officers' mess is also quite a sight; we are thirteen, all told. Searle who is working like a nigger all day building huts in the camp, is also looking after all the provisions for the mess, and I am mess president, looking after the food of course, and bossing the black boys and cook, and seeing that the water is boiled before distribution. I seem to be busy all day, and when night comes I feel that very little has been done. Last night we sounded the assembly, so as to get the men to their posts, just as if we were having a night attack from the natives; the men turned out well; they were all dressed and in their accoutrements and at their posts in about two-and-a-half minutes, which is considered very good. After inspecting them to see that they had come to their proper places, we dismissed them to their quarters. The gunners under Searle were prepared for action in the short space of two-and-a-quarter minutes, all fully equipped.

It seems strange to sit under a thatched roof on four posts, and eat our food in the open, and then after dinner to clear away and write letters. As I sit here at the present moment, a big ant walks calmly over my paper, or some insect drops from the roof down my neck; as of course we all wear shirts unbuttoned at the neck, we give the insects etc., every chance. Then again the chattering of the native troops is rather astonishing; one would think we were really amongst a lot of women. Unfortunately we are not, God bless them all the same. Many amongst us will wish for their tender care to nurse us as we go down with the fever or by the enemy's shot.

February 10th
Ceri.

I have had a talk with Locke and Boisragon, and from this conversation I gather it seems that it is rather Phillips fault that the massacre took place. The members of the expedition all tried to persuade him to give up the idea of going, even Crawford who was a sort of dare-devil, was against his going up, and several of the friendly chiefs went down on their knees, begging him not to go, as they felt very certain all would be killed. Yet after all this warning, Phillips persisted in attempting to go to Benin, and even gave orders that no one should wear arms, except well concealed ones. But as the members of the expedition wore only shirts and trousers they could not even carry revolvers, and so left them in their boxes, which the carriers had on their heads. Yet there must have been some sort of treachery, as the King of Benin, to a certain extent, was willing they should come up and see him. Besides the Bini did not attack them at once, as they wished to find out if the expedition were armed or not, and also have time to make an ambuscade. All the white men who were massacred behaved well. Dr Elliott again and again rushed in among the natives, who were several deep, and who were armed with long flint-locks, and although he was fired at, he struck right and left at them with only a stick. Poor Maling too, did his best, and like Crawford, while dying, told the others to run for their lives and leave him. A pity such fine men should fall in such a treacherous manner. Little Chumpy Lion has a seven year old nigger servant, who has been taught, when he brings a drink to anybody, to say the following:- "God bless the Queen, and I hope you will knock hell out of the King of Benin." He says this while saluting, with a most serious face. The Admiral and Staff, with our Consul-General, came up to-day to look about the place; it was astonishing how he managed to walk the distance from Warriga to Ceri, it was so very hot. He will be carried back, and quite right too, as he is rather a heavy man. Captain Egerton, who is at the head of the staff, decided in consultation with the others, to build a bridge across the Ologbo Creek, about half a mile higher up the creek than this village of Ceri. It will be a swinging one, made of steel wires, and attached at each end to trees on each side of the creek, which we find is about 120 feet across, something like the old chain pier at Brighton, the footpath being swung in the same manner. The gear for the same will be brought down the river to-night, and to-morrow the engineers start work in earnest.

While this is going on a party of black troops, over one hundred strong, with a seven-pounder and a Maxim, will reconnoitre inland for about a thousand yards. We shall have scouts in advance, and I am to accompany them as medical officer; I hope the natives will not spot any of us. We know of, and also notice, natives in hiding opposite Ceri. We are also to be supported by an armed launch, and surf boats full of men well armed with Maxims and rifles. I heard to-day we are most probably to make a start for Benin on the 11th, but I think it must be later. Before I proceed I must mention that a column called the Sapoba Column is to go to Sapoba, and is to consist of men from H.M.S. Phoebe, Alecto, and Widgeon. Another column, the Gwatto, is to consist of men from H.M.S. Philomel, Barrossa, and perhaps the Magpie. This last column is to destroy all the Bini towns on the eastern bank of the Gwatto Creek as far as Ikuro. Both columns are to be assisted by canoes, and are to patrol the river with their boats, and prevent fugitives from passing. Seven more men joined our mess to-night at a moment's notice. Their chairs were ammunition boxes – one dish, the piece-de-resistance, was a washing basin, containing an Irish hash. Being short of knives and forks, one man was obliged to have a mouthful, and then pass the table cutlery to the next man.

February 11th
Ceri.

The boat scouring party which started this morning, consisting of a hundred men under Colonel Hamilton, went up the river about a mile and a half, and landed on the other side, where a few huts were seen. From there a short trip was made into the bush, but the ground seemed very swampy, it was obliged to return after traversing only a few hundred yards. Another party under Searle, with the same number of men, a Maxim and seven-pounders, acted as a reserve on this side of the river. It is now found to be impossible to throw a bridge over the creek, and tomorrow a party is to make a start from Ologbo towards Benin. All the Protectorate troops, under Erskine and Turner, will cross the Ologbo Creek. The scouts to proceed first to see that we are not ambuscaded. Colonel Hamilton will be in command, and I am to go as medical officer. We have been busy all day preparing loads for the carriers. I am in charge of the mess and the mess gear, and, as the fellows are a hungry lot, it can be easily imagined what a work I will have to do to feed them. Up till now they have been very good, and have hardly grumbled or sworn at me at all. Captain Boisragon is invalided and leaves for home at once; we do not think he is fit for active service, as he is still suffering from a shock due to his very severe experiences during that awful massacre of a month ago. The weather is very hot and very dry for this country; it has not rained since we arrived here a month ago. I have asked Consul-General Moor, in case I am knocked over, to sell all my effects; we expect some heavy bush fighting to-morrow. A marine from H.M.S. Theseus died yesterday from heat apoplexy, but this is nothing, as many more will go down similarly. At present the men are in splendid condition. I have just heard that there has been a brush with the natives at Gwatto, four blue jackets and an officer wounded. I am too busy to write more news, but I hope to do so to-morrow. We had a little surprise to-night, as some shots were fired into camp, and the fellows got startled.

February 12th
Ologbo.

We started from Ceri yesterday at about 6 pm, in the launch "Primrose" and in surf boats, with 256 black troops, two Maxims, one seven-pounder, and half a company of blue-jackets, with one Maxim and a rocket tube. As I got my orders about half-an-hour before we started I was unprepared. Luckily, I always have my water bottle filled at night, but I had no rations. As I passed the Admiral's quarters I noticed a nice block of naval chocolate lying neatly in some paper outside his door. I stole the chocolate. We went up the Ologbo Creek for about three miles, until we reached Ologbo. We shelled the village, and cleared it of the natives. As the launch and surf boats grounded we jumped into the water, which reached to our waists, at once placed our Maxims and guns in position, firing so as to clear the bush where the natives might be hiding. We rushed on some hundred yards, again put our guns in position, and, in conjunction with volley firing again cleared the bush. We expect the second division to come up to our support in about two hours' time, as we sent the launch and surf boats back to fetch them. While holding the place the natives crept up on us several times, howling at the top of their voices, and firing at us. They attacked us first in the front, and then on each flank. Luckily we kept them at bay with volley firing and our Maxims, and only Captain Coe, of the N.C.P. Force, was severely wounded in the wrist. But luckily several other officers and men were hit by spent bullets only. After that we had drinks, and enjoyed the Admiral's chocolate. Soon afterwards more men came up, and we took our troops into the bush and cleared the natives out as well as possible.

This path to Benin City is only two or three feet broad, allowing sometimes two men to walk abreast, but as a rule are obliged to walk in single file. The natives showed some cuteness, for on one side of the road they had cut a track for some hundreds of yards, so as to be able to fire on us as we went up. Luckily for ourselves, we found this ambuscade at once, thanks to our scouts; and troops were sent up it. We went straight on for about three-quarters of a mile, with Maxims working in front and on the flank; at the same time volley firing was kept up by the troops, so as to clear the bush on each side of us. We arrived at a small village which we cleared with Maxims and rockets, and then rushed in, the natives clearing out right and left. We then put our pickets all round the place, and under their cover troops and carriers cut down the bush, so as to clear the place and allow us to see in case we were attacked by the natives. We camped here for the night, putting out double sentries everywhere. We shall remain here until we get our supplies, consisting of ammunition, rations for officers and men, and particularly water, which has always to be boiled. The usual routine of bush fighting is to use the Maxims in the front, and to keep up volley firing on the flanks by the troops. The men then rush ahead and again clear the bush, and so on. The first division is under Colonel Hamilton, a most charming man, very quiet and "all there", very energetic and cool, too; the climate does not seem to affect him much, although it has been very hot and very damp. The bush looks lovely: there are any amount of big trees about the place, and the green is of a rich colour, and it seems quite a mistake that there should be such a lot of hostile blacks about these quiet places. The village is, as usual, very straggling; still it gives us good shelter at night. We have been lucky so far; there has been no rain, and we all hope there will not be any before we get to Benin City. At Ologbo, Captain Campbell of H.M.S. Theseus, in charge of second division, is making a camp, arranging everything, getting our supplies over from Ceri, boiling the drinking water, building a hospital, and making sanitary arrangements and all ready that may be necessary for a good camp.

February 13th

We had rather a busy and exciting day yesterday. About 60 black scouts, under Turner of our force and Erskine of the Navy, came up to-day to scout in advance of us to find out the movements of the natives. The Admiral had been rather seedy after his walk in the sun from Warriga to Ceri; he got overheated; but he told me he was better yesterday, and I think he will be all right to-day. Our bridge could not be made as we should have had to walk three miles through the swamp opposite Ologbo. I had a chat with Moor, our Consul-General; he told me the following:- On February 10th Gwatto was attacked and occupied by naval men; one officer and two men of H.M.S. Widgeon severely wounded, one officer and one man of H.M.S. Philomel slightly wounded. On February 11th Sapoba and roads at back were occupied by naval men. Whilst stockading camp there

Pritchard and one man of H.M.S. Alecto were killed. So our column has so far fared the best; but it won't last long, and we shall have to fight our way up to Benin City. Some more men have gone down with sunstroke, but I have not seen or heard of any case of malarial fever yet. Smallpox has broken out among some of the Sierra Leone carriers; but it is of a mild sort of form, and somehow it has never been known to have been communicated by the blacks to the white men. We make another start late to-day or to-morrow; we have seen no natives since yesterday, but some have crept up and fired into us. We believe they are concentrating their forces at the next village or somewhere on the road to Benin City, for their final stand. Of course, they may ambuscade themselves, and try to stop us, but we will succeed in the long run, however many men we may lose. We are now in the Bini Country, and the houses in the village are thatched in a different way to the other villages we have passed so far. They are covered with leaves only, tied up in bunches, and not with big palm leaves. Then again the walls are made with split wood, and not of mud, as in the other places. We shall have great difficulty in getting water up here, and it is uncomfortable to be without it. We are dirty and dust-begrimed, unshaven, and sticky; our clothes are wet, and at night all the horrid animals of the bush crawl over us and sting us.

February 15th
Cross-Road Camp.

We left the Ologbo Camp yesterday morning at 6am, but a little before 3am, we had a night alarm, the natives came round part of the camp, beat the tom-toms for our edification, and kept us awake and on the alert, ready for our start. Allman, the principal medical officer, and myself, of the N.C. Protectorate, dressed and got pottering round, getting our carriers in order, and collecting hammocks and stretchers for the wounded. Well, we started at daybreak, Colonel Hamilton in command, with 260 black troops, one rocket tube, two Maxims, one Navy Maxim, two seven-pounders, a company of marines, and 40 scouts. We proceeded up the Benin road for about three miles, when the natives, who were in ambush, fired upon us again and again. We cleared them out with Maxims and volley firing several times, but they again came on and fired into us. We again cleared them out of the bush with Maxims, and forced them to retire, and after our column had done another mile or so, we formed camp for the night. Our firing was pretty hot, the rattling of the Maxims and rifles, the shouting of the officers, the howling of the enemy, and the excitement amongst our own carriers, is beyond me to describe. The excitement in the dense bush, the smoke, the working of the seven-pounders, and the whizzing past of our rockets, put the fear of God both into ourselves and the natives. I picked up one man shot through the thigh, and another through the lungs. Luckily, no white men were wounded; we all got off scot-free. We marched in single file, the scouts in front, followed by a half company of black troops under white officers, then followed a Maxim, with one in reserve; myself, with stretcher party were close behind them. We seem to be doing all the fighting up at this end of the column. I cannot tell the order of the middle and the rear part of the column, which is nearly three miles long, being much too busy at my end. We had now cleared the natives out of their camp, and the troops, in conjunction with my stretcher party, started to build a hospital. This consists of four upright posts, fixed into the ground, and lashed together at the top with cross-pieces, all tightly fixed together by a native creeper called "tie-tie". The roof consists of the hammocks laid on the cross-pieces. Being at the head of the column, where all the fighting takes place, most of the wounded come under my hands first. Every time a man is wounded the whole column stops, the path being so narrow we can only march in single file. It is impossible for me to do much for the wounded. If a man is bleeding badly I simply put on a tourniquet or a dressing, and leave him on the side of the path, to be picked up by Allman and his stretcher party, who are at the rear of the column. By the time I have built my hospital Allman comes up with the wounded and the field cases, and we at once start to do our best for them. Everybody has complimented us on our arrangements, and the quick way we erect our hospitals. We make the poor wounded chaps as comfortable as possible, and dispatch them at once to our base at Ologbo. We sent a batch down to-day at 3 p.m. I must mention that our black troops with the scouts in front and a few Maxims do all the fighting. I am the medical officer, with them in the thick of everything. My black boy Charles carries my bag, which contains a few bandages and tourni-quets, and I have also with me four hammocks and four stretchers. In fact I am the first aid to the wounded. Allman follows up with a field case and another stretcher party. We extracted the bullet from the wounded man's thigh, but could do nothing for the man shot in the lungs. These black men heal wonderfully well, and take everything as a matter of course. At about 3 pm part of the column started to burn a village, but after nearly losing ourselves in the bush, and struggling through the same for seven miles, we were obliged to return before dark, accomplishing nothing. Our camp is a great clearing made by the natives; the trees are nearly 120 feet high, with much foliage at the top, the sun hardly being able to penetrate down to us, which is lucky, as the place is thus kept cool.

February 16th
Obarate.

We have to-day had a real lively and hot day, fighting our way through the bush. We left the camp at the Cross Roads at 11.15 am, as the first division entered it. After advancing for about two hours, at the rate of one mile an hour, the enemy commenced firing at us along the whole line, which was in single file, and nearly a mile long. At two places the natives broke into us, but we soon cleared them off. At the head of the column, where I was, the firing was very heavy. Luckily, no white man was hit, but I do not know what may happen further on, as we get nearer to Benin, where we are certain to meet with much greater opposition. One black soldier was shot in the head and killed, one native scout was shot right through the neck, below the jaw, and one little carrier was shot in the cheek. These men were dressed, and brought along with us, and ultimately sent back with an escort to the base. But I am digressing; time after time the natives came on us, but our Maxims and volley firing cleared the bush, and we advanced steadily until we came to a clearing. It was a native camp, which the natives had just left, and part of the advance guard, going on, occupied the village of Obarate. It was soon taken, hardly any firing being necessary, as the natives had cleared out, and the rest of the advance guard coming on, we encamped there for the night. We were all very tired and slept well, although we first cut down the bush, and put sentries all round the place. It has never been known that the natives attack at night; this holds good all the world over, still we always take precautions. We have been short of water, and are sending some hundreds of carriers out to get some, and if it comes back in time we will proceed to take the next village on the road to Benin. We can only get about two quarts of water daily per white man, so there is no washing to be done, and we keep away from each other as far as possible, and as we have no change of clothes, or very little, and as the weather is very hot, one can imagine what a beautiful state we are in. From the last camp to this village is only about four miles, but fighting and stoppage kept us on the road from 11.15 am, to nearly 4 pm. The village we are in is rather pretty. There is an avenue of cocoanut palms about 40 feet wide, the road running between them; outside this again are the native huts, extending two and three deep, the avenue being a third of a mile long. We have had no orders about starting yet. One of the officers went away with some troops to look for water, and just now we hear firing, so I suppose the natives have been coming on again. I shall be glad when I am well out of this. We all think that it is a settled affair that we shall get medals and clasps. I had to stop just now at about 1 pm, as the natives kept crawling up and potting at us, Colonel Hamilton ordering us to get under cover; I take advantage of it, and write a few more notes. We have been busy all day; the Admiral and the Consul are coming up from the Cross-Road Camp. I hear we are to start to-morrow, the 17th, with the advance column, part of the first division, and some of the staff, as it will be a long one, extending over several miles, the men being in single file. The intention is to do the next seven miles to Benin as quickly as possible in two days, but it is hard to say whether we shall succeed, as we do not know the position of Benin City, and all the information we can get is from a dumb man and a slave boy, who has only been there once. I think we are in a fairly safe condition now. We have just heard that a number of dead natives were found near Ologbo, who were shot down by our volley firing and Maxims, when we landed there for the first time some days ago. This morning I was sent out with a hundred men and officers and two stretchers to reconnoitre about a mile off. We got to a clearing and rested. Suddenly the natives started potting at us. We returned the fire, but one of our scouts was shot through the head and killed ten yards from the path. The Admiral is not in very good health. In chatting with me he informed me he was all right bodily, but that he could not sleep at night, as he had so much in his mind with respect to the expedition. Moor looks very fit, perhaps a bit anxious, but otherwise very cheery, and always chaffing me. O'Farrell went down with fever as soon as he arrived at Ologbo, so he was sent back to base. I am up with the advanced column and at its head continually under fire, so shall not be astonished if I come back with a bullet or two inside me. Considering the bush we have to get through we have lucky so far. We have lost no white men yet as they did on the Sapoba and Gwatto routes. We get no water for washing, and hardly any to drink; what an awful lot we will look in a day or two. I hear that when we get to Benin City the N.C.P. Forces will hold the place, while the naval men will return to their ships and will divide all the honours with the few Special Services officers who have been sent out here to help us. We poor devils will be out here for another twelve months, and get no kudos when we get home, though we are doing and will be doing all the heavy work! But such is life! We are completely cut off from our base for the next few days. It is wonderful how thirsty all the men are here. There has been no rain; marching in the sun is dry work, and all the native wells we have passed are empty.

February 17th
Awako Village.

We left Obarate this morning with the Admiral and staff and the Consul-General. Colonel Hamilton led the advance. Our scouts and black troops, under English officers belonging to the N.C.P. Force, with a Maxim or two cleared the bush with volley firing at the head of the column, as usual. Admiral Rawson, Moor and staff are in the middle of the column, which is about three miles long. The carriers who number about a thousand, carrying principally water, ammunition and food, are well sprinkled with marines and blue jackets. The column consists roughly of 250 N.C.P. troops, 120 marines, 100 bluejackets, 30 scouts, 5 maxims, 2 seven-pounders, 2 rocket-tubes, and about six medical men with stretchers, hammocks and field cases. I was as usual at the head of the column and continuously under fire. We left at about 6.15 am. At 7 am we came in contact with the enemy, a running fight being kept up until 10 a.m., when Agage Village was taken. We rested here for one and a half hours and made another start at 11.30 am. Again a running fight was kept up, on and off, until 3 pm, when we reached the village of Awako, which the enemy had deserted. En route we dislodged the natives from their camps. It is hard to imagine what our nerves are like after firing away and being fired at for so many hours on a blazing hot day in dense bush, where the path is only broad enough for men to walk in single file, and so dense that one cannot see more than a few yards on each side of one's self, and where we never get a glimpse of those who are potting at us. Anyhow, we are all getting accustomed to it. One man was shot to-day, and while making our camp to-night another was shot in the stomach and one in the face, but not seriously. We reckon we are about six miles from Benin City, and ought to take it to-morrow.

February 18th
Benin City.

We are now settled down in the above place. It is a misnomer to call it a city; it is a charnel-house. All about the houses and streets are dead natives, some crucified and sacrificed on trees, others on stage erections, some on the ground, some in pits, and amongst the latter we found several half dead ones. I suppose there is not another place on the face of the globe so near civilisation where such butcheries are carried on with impunity. But to continue my narrative, we left Awako, with the whole force, our black troops leading. At 1 p.m. we came to a clearing in the path and about a mile ahead was the city. We put some rockets and shells into the place and then started off again. Again and again we were fired into. The enemy collected on the opposite side of the road, the main thoroughfare leading into Benin. They made a sort of embankment which owing to the dense bush could not be seen; they fired over this so that when some of our troops passed this place they were afraid of being cut off. I was in the middle of it and feeling most uncomfortable, dressing the men's wounds, and stopping their bleeding to the best of my ability. I did not like it at all, and I noticed by the ping of the bullets that the natives must be using repeating rifles, the firing being so heavy and quickly delivered. I have never seen anything like it before. The grass was only about two feet high and I was obliged to crawl with my black boy Charles from one wounded to another. Luckily the very severely wounded had been carried under cover by their comrades and although I found several slightly wounded, with a little persuasion I managed to get them to crawl under cover by themselves, my stretcher party having disappeared, with the hammocks and stretchers as soon as the firing commenced. Poor Captain Byrne and his company of 60 men were the ones that suffered most, the former being severely wounded in the spine and sixteen of the latter killed and wounded. There was no naval doctor with them and I was up in front and seeing how they got bowled over, I was obliged to fall back and do my best for them. While attending to the wounded I was informed that several more were lying out on the road, and as nobody offered to bring them in, I told my black boy Charles to do so. I could not go myself, as I was too busy tying up wounds, so Charles went out and brought in a wounded carrier. Shortly afterwards he again went out, followed by Lieutenant Beamish, and brought in a wounded marine. It was lucky neither of them was hit as the natives tried to pot them from the ambush. All of us believed that Charles behaved splendidly; he was very cool, and did not seem to mind the bullets at all, although they were hitting the ground and throwing up the sand around him. While under cover I noticed three of the men in a dying condition; others were shrieking, cursing and damning the natives. One man implored me to let him have his revolver back, that he might shoot himself, the agony he suffered being so great. As I was leaning over him, trying to relieve his pain, unseen by me he pulled my loaded revolver out of its case but I was just in time to knock it out of his hand. Afterwards he tried to get hold of a marine's rifle. The poor chap must have been suffering agonies, while all around him the wounded were shrieking for water, blaspheming the natives and crying for help; others again were helping one another, tying up their wounds, and trying to staunch the bleeding. It was a curious sight to see the unwounded, with their arms around the necks of the wounded talking to them in tender womanising words. Every now and again I could hear one man saying to another softly – "All right, don't give way, I'll look after you – I won't let the natives get at you – I'll kill and revenge those brutes," etc., etc. I wish I could express here what I saw the men must have felt for one another. The whole thing was most heartrending. Shortly afterwards the rear of the main column came up to us, and the poor wounded men felt somehow safe again. After dispersing the natives with Maxims and volley firing, Benin City was ours.

As we neared Benin City we passed several human sacrifices, live women slaves gagged and pegged on their backs to the ground, the abdominal wall being cut in the form of a cross, and the uninjured gut hanging out. These poor women were allowed to die like this in the sun. Men slaves with their hands tied at the back, and feet lashed together, also gagged were lying about. As our white troops passed these horrors, one can well imagine the effect on them – many were roused to fury, and many of the younger ones felt sick and ill at ease. As we neared the city, sacrificed human beings were lying in the path and bush. Dead and mutilated bodies seemed to be everywhere – by God! May I never see such sights again! In the King's compound on a raised platform or altar, running the whole breadth of each, beautiful idols were found. All of them were caked over with human blood and by giving them a slight tap, crusts of blood would, as it were, fly off. Lying about were big bronze heads, dozens in a row, with holes at the top, in which immense carved ivory tusks were fixed. One can form no idea of the impression it made on us. The whole place reeked of blood. Fresh blood was dripping off the figures and altars (months afterwards when we broke these long altars we found that they contained human bones). Most of the men are in good health but these awful sights rather shattered their nerves. We are 300 white men and will pull through somehow, you bet. I must mention that both black troops (which led all the way, by the by) and all the white men behaved splendidly. All of you at home can be proud of them. Of course our great enemy was the want of water, and this was a great trial to the men, in the hot and blazing sun. I must not forget to mention that when we left Awako yesterday morning, the natives attacked the rear part of our column, the casualties being (or the eight hours till we took the city) four white men killed, one being Surgeon Fyfe, R.N. and sixteen white men wounded, Captain Byrne being one of them, three N.C.P. black men and three carriers killed, one Court Messenger and one guide wounded. This was rather a heavy loss for such a small force.

February 19th

We are getting the place into ship shape to-day, and trying our best to make it defensible. We are all right for ammunition and can hold the place if we get enough water, till the second division comes up. We buried our dead to-day. Captain Byrne is better, but there seems very little hope for him. Three hundred yards past the King's compound, the road is covered with bodies, skulls, bones etc., most of the bodies being headless. The King's house is rather a marvel – the doors are lined with embossed brass representing figures, while the roof is formed of sheets of muntz metal, and the rafters to support the same artistically carved.

February 20th

In front of the King's compound is an immense wall, fully twenty feet high, two to four feet thick, formed of sun dried red clay. In front stakes have been driven into the ground, and cross pieces of wood lashed to them. On this framework live human beings are tied to die of thirst or heat and ultimately to be dried up in the sun, and eaten by the carrion birds. Black troops heard faint cries coming from some pits and came upon some live captives, there for many days without food or water intermingled with the dead and rotting bodies. Some of these poor fellows had been carriers with the Phillips' party some weeks before. All the white men had been killed on the Gwatto Road and none had been brought into Benin City to be sacrificed as the British public were led to believe. One of the saddest sights as we entered the big palaver house was to notice the effects of the massacred white men. Amongst them we noticed Phillips' helmet in its case, a doctor's bag complete which belonged to poor Elliot.

February 21st

About 3 pm a good breeze sprang up and two carriers carelessly set fire to a hut. Even the things we had placed in the middle of the compound caught fire. In less than an hour the conflagration had burnt itself out and the whole place was strewn with ashes. The next day we found what a blessing had come to us for the fire, smoke and charcoal removed all the smell and the city became sweet and pure again.

February 22nd

At 8 am the Admiral and staff left Benin City with all their troops and wounded. Our black troops and officers lined the road and gave him three hearty cheers. To-morrow the N.C.P. Forces start their heavy work again. The King has to be followed and caught.

I cannot help closing this article with a word of praise for my black Accra boy, Charles Nartey. He is about eighteen years old. Throughout the expedition he behaved splendidly under fire. Consul-General Sir Ralph Moor ordered me to put his name down for a medal and clasp, for behaving so well, and bringing in two wounded men under heavy fire.

(The expedition brought back as booty several thousand art objects and antiquities. Most striking were the magnificent bronze castings and ivories. Benin art, which ceased after the sacking of the city is now acknowledged throughout the world as being amongst the finest examples of African culture.

From 1902 to 1921 Felix Roth gave his address as The Sports Club, St James Square London S.W.)

CHAPTER 2

The Inoculation Department of
St Mary's Hospital

It is remarkable that the outcome of two major world wars and subsequent conflicts was influenced by the Inoculation Department of St Mary's Hospital, Paddington. The driving force in the creation of this department was Almroth Wright, a unique man. He influenced a singular group of medical research workers, Stewart Douglas, John Wells, John Freeman, Alexander Fleming, Parry Morgan, Leonard Colebrook, John Matthews and Carmalt-Jones. Among these high academic achievers the best remembered by history are Wright and Fleming. The Inoculation Department had its origin in the Clarence Wing of the hospital in 1908 and eventually moved to premises adjoining the Medical School. It is known today as the Wright-Fleming Institute. Wright found in Fleming an apt researcher and eventually a worthy successor. Many accounts of their lives have been written, and we have quoted here from some of them, ie *The History of St. Mary's* by Zachary Cope, *The Plato of Praed Street* by Michel Dunnill, and *The Life of Alexander Fleming* by André Maurois. The texts give an insight into the personalities of these two men and paint a picture of how different they were. Perhaps it was this difference in character that permitted two such successful men to work and foster together in the same institution.

Almroth Wright was born on 10 August 1861 in Middleton Tyas in Yorkshire. His father, Charles Wright, was an ordained minister descended from the Wrights of Donnybrook, Co. Dublin, Ireland. His mother, Ebba, came from the Almroth family of Sweden, distinguished and financially secure. Her sister, Emma, also married a curate in the Anglican Church. Both ladies had a strong religious faith and volunteered to join Florence Nightingale in Constantinople and Scutari, during the Crimean War.

Almroth's father, Charles, preached a strong evangelical Christianity, believing vehemently in the literal translation of the Bible. His preaching extended to a declared opposition to Roman Catholicism. Despite this background, or because of it, Almroth criticised Christian dogma and refused to accept the virgin birth and questioned seriously the Resurrection. This led to him embracing atheism. This is not surprising as he had a critically analytical mind and remarkable self assurance. It would appear he did not need the help or support of a heavenly deity. The family moved from Yorkshire to Belfast in Northern Ireland in 1874 and Almroth was

16

schooled in the Belfast Academical Institution. It was here he obtained his basic knowledge of Greek and Latin. Leaving school he read for an arts degree in Trinity College, Dublin, in Southern Ireland and graduated in 1882 with first class honours and the gold medal. He began to study medicine at the same time. He spoke French, German and Spanish fluently in addition to his familiarity with the Classical languages. His far-reaching knowledge included European literature and poetry. An interest in philosophy was to occupy much of his time throughout his life and to constitute much of his writing. He was unsure of where his future lay and asked advice from the Professor of Literature at Trinity. The professor said, 'If I were you I would go on with medicine. It is the finest possible introduction to life, and if you have the gift to write afterwards, it will give you an invaluable background.' That this is true is seen in the large number of doctors who have turned to writing, among whom are Oliver Goldsmith who studied in Trinity, Keats, Sir William Wilde who practised in Dublin and fathered Oscar Wilde, Chekhov, Maugham, Conan Doyle, whose son was a student at St Mary's Hospital Medical School, and Oliver St John Gogarty who practised in Dublin, and countless others equally or more prestigious.

Almroth Wright qualified in medicine in 1883. His future distinction was not to be in writing. When he qualified he travelled to Leipzig to a school of physiology on a scholarship of £100. Returning to England still uncertain of his future he obtained a law studentship, passed an examination for the Civil Service and in 1885 entered the service of the Admiralty. There followed a period in the Brown Institute where he assisted with work on thyroid disease. In 1887 Dr Charles Roy, superintendent of the Institute invited Wright to take a post as demonstrator in the pathology department in Cambridge, to which Roy had been appointed professor. This was a pivotal move in Wright's career leading to his specialisation in pathology and bacteriology in particular.

Wright married on 8 January 1889. His wife was Jane Georgina Wilson, an Anglo-Irish girl from a wealthy family in Kildare in Southern Ireland. Shortly after the marriage they sailed for Sydney, Australia, where Wright had accepted a post in the medical school. Jane did not take happily to life in Australia, and disliked the lack of servants. Dunnill in his book writes that the marriage however was uneasy from its earliest days. They sailed for England in 1891 where fate provided another pivotal move in Wright's career. He obtained the post of pathologist to the Royal Victoria Hospital, Netley, the Army Medical Hospital. It is surprising that he was appointed to this post as his rival was David Bruce, a regular Army medical officer who was a bacteriologist with an excellent academic background and who had published more than Wright at the time. Bruce proceeded to a distinguished career describing brucellosis and the trypanosoma brucei, and was elected a Fellow of the Royal Society in 1899. Wright's appointment was not welcomed by many in the Army Medical School at Netley and Bruce and Wright displayed mutual personal antagonism for most of their careers. It was at Netley that Wright's fame as a bacteriologist began. Pasteur had demonstrated that some immunity could be given to anthrax by injecting attenuated anthrax bacilli and Jenner had produced immunity to smallpox by vaccination. Wright at that time nurtured the seeds of his life-long belief that the most effective way to treat infections was to increase the body's immune reaction with the development of antibodies. These antibodies weakened the bacteria and increased the power of phagocytosis to destroy them. Wright continued throughout his career to believe in the primacy of the immune reaction in combating infections and even to harbour a suspicion of the value of antibiotics when later they were discovered.

In their experiments Wright and David Semple, a bacteriologist working with him in Netley, injected themselves with doses of dead bacteria. Wright concluded that the power to destroy bacteria lay in the plasma, and he called this the Opsonic power, produced by Opsonins. He even measured this power and termed the result the Opsonic Index. He stated this Index was a measure of the patient's resistance to infection; this was the basis of his work on vaccine therapy and his reputation in immunology.

He soon turned his attention to typhoid, at the time a serious infection causing numerous epidemics and many deaths. He developed a vaccine which he tried in 1897 on the inmates of a lunatic asylum in Maidstone, Kent. It is not hard to imagine what a hue and cry such an act and such a choice of recipients would raise, both inside and outside the profession today. Soon he had another opportunity to test it again, and this time more ethically. In the Boer War of 1899 the effect of typhoid was devastating and more men were incapacitated and killed by typhoid than by enemy action. Dunnill in his book on Wright states that the figures given for injury and death from enemy fire and those stricken by illness vary according to the sources consulted, but the trend is much the same. Thus one source quotes 8,000 soldiers killed by enemy fire out of an average strength of 209,404, but 13,000 died of typhoid fever and 64,000 had to be invalided home. In the nineteenth century, the mortality rate for typhoid was 20% of those afflicted. Wright fought strongly for anti-typhoid vaccination to be performed on all those serving in South Africa, but it was only offered to volunteers. At the time the vaccine was causing severe reactions in the recipients, incapacitating them for days and even weeks. So its use was opposed by David Bruce and the Army hierarchy. Following numerous Army committee meetings, vaccination was stopped. Wright was disappointed and furious. He resigned from his post in Netley and applied for the post of pathologist and bacteriologist at St Mary's Hospital, Paddington. His long career at St Mary's began on 24 October 1902, the year the Boer War ended. His work on the anti-typhoid vaccine continued.

In 1903 a committee of the Royal College of Physicians concluded in favour of vaccine therapy saying it lessened susceptibility and case mortality. This was not however, universal medical opinion at the time. From his post in St Mary's Wright continued to fight with the Army hierarchy.

He was an impressive man, heavy in build and with a large bushy moustache. He was described as fascinating and formidable and was a brilliant lecturer. Although popular with his staff, he was blunt and dictatorial, disliked any form of criticism, and would defend his beliefs vehemently. Men of medical stature on his team were not easily intimidated but they knew who was in charge. Wright was familiar with influential men of the time such as Balfour and other eminent politicians, Kitchener, society hostesses and Bernard Shaw. He and Shaw liked to debate together and Shaw used Wright as the model for Sir Colenso Ridgeon in *The Doctor's Dilemma*. It wasn't only in medical matters that Wright was controversial. He was strongly opposed to women suffrage and wrote against it. It was said he was a misogynist. This he wasn't as he developed strong attachments to several women in his life, but he did think that women's minds were inferior to those in men. He opposed women studying medicine in St Mary's Hospital Medical School and would not employ women on his staff in the laboratory. Perhaps his influence was too strong in these respects for apart for a short spell during World War I, it was years after that war that female entry into the Medical School was accepted and then only in a small percentage of the intake. It marks the change of time that today female entrants into the medical school make up *circa* 60%.

It was in Wright's character to fight for what he believed with remarkable self-confidence and having purified his anti-typhoid vaccine he continued his battle with the army authorities, as he was to do later over army medical organisation in World War I. On 11 May 1904 a further committee recommended that the practice of voluntary inoculation against typhoid fever in the Army be resumed. So it was that in 1914 at the outbreak of World War I, inoculation against typhoid was given on a voluntary basis. Wright thought every soldier should be inoculated and spoke to his friend Lord Kitchener to convince him and get his support. At the time the War Office did encourage medical officers to recommend it to soldiers in their charge, but in the short term Kitchener ruled that no soldier was to be posted overseas without being inoculated. This increased the number protected enormously. Sir Arthur Hurst in his book, *Medical Diseases of War* published in 1940 stated,

There is no doubt that the almost universal inoculation practised in the last war (1914–18), is the explanation of the very small number of cases (of typhoid) which occurred. The admission rate for typhoid fever amongst the troops in France who had not been inoculated was fifteen times as great as amongst those who had been inoculated and the death rate was seventy times as high.

In his book on Fleming, Kevin Brown states that: 'It has been argued that without vaccination in World War I there would have been closer to 120,000 deaths in the British Army from typhoid rather than the 1,200 actual deaths.'

Wright continued his work on vaccines against all manners of infections on the basis of increasing the body's natural defences. During the First World War the death rate from wound infections was extremely high and particularly from gas gangrene. Sir Alfred Keogh, Director General of the Army Medical Services proposed that Almroth Wright should set up a laboratory to investigate wound sepsis. Wright set up such a laboratory in Boulogne in Northern France and took with him several of his staff from St Mary's Hospital, among whom were Leonard Colebrook and Alexander Fleming. Unlike the battlefields of the Boer War, the wounds in the fields of France were heavily contaminated with pyogenic organisms including the tetanus bacillus and the clostridium of gas gangrene from the fertilised farmland soil. The wounds were more complex and contained foreign bodies, bullets, shell shrapnel and bits of contaminated clothing; such wounds were seldom simple, but had numerous cavities and crevices. Many of the wounded could not be removed from the battlefield during the day and lay for hours. Treatment was delayed sometimes for days and this allowed infections to become established. The value of antiseptics for prophylaxis in infections was well-known but the practice was extended to the treatment of wounds already infected; if they failed then a larger dose of antiseptics was recommended.

This was the general policy among the Army medical officers at the time. Wright and Fleming working in their laboratory in Boulogne showed that the presence of foreign bodies in the wounds and the presence of devitalised and dead tissue facilitated the growth of pyogenic bacteria and moreover that the application of antiseptics had an adverse effect on the tissues, encouraging the growth of organisms and the development of sepsis. Many of the pyogenic bacteria also utilised oxygen and permitted the growth of anaerobic organisms including the organisms of gas gangrene and tetanus, which found a perfect growth medium in the dead tissues. They recommended that all dead and devitalised tissues should be removed surgically from the wounds as soon as possible. The wounds should then be thoroughly irrigated with hypertonic saline. This would encourage an outflow of lymph with its natural bacterial defences. The wounds may be drained surgically, but often could be treated by primary closure. This required skilled surgical help. Many Army medical men opposed these new ideas. Watson Cheyne, President of the Royal College of Surgeons at the time also opposed Wright and Fleming's view that antiseptics could be harmful to the tissues. So again Wright found himself in opposition to the medical opinion of the time. A lesser man would have been discouraged. However Wright also criticised the organisation of medical treatment which over days shunted men back from the front line before treatment was begun. He accused the Army authorities with being more concerned with evacuating the wounded rather than treating them at the front and advocated surgical treatment as near to the front line as possible. It was a long time before Wright's advice was implemented but improved results were convincing and his recommendations were acted upon.

During World War II surgery for wounds was performed as early as possible and as near to the front line as possible from the onset. By then chemotherapeutic agents were being developed. It is remarkable that the name of Sir Almroth Wright is not more familiar to the public, yet his inspired work in wartime was crucial for the saving of so many lives and the success of the armed forces.

Alexander Fleming was born in Lochfield in Ayrshire, Scotland and educated at Kilmarnock Academy. His brother advised him to study medicine. Much of Fleming's career was influenced by chance. He choose to go to St Mary's Hospital Medical School because he was a good swimmer and had played water polo against St Mary's who had a very strong team. He was an ardent student and successful in examinations, qualifying with honours and obtained the Gold medal. His choice of bacteriology as a career was because of his excellence in shooting. John Freeman worked in the Inoculation Department and was a crack shot in the team that competed in Bisley. He persuaded Fleming to join the department for this reason and he was accepted by Almroth Wright. Thus Fleming worked with Wright for the greater part of his career, yet they couldn't have been more different. Fleming was a dour Scot. Wright had flair and was anything but dour. Fleming was quiet, reserved and had difficulty in expressing himself; he had none of Wright's skills in lecturing. He accepted the authoritarian attitude of Wright without question, even when he disagreed with his views. It has been said that his strongest feelings remained unuttered. Along with Wright he did sterling work in Boulogne during World War I on the treatment of war wounds, and shared with him the recommendations to the War Office.

Fleming married while on leave on 23 December 1915. His bride was an Irish nurse, Sarah McElroy, one of twins, who ran a nursing home in Baker Street, London. Kevin Brown in his book *Penicillin Man*, says that it was the marriage of opposites. Sarah McElroy trained in nursing at the Richmond Hospital, Dublin. Fleming's first great discovery (and indeed his second), was by chance contamination of a culture plate: while handling it he sneezed over it and this led to his discovery of lysozyme in nasal secretions and later in tears. Lysozyme had bacteriocidal properties, but with limited effectiveness. This was in 1921 and soon his aim was to find some chemical substance that would kill bacteria without damaging the tissues or weakening the phagocytes in the blood.

It is common knowledge that chance again played its part in the discovery of penicillin: he was an untidy man and left some culture plates overnight on his desk in the laboratory, near an open window. Clearing up he noticed a mould had landed on one plate. Astute in his work and careful in his methods he saw an absence of bacterial growth in the neighbourhood of the mould. This mould was penicillium notatum. He explored the mould further, proving its ability to destroy bacteria and also its safety in the tissues and the blood. He called the active ingredient in the blood 'penicillin'. This was in 1928 and his report heralded a discovery of pivotal significance which was to change the practice of medicine worldwide. The problem that Fleming then faced was to isolate the active ingredient in the mould if it was to be of any use in treating vast number of patients; this needed the skills of dedicated chemists. Fleming, being a bacteriologist did not have these skills, nor unfortunately did he have at his disposal a team of chemists, so his work and his success remained confined for some time. Indeed it remained static for a remarkable number of years.

In 1935, prontosil, a sulphonamide was manufactured and had bacteriocidal properties. It was stated in *The Life of Alexander Fleming* by André Maurois that Fleming said to Douglas MacLeod, an obstetrician and gynaecologist, that he had something much better than prontosil to offer, but nobody would listen to him, and he could not get anyone interested or a chemist who would extract the active ingredient for him. This fact raises the question whether or not he had effectively pursued the follow-up or whether his retiring personality failed to get across to others the enormous significance of his discovery. It was not until 1939, eleven years later, that Chain and Florey in Oxford having read the papers on penicillin written by Fleming became interested. They embarked on the difficult task of isolating and purifying the active ingredient and succeeded magnificently.

The significant test of their penicillin powder was made in 1940 when three groups of mice were injected with streptococci, staphylococci and clostridium septicum. Those treated with penicillin survived while the controls all died. Penicillin was tried clinically, and allowing a few setbacks, the results proved beyond doubt its clinical safety and its efficacy in the treatment of numerous infections. Florey and Chain built up a small stock of the precious penicillin powder, but there was a demand to produce vast quantities of this new therapeutic agent. Information was shared with the major manufacturing drug companies in Britain and America and in 1943 their factories began to produce penicillin on a large scale. This was originally used only for the armed forces and revolutionised the treatment of war wounds as well as other infectious ailments. Universal use followed. Medicine entered a new era – the antibiotic age.

Fleming was lauded worldwide and surprisingly this quiet, dour man took readily to the adulation heaped on him. He was knighted in 1944. The Nobel Prize Committee recognising Fleming's discovery but conscious of the work of Florey and Chain in isolating the active ingredient, argued over to whom the award should go. Almroth Wright, even though maintaining his belief in natural immunity and suspicious of chemotherapeutic agents, argued strongly in favour of the prize going to Fleming. It also was not surprising that Lord Moran, Dean of St Mary's Hospital Medical School and President of the Royal College of Physicians at the time, spoke publicly of Fleming's right to the prize. The decision of the Nobel Prize Committee was to divide the prize between all three. Fleming travelled to Stockholm to receive it in December 1945.

Although married, it has been said that Fleming had the air and the mannerisms of a batchelor. He liked the company of his male colleagues when drinking pints of beer in the pub close to the hospital. However after the death of Lady Fleming he married Amalia Coutsouris-Voureka, a bacteriologist whom he employed in his laboratory and who developed an affection and an unwavering dedication to Fleming from her earliest days with him. Sir Alexander Fleming died on 11 March 1955 and his ashes lie in St Paul's Cathedral. Professor Pannett, a St Mary's surgeon said in his oration at the funeral,

> He has saved more lives and relieved more suffering than any other living man, perhaps more than any man who has ever lived. This by itself is enough to alter the history of the world. His choice of a profession, his selection of a medical school, his deviation into bacteriology, his meeting with Almroth Wright, the nature of the work with him, the chance drop of a tear, the chance fall of a mould, all these events were surely not due to mere chance. We can almost see the finger of God pointed to the direction his career should take at every turn.

(Quoted in *The Life of Fleming* by André Maurois.)

CHAPTER 3

The Boer War 1899–1902

In 1652 the Dutch East India Company established a shipping station at the Cape of Good Hope in South Africa. The settlers were mainly Dutch Protestants, with some German and French Huguenot refugees. They called themselves Afrikaners and among them were the farmers, the Boers who moved into African territory in search of land. In 1806 the British took over the colony as the Cape gave a naval base on the route to India. The Dutch settlers remained the majority and most were content with the British rule, but not so the Boers. Antagonism to British rule increased in 1834 when Britain ordered slaves to be freed in every part of the Empire. This precipitated the Great Trek when 5,000 Boers and about 5,000 black servants moved across the Orange and Vaal rivers beyond the frontiers of the colony between 1835 and 1837. Following the Great Trek the Afrikaners established two republics to the north of Cape Colony, the Orange Free State and the Transvaal. In the early 1850s the British Government recognised them. In 1869 the discovery of diamonds in Kimberley, made Cecil Rhodes, a young Englishman, and Alfred Beit millionaires. Gold deposits were discovered in the Transvaal in 1886 and led to large numbers of British citizens flooding into Johannesburg. These immigrants were known as Uitlanders. They presented a problem for Paul Kruger, the President of the Transvaal, who refused to give them full civil rights including the vote.

By 1890 Cecil Rhodes was Prime Minister of the Cape Colony and had formed the Rhodesias and crushed the Mashona and Matabele tribes. In 1895 he attempted to overthrow Kruger's republic by an armed raid led by Dr Starr Jameson. Rhodes and Jameson hoped that their attack would coincide with an uprising by the Uitlanders, but this proved to be half-hearted and the invasion force was routed. Rhodes had to resign his premiership and Kruger's reputation was enhanced. The German Kaiser sent Kruger a congratulatory note and Afrikaners throughout Africa, including in the Cape where they accounted for two-thirds of the population, rallied to him. Within four years the Uitlanders were presented as an unjustly persecuted group as Kruger refused to make any concessions for them and they were still denied civil rights including a vote. The British public were prepared for war on their account.

On 9 October 1899, Transvaal issued an ultimatum to the British to withdraw their troops from the frontier. This was rejected and war was

declared by the Boers on 11 October 1899. The British public expected it
to be over by Christmas but it lasted until 1902. At the end of the war
Britain had lost 8,000 soldiers killed in action and there were 21,000
wounded, but 13,000 died of enteric fever and 64,000 had to be invalided
home.

In October 1899 an article appeared in the St Mary's Hospital *Gazette*
headed 'Government Service', written by the editor at the time. It stated
that:

With the outbreak of the war in South Africa against the Transvaal and
the Free State Boers, the call upon the resources of the Royal Medical
Corps has been one it has been found impossible to meet without calling
upon civilian practitioners as volunteers to proceed to the seat of strife, as
well as to fill vacancies occurring in garrison towns at home. Though
regiments may call up a certain number of Reservists to fill their battalion
numbers up to war strength on foreign service, no such arrangements are
in force to make the Medical Corps elastic in a similar emergency, since
one of the regulations of the Medical Reserve expressly states that the
medical officers may only be employed on home duty. Such being the case,
the Government can only trust to inducement of pay, the glamour of
campaigning, and, last but not least, patriotism to attract young surgeons to
give up, on the shortest notice, six months or perhaps a year to attending
the sick and wounded in the service of the Queen. As at first announced
the numbers of civilian practitioners going out to the Cape were but few,
and the Government invited applications only for civilians to take garrison
duty in England at £270 a year. Now owing perhaps to the larger scheme
of operations, and the heavy lists of casualties reported, it is announced that
fifty-six extra men are wanted to go out, with the remuneration of £1 per
day and a donation of two months pay, or £60 at the end of service. Such
terms ought not to go begging for want of capable men to fill the posts,
and in addition comes the announcement that Sir William McCormac,
President of the Royal College of Surgeons, has offered, and has been
accepted, to go out to South Africa to place his services at the disposal of
the Army. Two or three other first class surgeons will probably go with
him, and their presence, with the distinguished President's unique experiences as an Ambulance Surgeon in the Franco-Prussian War to guide them,
is likely to be an invaluable stimulus and help in the rendering of the best
surgery and science possible to the wounded brought from the front. In all
probability the lack of knowledge of military arrangements, bearer and
stretcher drill, and the like, on the part of the civilian volunteers will not
be any hindrance to the execution of their work, for no doubt their chief
employment will be in the larger hospitals at the base, while the trained
Medical Army Officers will be available for service at the front, and in the

field hospitals. Should casualties or other vacancies occur, however, among the latter, the civilian may get his chance of seeing actual fighting, and, maybe, of proving himself also to be something more than a non-combatant. This, we fancy, will be the wish uppermost in the minds of all who volunteer for this special service, but probably to few only will the possible chance be given of earning the soldier's Blue Ribbon, the Victoria Cross. Boer as well as Briton, soldier and staff officer, each alike will need attention, and to each impartially alike will the best skill of the surgeon be given. A chance such as this does not often come of widening one's view of life, of foreign travel, of active service, and good pay into the bargain. Life long friends are made of men under circumstances and conditions of active warfare, in a few days of close comradeship, in whom no amount of ordinary introduction in society would thaw those who are fortunate enough to be accepted, we wish good luck and God speed, in the hope, nay knowledge, that their every endeavour will be to use their opportunities not only for their own advancement and emolument, but to shed lustre on the name of their profession.

(This unusual editorial urges St Mary's doctors to join the forces fighting in South Africa. It reflects the thinking of the times and the lengthy sentences are heavy with the emphasis on patriotism and duty. It would be surprising for an equally emotive script to be written in the United Kingdom in the twenty-first century.)

A letter undated, but signed 'A Civilian Surgeon' was sent to the *Gazette* and published under the title 'Letters from South Africa'. It deals with the difficult problem of inoculation against typhoid fever and it seems appropriate to consider it now in the early stages of the war.

'S.S. Sicilian', off Capetown

Dear Sir, 'Many are called but few are chosen'. I dare say that many old students have promised to write a short description of their experiences to you, but I am convinced that few will do as they promised. Let us begin at the start. We paraded at the R.H.M.C. Guard Room, Aldershot at 4 a.m. on the morning of 7th February, and after roll call started for a mile and a half march through the muddy roads, we were fortunate enough to have the struggling moonbeams misty light as our guiding star, but at times it became obscured by clouds, and we "sploshed" on to the station. We went by train round Hounslow and London to the Royal Albert Docks where we embarked, finishing at 4 p.m., 400 men, 300 horses and war material leaving punctually to time. Soon after starting we began to feel the swell which gradually increased for about four days, when we had to slow down to give the horses a rest. For the next three days we were not rocked so much, but quite sufficient to make a good number feel uncomfortable. We reached Las Palmas on Sunday evening, eight days after leaving London, but were not allowed to land as we had no pratique; we received orders for Cape Town, and heard of Lord Robert's advance which cheered us very much. Three days later out of Canary it was decided to inject serum into those who were willing, as a prophylactic against enteric fever. All hands were assembled for the head medicine man, Major R.H.M.C., to explain its advantages etc. He quoted from Prof. Wright's (Netley) schedule. About 200 volunteers came forward to be injected the following day. 120 were injected and suffered accordingly. Three days later the remainder were done, and likewise suffered. As in civil life one does not see much of this kind of thing, I will endeavour to explain what happened. The men were washed, carbolised and injected with 1cc of the serum, into the flank. Two fainted at once, but this was with fright. About an hour to an hour and a half after inoculation nearly everyone began to feel "ill", some were seized with cramp in the abdomen, some with nausea, some with vomiting, and some with fainting, some diarrhoea, all had a rise in temperature from 102 degrees F. to 104.5 degrees F., and so the long night passed; next day very few of those who were injected were able to go on duty, and some were in a condition of great collapse; towards evening they began to recover, but were not able to resume duty until three full days had passed. Notwithstanding all this, nearly all the remaining volunteers came forward to form a second batch, I amongst them. After I was done at 5.30 I went straight to bed, and had my dinner brought in at 7 p.m. A little soup was all that I could manage, as I was beginning to feel sick. An hour later my temperature began to rise, and continued to do so until it reached 104.5 degrees F. at about 11 p.m., and I was very light-headed. At 9.30 p.m. I got up to get a drink, but was for some time unable to do so; when I had done so, my servant caught me in his arms, as I had fainted. My servant got me back to bed again. I slept very little during the night, and the next day was unable to move hand or foot without assistance. Diet (all retained), Breakfast, porridge; Lunch, soup; Dinner, soup. The next day I was a little better, but still unable to leave my bed, the day after I got up to my dinner, but had to return to bed again. For the succeeding two days I was very weak and suffered from a continuous headache. I quite forgot to add that many developed buboes. Two glands in my groin were swollen to the size of pigeon's eggs, and two were swollen in the axilla. There were red streaks passing from the inoculated point to the glands. The area round the point of inoculation, about six inches in diameter, was red, swollen, extremely tender, and almost brawny; one could hardly bear to have it touched. We have now nearly all recovered, though everybody looks and feels seedy. I must ask you not to pull the style of my description to pieces as I am writing with many voices around me, and a ship rolling to 20 degrees every few minutes. The wonders of the deep, the monotony of a sea voyage etc., I will not bore you with. We are now off Capetown and are all anxiously waiting for news of the advance, and where we are to go.

A Civilian Surgeon

P.S. One man who was injected had had typhoid about 4 years ago; it had no effect on him.

(Interesting points in the letter are the use of unusual punctuations and the social history of the time, eg the servant's role for the officer rank.)

CHAPTER 4

The Siege of Ladysmith

Ladysmith was a major training ground and principal supply base for the British Army in the South African War. It was surrounded by hills which dominated the landscape. For this and other reasons it was unsuitable for being a garrison town in times of war. The Boers occupied the hills surrounding Ladysmith, fortified themselves and trapped the town and its inhabitants. This siege began in October 1899 and lasted until February 1900, 120 days in all. The garrison was shelled from the hills, principally by a cannon known by the British as 'Long Tom'. However the Boers usually ceased shelling on Sundays. During this lull, the sounds of hymn singing in the hills reached the besieged town. The singing was lusty as the Boers were convinced that God was on their side (in so many wars God must get confused!!!) Apart from the shelling there were frequent raids by the Boers but these were repulsed by the British each time. It was a matter of discontent among the officers and men that few retaliatory raids were made by the British into the hills held by the Boers. By and large the senior army staff waited to be relieved by General Sir Redvers Buller who was advancing with a force to do so. The besieged garrison suffered many disappointments as General Buller postponed his attack on occasions and was repulsed on others. Inside the town the mood was one of despair and boredom. In an account by Thomas Packenham in *The Boer War*, he states that George Stevens in a dispatch to the *Daily Mail* wrote, 'it is nothing but a weary, weary, weary bore – relieve us or we die of dullness'. Stevens did die – but of typhoid fever. In the same book, Gunner Netley is quoted – 'boots worn out, clothes in tatters, living in a hole in the ground for six weeks it was the worst experience of my life'. He wrote in his diary of church parades and cricket matches. Many of the officers played polo. These activities may have eased the boredom and the monotony of the siege but the facts are that this garrison was a place of starvation, hell and death. The deaths were mainly from the effects of typhoid and dysentery.

Referring to the siege Captain Gough wrote, 'the whole thing is a disgrace which will take some time to get over'. Trapped in Ladysmith were 13,745 white soldiers, 5,400 civilians including 2,400 African servants and Indian camp followers. The major hospital was in Intombi built to house 300 patients but within the first ninety days was trying to cope with 2,000 sick and wounded patients of which 842 cases were due to typhoid fever and 472 dysentery. There were fifteen to twenty deaths each day. There was a disastrous shortage of medicines and medical and nursing staff. As the food fell to starvation levels the army horses were sacrificed. According to Packenham the poor conditions within the hospitals were partly due to the inadequacy of the Principal Medical Officer, Lieutenant-Colonel Exham. He appears to have been more interested in the tidiness of the soldiers than in their health. Major Donegan in charge of the 18th Field Hospital clashed with Exham on many occasions. After one such encounter Donegan said 'God Almighty! We have four doctors and 120 patients in 3 churches and 36 tents and the Principal Medical Officer only worries whether the men's clothes are neatly folded or if their boots are in line. Why can't the Head Quarters Staff intervene.' However Sir George White the Senior British Officer in charge of the garrison, never once visited any of the hospitals.

Among the letters written to the St Mary's Hospital Medical School *Gazette* was an account taken from the diary of Miss Charleson, a St Mary's nursing sister. This account gives a rare insight into the hardships suffered by the inhabitants of Ladysmith and the staff and patients in the hospitals.

Recollections of the Siege of Ladysmith
From the diary of Miss Charleson

On the morning of the 21st October I arrived at Ladysmith for duty at the Station Hospital. It was half past six, and I found myself amid a scene of great excitement. War! The atmosphere around us was heavy with war – and an armoured train was leaving for the north as I entered the town. It was a great relief to have reached Ladysmith in safety; for weeks we had dreaded lest the Boers would cut our communications; they knew well enough that we had not sufficient troops to guard our communications. Why did Joubert delay? Who can say? Yet it was our salvation, for during that strange delay, our Indian troops were landed at Port Natal. In the city also the scene was one of wild excitement. All day long troops were galloping along the Newcastle Road, and the roar of artillery in the distance told us of a great battle – the desperate fight of Elaandslaagte. Then towards evening the rain commenced, a chill, deathly drizzling mist, the guns ceased and a silence worse than the thunder of artillery completed the dismal picture.

I had been travelling all the previous night, and at once went to bed, to be roused at nine in the evening with the order to be in readiness by ten o'clock. But when ten o'clock came I was told to lie down in my clothes and rest, for the wounded would not arrive until one o'clock. Just before one o'clock I stepped out into the drizzling rain; trembling from want of rest, strangely excited at the thought of seeing – for the first time – the wounded from a field of battle. I shall never forget that scene, by the dim light of many lanterns, I traced a moving mass of ambulances, carrying the wounded and the dead. The Town Hall was fitted up as a hospital, and within a few minutes every bed was full, and the floor covered with stretchers. The wounded were cold and collapsed, and so at once we handed them cups of hot Bovril. One of the wounded had seen me earlier in the day, on my arrival, and remarked, "I little thought I should see you so soon, Sister!"

The hospital accommodation was excellent, and every comfort was at hand, but I was not to stop long in this part of the hall, for Sister B— came to me, and asked me to help in the operating theatre. That was a terrible night – case after case came in, some past all hope, and alas for the brave Gordons, many of them with their heads shattered by shells, or with hair matted with gore, and faces grey with suffering. Several of those who came in looked up at the operator, and said, "Hullo, don't you remember me?" "No" "Don't you remember D—P—?" "Yes, to be sure, but you were then only a lad in kilts."

Others on being asked if in pain, said "Very little", and always Tommy was very anxious to get his bullet "for the missus."

Hour after hour passed by, and by seven o'clock in the evening we were dead tired, but still the cases came in, and with little food we continued until midnight, and then at last we rested.

Our quarters were novel; our bedrooms with canvas walls, with mattresses, blankets but no sheets had been prepared for us in the upper storey of the Grand Stand erected in the Square of Ladysmith.

Next morning operations commenced again at seven o'clock, and as many of the wounded as possible were moved to Maritzburgh each day, to leave our hospital ready for new arrivals; our nursing staff I should say, consisted at first of three Army Nursing Sisters and seven volunteers, but by the 1st of November the number had been increased to eighteen.

After the battle of Elaandslaagte there followed that of Modder Spruit, and some others, so that we had for many days the same heavy work in the operating theatre and many more examples of the splendid bravery of the English officer and private. The next event that roused great excitement was the first journey made by the military balloon. This was on October 28th, and how much we expected from this balloon, who shall say? Then on the 30th came "Black Monday", for on that day some of the Gloucesters, the 16th Mountain Battery and Royal Irish Fusiliers were captured at Nicholson's Nek. That morning a loud report followed by a shrill whizzing scream awakened me. It was the first shell from a "Long Tom" that fell in Ladysmith. I jumped from my mattress and looking out of the window I saw it fall among a group of mules, scattering the dust in every direction.

All day till sundown the shelling continued, and we sisters as we crossed to our quarters involuntarily ducked our heads to avoid them. Some pieces fell within two feet of me, making holes in the ground a yard deep.

Our dismay at this bombardment was much lessened by the good news that the Naval Brigade of H.M.S. Powerful had arrived with their big guns, but it was not until the 2nd of November that they were able to fire their first shot, and meantime the shelling that we endured was incessant.

On 1st of November I met while crossing the square a young R.A.M.C. officer who smilingly saluted me. I was puzzled, for though I knew the face I could not recall his name, and thought he must have made a mistake. On my return I passed him again, and then he said, "Do you not come from St. Mary's?" I answered in the affirmative, but was obliged to say that though I knew his face, I did not remember his name, but the moment he told me I recalled him as a dresser at the time I was a "pro". He was full of enthusiasm, and many times afterwards when I met him used to tease me, because involuntarily I had put up my sunshade to protect myself from the shells that were whizzing and screaming overhead. He had been among the prisoners on "Black Monday", but, being a medical officer, had been released; now he was attached to one of the British field hospitals, and was full of brave hopes for the future. Alas, that future was all too brief!

The long expected news arrived on November 2nd that the railway had been cut, and now we were surrounded by Boers, and the famous siege of Ladysmith had commenced. On this day also the news arrived that one of our naval officers had been severely wounded by a shell, and that he was to be operated on in a few minutes. I shall never forget this officer as he was brought in on the stretcher, with both his legs shattered, and placed on the operating table. His face was pale and peaceful, a tender heroic smile was on his lips, and his eyes had no pain in them, only a look of satisfaction for having done his duty, and a glory for dying for his country. He looked around kindly and calmly, and his great fortitude seemed to be-little us all. On being asked if he was in pain he said, "No, only bad luck!" And expressed a wish to see a medical officer he knew. This request was quickly granted, and the poor old doctor seemed deeply affected, yet the sufferer remained calm. Then we were told he was ready for chloroform, which he took easily and went to sleep like a tired child. His mangled limbs were skilfully attended to, and although it was a long and tedious operation, he stood it well, and was afterwards removed to his bed in the ward. He did excellently, and great hopes were entertained for his recovery, when at seven o'clock in the evening he suddenly collapsed, and was no more. This brave officer was Commander Egerton of H.M.S. Powerful. A more serenely brave soul I have never seen approach the gates of death. His glorious fortitude, his pale, smiling face, with the clear fearless eyes, I shall never forget; and England may rightly feel proud of such a son. He was tended with the utmost care, and although so short a time with us, he inspired all who saw him with admiration and respect above the ordinary sufferer.

This is one of the sad incidents of the war, and it affected me more than I can express. It seemed good to have lived to see such a brave man. Death, with its "great stillness" approaching, had no fears for that valiant soul. Truly of him it could be said, "Death where is thy sting, and grave, where is thy victory". Very soon after this sad incident, the danger to the hospitals from the continuous shelling, became so great that arrangements were made for the removal of the sick and wounded to a neutral camp at Intombi Spruit. It was a dismal spot, its extent marked out by white flags, and our hearts sank as we passed to it over the bridge, past our outposts below Caesar's Camp, into the shadow of Bulwana. There was no station, no platform, and many of us fell over the ant-heaps on our way. This alone kept our spirits cheerful – that very soon we should be released from this grim imprisonment. Here again I met my old acquaintance at St. Mary's, who had come here with the field hospital. He was very kind to me, helping with my baggage to our tents. We little thought he would find his last resting-place beneath the shadow of that mountain!

Upon the 9th of November, Captain Lampton, R.N., celebrated the Prince of Wales' birthday, by firing a royal salute, and afterwards, so rumour goes, he, with Sir George White and his staff, drank his health.

One day in the middle of November, a doctor of the commando came into our camp in a highly peremptory manner, and demanded to see the Boer wounded, whom he declared were being neglected. Needless to say, this was absolutely untrue, but the chief interest in the visit was, that he was overheard to say to some prisoners, that the town would be taken within three days. After this, rain set in, and the camp became almost a swamp; so much so, that I was obliged to wade from one marquee to another in a very short dress, shod with long gum boots, and with an old waterproof bag on my head.

About St. Andrew's Day we became anxious; there was no good news of relief, and in every direction we could see nothing but Boers. An armoured train from Estcourt was captured by the Boers about this time and among the prisoners were Captain H and Mr. Winston Churchill. Enteric has now also commenced to make an appearance.

It was not until Dec. 1st that we heard that Sir Redvers Buller had heliographed to Sir George White to know how long we could hold out. Needless to say we did not know the reply that was sent, but we knew we had food for eighty days, and that the forage for the horses was already beginning to fail.

On Dec. 6th we noticed Buller signalling on the clouds, and the Boer searchlight on Bulwana above us was turned on to try and destroy the signals. Dysentry and enteric were on the increase, and our work was very heavy now. Cooking in the blazing sun and down-pouring rain was no slight task, but nothing in comparison of what we were to suffer from scarcity of food and scanty fuel. In the early morning of December 7th I heard what sounded like a great explosion; so, striking a light, I looked at my watch, and found the time was half-past three. When I got outside I found there was some disturbance in the neighbourhood of Lombard's Kop, and the "Ping"! of the rifles reached us very clearly. Afterwards we learnt that our people had blown up a "Long Tom", and also taken a Howitzer and Maxim, which they had brought back to the town. The next day 17 wounded arrived.

December the 9th or 11th we took two guns on Surprise Hill, and amongst the wounded in this attack were two young officers, both having fractured thighs. An attack was made on one of these wounded officers by a Boer, but another, seeing the cowardly act, stepped between them, and thus saved his life. I well remember these two young officers, in the first flush of youth, both so cruelly wounded as to almost demand the necessity for removing their limbs. Happily they both recovered, and, most miraculously, both limbs united, without much shortening of the legs. These good recoveries were most noticeable, for daily the camp was becoming more unhealthy, and the food rations were decreasing. Nothing but a good, sound constitution could have possibly overcome these obstacles to recovery. There was very bad news for us on December 13th. For some while we had heard in the distance heavy firing, and upon this day we were told, what seemed to us as almost incredible, that Buller had failed. We were expecting him, and as many as our medical officers and orderlies belonging to the bearer company had gone into town to receive the wounded, 1000 beds had been put in readiness in old camp to receive them. On this day also 86 sick arrived, rumour having it that Sir George White had sent out all the sick to prevent his being hampered with them. The heat had become very oppressive, and our camp, with no trees near, was very exposed. The glare of the sun and the increase in the number of sick made the work very difficult and hard to bear; yet the excitement of the hope of relief kept us up, and we had no time to think of our fatigue.

All day long on the 14th we again heard heavy firing, and we knew that Buller was not far off. But alas, the firing ceased and no relief came! Our medical officers and the bearer orderlies returned in a few days; their services had not been needed. The silence that follows a battle is very terrible, and especially when expecting to be saved. No relief comes! Shut up in that hollow with so many sick and wounded, surrounded by high mountains in which our enemies were seated with their long-reaching guns, we were indeed to be pitied. Can any who has not experienced this truly realise it? I doubt it. We looked helplessly to the mountains, but they preserved their impervious silence! No hope from them: they were coldly indifferent in their grandeur.

For our readers thoroughly to recognise the bravery of the gallant generals and troops in holding out so long, against an enemy four times their number, and occupying every position of vantage, they should have visited Ladysmith. This town lies in a hollow, exactly like the inside of a soup plate. Our troops occupied a few kopjes on the very inside of the rim, whilst the Boers occupied the outside part of the plate all round. Guns were mounted on every mountain. It was a gloriously brave defence!

From this date onward I have no diary to refer to for notes, and must trust to my memory. So far as I can remember we were put on half rations before Christmas. The quantity of tinned milk was rapidly decreasing, and as the cows' milk had been at all times scarce, we began to feel badly off for feeding the sick. We ourselves had not seen milk for many weeks.

Christmas day dawned, but with it no pleasurable feelings. I was thankful that I had not one patient on a full diet, for I had no extra dainty to give them. Sir George White most kindly sent us sisters a gift of some groceries. Our mess orderly tried to make us a plum pudding, but it was a great failure – for there was no fat or suet in it. On the whole, Christmas was very disappointing. Our faith in our soldiers alone kept us from despair, for we felt if we could wait patiently, and suffer sickness and hunger, our garrison would never surrender, and the day must come when we should be free once more.

It was at this time that volunteers were called upon, for some of the limited number of sisters were ill, and also many Medical Officers and orderlies. Among these volunteers was young man named T—, whose services to *me* can never be too highly estimated. He was an Englishman from the Transvaal, who had done much wandering in South Africa; he was trying to do some business in Ladysmith when it became invested and could not get away. There was nothing this man could not do, from digging trenches to making puddings. New Year's Day passed uneventfully.

Upon January 6th I was awakened by the noise of heavy rifle firing. "Ping-ping!" the double "ping-ping" of the Mauser. On striking a light I found it was a quarter-past three o'clock; I quickly got into my dressing gown, and went outside the tent. The sound of the rifle firing came from the side of Waggon Hill, our only position of importance near Ladysmith, lying on our left looking towards the town. It was not very far from our camp, so I could see the flashes of the rifles, and what appeared to be an attack by the Boers on our position. I watched these rifle flashes and reports increasing, and getting higher up the side of the mountain, and knew now for certainty there was to be a severe day's fighting. Knowing the hungry condition of our men, I felt grieved for them, but felt sure that in spite of all they would succeed in holding the position. Chilled by the cold morning air, I went back to bed; but the firing never ceased, so shortly after dawn I got up again and went out to watch the progress of the fight. To me rifle firing is much more gruesome than that of big guns. The sound of those "Long Toms" was to us by this time such an ordinary noise that we could sleep through it, although Bulwana "Long Tom", right above us, made a loud enough report to alarm anyone; but the sharp sound of the rifle made us jump. By breakfast time the fight seemed growing fiercer; we could see everything going on quite well, for we were practically in the Boer lines. By midday the enemy had reached the first ridge. Already their heliograph was up, and the Boers above us on Bulwana were replying to them, whilst "Long Tom" was assisting to the best of his ability, continually roaring, whistling, and screaming over our heads. All day the battle raged, but by seven o'clock in the evening not a Boer was to be seen on Waggon Hill. The day was ours and a thanksgiving arose in our souls for the brave defence our poor tired troops had made. The total defeat of the enemy was quite apparent to us, and that was the last attack made on our people. The newspapers have chronicled the particulars and statistics of the brave fight, of the loss of the gallant Colonel Dick-Cunyngham, Lord Ava, and other valiant soldiers; of the gallant defence of the position by the Manchesters; of the dashing charge of the Devons; and anything I might add would only be superfluous. It is strange to witness a battle, but stranger after it is over, in the stillness, to see the groups bearing white flags, searching for their wounded and dead; and later to see the numbers of vultures soaring round.

To look at the glorious mountains round us, it was sometimes difficult to imagine a hostile foe sat there, watching us as a spider does the fly he has in his net. At other times it seemed wonderful to imagine we should ever be free and able to go beyond the present boundaries. The sunsets were beautiful, and behind Ladysmith rose the Drakensberg mountains, on whose lofty crags the departing sun shed his warm beams as if loath to leave them. My acquaintance from St. Mary's always admired these sunsets, and told me how much he liked South Africa. I often told him that Ladysmith could give him no idea of the grandeur of the vast expanses of the Transvaal. But he was never to see that land, for he developed enteric fever of a very virulent type, and not all that medical skill and nursing could do, saved him. His resting place is within sight of his beloved mountains. After the siege was raised I sent for flowers to plant on his grave, but before I got them, I was also a victim to enteric, so did not get the work done. I shall return later and do as I intended, for I know his friends would be glad to know that a friend's hand adorned his last home. After the battle of Waggon Hill, each day became more monotonous, and medical comforts rapidly decreased. Fuel was very scarce, and would have been an impossibility for me, if the orderly T— had not sent daily "Coolies" to fetch green thorn branches. But how the smoke from the green fuel tried our eyes! In January we once more heard the firing of Duller's column, and we prayed for relief, but the firing ceased, and for days silence followed. We knew another failure had taken place. More and more scarce became the food, the lack of bread was the greatest trial for those that were well, and the scarcity of milk for the sick. At last we were reduced to a quarter of a small bun of "mealie" meal held together by starch and then baked. The result of this bread was that dysentery became more prevalent, then instead we got a biscuit and a quarter for daily allowance. I was obliged to keep the meat that made beef tea and stew it over again, adding a little flour and horse sausage-meat for flavouring, and give it to my convalescent patients for supper. It is needless to say they relished it. Stimulants also were very scarce, and it is now a long time since a candle or match has been seen in the camp; men wanting to light their pipes of dried tea leaves, which many were now smoking, had to do so by putting twigs into any fire they could see.

There were some lamps for use in the wards in which the worst cases were placed. I personally, went to bed for a long time in the dark, stumbling over tent ropes, cold, wet, fatigued, and hungry. Sometimes the Boer search-light used to play upon our camp, and by its light I many times was aided in making my night toilette. Food, as the figures below bear witness, was fast becoming a luxury. These privations took effect on me, and about ten days before the relief, I took to my bed, laid up by an attack of dysentery. For the first few days I was too ill to care about anything, but after a little rest I got over the attack, and by the time Buller arrived, was out of bed again.

Siege of Ladysmith 1899–1900

I certify that the following are the correct and highest prices realised at my sales by Public Auction during the above Siege. Joe Dyson Ladysmith,

February 21st 1900	Auctioneer		
	£	s	d
14 lbs. Oatmeal	2	19	6
Condensed Milk, per tin	0	10	0
1 lb. Beef Fat	0	11	0
1 lb. Tin Coffee	0	17	0
2 lb. Tin Tongue	1	6	0
1 Sucking Pig	1	17	0
Eggs per dozen	2	8	0
Fowls each	0	18	6

4 Small Cucumbers	0	15	6
Green Mealies, each	0	3	8
1 Small plate Grapes	1	5	0
1 Small plate Apples	0	12	6
1 Pkte Tomatoes	0	18	0
1 Vegetable Marrow	1	8	0
1 Eschalots	0	11	0
1 Plate Potatoes	0	19	0
3 Small bunches Carrots	0	9	0
1 Glass Jelly	0	18	0
1 lb. Bottle Jam	1	11	0
1 lb. Tin Marmalade	1	1	0
1 dozen Matches	0	13	6
1 pkt. Cigarettes	1	5	0
50 Cigars	9	5	0
¼ lb. Cake "Fair Maid" Tobacco	2	5	0
½ lb. Cake " Fair Maid" Tobacco	3	5	0
1 lb. Sailors' Tobacco	2	3	0
¼ Tin "Capstan" Navy Cut Tobacco	3	0	0

On Sunday, February 25th, we could hear heavy firing beyond the hills south of us, in the direction of Pieters. The firing continued all day and all the following Monday, sometimes sounding near, sometimes far away. It was a hopeful sign, but on Tuesday we could not hear the sound of a single gun. Our hearts sank low – and you cannot imagine how low your heart can sink unless you are faint from fatigue and hunger – and so passed another day of anxious thought.

On Wednesday, the 28th, we were still convinced our people had failed again. The stillness of the afternoon was broken by one gun on Caesar's Camp firing persistently at "Long Tom". There appeared to be something unusual happening, for our guns did not waste ammunition. About 5 o'clock, what we most prayed for, but what we have nearly despaired of, we discovered had happened, for suddenly on the hills, a little to our right looking towards Colenso, we saw horsemen appearing on the skyline coming towards us. We were free at last! It was sufficient reward for all we had gone through, that moment of supreme joy! Everybody knows this was Lord Dundonald accompanied by some of the Natal Carbineers and I.L.H. who first reached Ladysmith.

Thus ended the Siege of Ladysmith in no dramatic manner, but words cannot express the delight of the famished victims of the siege, the welcome that was given to Duller, or the joy that we felt at having endured unto the end.

CHAPTER 5

Spion Kop

As the relief column, led by Sir Redvers Buller moved towards Ladysmith it was impeded by the Boers at Spion Kop, a hill 1,470 feet high commanding a view over the surrounding countryside. Buller gave authority to General Warren to attack on 24 January 1900. This turned out to be an enormous blunder and the loss of lives on both sides served little purpose. One thousand eight hundred men of the Lancashire Fusiliers climbed the hill in darkness, taking seven hours to do so. In the morning as the mist cleared, they found they were not at the top of the hill, as they had thought. The Boers above them with the vantage position, fired effectively into the Fusiliers. Pakenham in his book says, 'the battlefield was hardly bigger than a large theatre, but the two armies were stumbling about as though blindfolded.' The British lost 243 dead and the Boers 335. Although the Boers seemed to have the victory, both sides retreated without each other knowing so and while little good came from this skirmish, Buller said he learnt something of twentieth-century war!!!

An editorial appeared in the St Mary's *Gazette* dated February 1900 and headed:

The Hospital and the War

Twenty-five medical officers, ten of whom belong to the R.A.M.C., is a very respectable total to be representing St. Mary's at the front. Two names must however already be withdrawn from the list, since death has claimed Captain R.H.E.G. Holt, and Lieutenant G.W.G. Jones during the last week, the former succumbing to wounds received with General Buller's force on 21 February, and the latter dying of enteric fever in Ladysmith two days later, just when the prospects of relief of the town were becoming brighter. (*Authors Note*: Lieutenant Jones must be the name of Sister Charleson's friend, the young medical officer from St Mary's Hospital, mentioned in her diary.)

Three Volunteer Medical Officers and twelve other Civilian Surgeons, the last of whom has not yet started, bring up the numbers to five and twenty. Three members of the V.M.S.C. (Volunteer Medical Staff Corps) also go out shortly, and, in addition to those serving in a medical capacity, C.R. Worthington has gone with the Cambridge University Volunteers,

H.H.B. Cunningham has gone to do garrison duty at Malta with a militia battalion, and G.L. Soames, until recently a student in the school, has obtained a commission in the 3rd Militia Battalion of the Essex Regiment. The Nursing Staff too is represented by Sister Thistlethwayte and Sister Kitching, who went out about a month ago, and Nurse Nicholson and Nurse Charleson who have endured the trials of siege in Kimberley and Ladysmith respectively. On account of the war, too, Lt. Col. Aylmer Hayes, R.A.M.C., although retired, has returned to duty, and is now in charge of the Connaught Hospital, Aldershot. Attached is a tabulated list of St. Mary's men at present employed with the forces in South Africa.

Royal Army Medical Corps
Lieut. Col. R.D. Davies
Major G.E. Hale D.S.O.
Major J.P.S. Hayes
Major A. Baird
Capt. E.G. Anderson
Capt. R.H.G.E. Holt (died of wounds in Natal Feb. 21st)
Lieut G.B. Crisp
    "   E.P. Hewitt
    "   G.W.G. Jones (died of enteric fever in Ladysmith)
    "   J.H.R. Bond
    "   H.B.G. Walton
    "   B.F. Wingate (with Lord Roberts' force)

The Imperial Yeomanry
W. Ashdowne F.R.C.S., Surgeon to the Yoemanry Base Hospital

The City Imperial Volunteers
Capt. Atwood Thorne, M.B.
Capt. R.R. Sleman
Civilian Surgeons J.H Brinker M.B., B.C. Camb.
R. Corfe M.B. M.R.C.S.
H.L. Hatch M.B.,
A.E. Horn M.B., B.Sc. M.R.C.S.
H.H.G. Knapp M.D. Oxon.
P. Lelean F.R.C.S.
J.T. Leon M.D.
V.W. Low M.D. F.R.C.S.
E.A. Nathan M.D.
B. Pares M.R.C.S. L.R.C.P.
A.E. Priddle M.R.C.S. L.R.C.P.
C.C. Parsons M.R.C.S. L.R.C.P.
A.W. Sanders M.D., F.R.C.S.
J.O. Skevington F.R.C.S.
S.M. Smith M.R.C.S. L.R.C.P.
J.W. Summerhayes M.D.
E.C.Taylor B.C. Camb.
W.W. Walker M.R.C.S.

C.B. Whitehead M.R.C.S. L.R.C.P.

Volunteer Medical Staff Corps
Surg. Lieut. E.W. Herrington
Staff-Sergt. W.G. Speers
H. Cadwaladr Jones
R.H. Preston
A.B. Tytheridge
G.E. Wood.

Paget's Horse
O. Heath
C. Speers

In March 1900 a letter was published in the *Gazette* written by Alfred. W. Sanders M.D. F.R.C.S. and titled:

Civilian Surgery in South Africa

On December 21st, a dull, foggy, and dirty day, I left Euston for Liverpool, and early next morning made my way to the docks, where I found the S.S. Ottoman, a hired transport belonging to the Dominion Line, and usually engaged in the North Atlantic Cattle trade, which was to take me and others to Cape Town. Making my way through the lines of policemen guarding the entrance to the wharf, I reported myself to the Commanding Officer, Prince Francis of Teck, who was superintending the embarkation of the men and horses. Going on board I found a comfortable cabin ready, and learnt that we were to take 103 men and 410 horses. By four o'clock all had come aboard, and the spar and main decks newly fitted up with stalls were full of our four legged fellow travellers.

Soon we were out in the Mersey, but could see little of our surroundings because of fog. Early next morning we rounded Holyhead, and were soon out of sight of land. Having enjoyed excellent weather, we reached Las Palmas on the 29th, and went ashore for a few hours. Most of our interest during the voyage centred on the horses. For these there was plenty of work to be done, and everyone from the Commanding Officer and Captain downward worked with a will. Almost every day the horses were taken out of their stalls, and exercised in the narrow gangways, while the former were cleared out. In spite of all 32 died, the majority of pneumonia, which in many cases went on to gangrene of the lung. Had it not been for exceptionally good weather, and the great care taken, we must have lost more. Possibly some of these cases were influenzal in character, as we had several cases of this disease among the men. On January 14th in the evening we sighted land again, and, at 2 o'clock in the morning, going on deck, I found we were at anchor in Table Bay, five great mountains capped with clouds looming in the background, while all along the base a line of lights showed us the town. All day Sunday we remained at anchor, a strong breeze keeping us off the land, but early Monday morning we went alongside the wharf, and soon a crowd of colonial men and boys were getting our cargo, living and otherwise over the side. Of medical work on the voyage there was but little; in fact I saw by the courtesy of the Veterinary Surgeon more of his kind of work, than of my own. Cape Town is a flourishing city, containing a number of fine new buildings, and with its suburbs is a large place. The population is as varied as could well be found. Whites, Blacks, Hindoos, Malays, of all colours, costumes and features. Electric cars run through the town, and out for several miles on either side, in the South to Woodstock, Rondebosch, and Wynberg; to the North to Green Point and Sea Point Camp, situated on a wide sandy common facing the shore of Table Bay. The camp was at this time occupied by men of various regiments, waiting opportunities to fill vacancies at the front. Here also was a non-dieted (sic) hospital, to which were sent a few convalescent wounded. There was but little to do here, and a few days later orders reached me to go to Victoria West Road, a station on the line from Cape Town to Kimberley, and about 400 miles from the former. I travelled up with a battalion of the recently enrolled Roberts' Horse, largely recruited from Colonials, but contained a number of men who had come from far and wide to enlist; one from Canada, another from British Honduras etc., all very keen on getting to the front. The railroad having climbed up through the passes of the Drakenstein mountains, emerges on the Karoo desert, and for 300 miles one travels across a great tableland rising in steps to a height of 4,000 feet, studded by hills varying greatly in height, but all rocky and barren; some are long and flat topped, others more rounded and conical in outline, but all covered with stones, varying in size from pebbles at the basis to great boulders at the summit. For the most part at this time of the year, the whole of the district is treeless and barren, except for dried up karoo shrub, or thorny mimosa trees, and is practically waterless, though water can always be obtained by boring. The sharp-cut banks of the now dry river beds, show how rapidly these African rivers rise in the rainy season, wasting away the sandy banks, and then as rapidly go down again, leaving nothing but the dry bed and a few green spots along the banks to indicate their existence. All parts of the Karoo at this season are swept by dust storms, great clouds of brown dust driving along, obscuring everything, penetrating everywhere, and covering everything with a thick layer of brown dust. I spent a few days at Victoria West Road, and then was ordered to De Aar. De Aar is, as you know, a place of importance, being a junction on the line running from Cape Town to Kimberley. Here I was to join the staff of No.3 Stationary Hospital, and found it consisting of three R.A.M.C. men, with

Major Marsh as C.O. and six civil surgeons, several of whom were from London schools, Richardson of St. Thomas'; Burton of St. George's; Fairbank of Charing Cross; Granville of St. Bart's; Dent of Birmingham; and Goldschmidt of Manchester; quite a representative body. Our hospital is formed partly of the local school house, and partly of large corrugated iron huts lined with wood, a good many mild cases occupying tents and marquees.

At present most of our sick are medical cases, of which a fair number have enteric fever. We are at present however, sending as many cases as possible down to the base, in anticipation of receiving wounded from the front, for, although things have been quiet there for some time, a forward movement is shortly expected. Situated as we are, a good way from the front, our occupation is perfectly pacific, and we are kept in mind of the war chiefly by the number of men, horses, mules, transport wagons etc., which have been going through in an almost uninterrupted stream for the last 10 days.

The climate is splendid; very hot in the day-time; 102 degrees F often in our tents, but the mornings and evenings are grand. The air is very clear and dry, and distances are most deceiving; hills that look so clear, that we think them but a moderate distance, are 12 to 16 or more miles off, and when one climbs a hill, often it is to see 20 to 30 miles in either direction. Some of us have ponies, and some of the country around is well worth a ride through it. Skevington and Pares must be out here by now, but I have seen or heard nothing of them yet.

No.5 General Hospital has been broken up. Sister Thistle, whom I saw on the Moor the day she arrived at Cape Town, having spent a little time at Rondesbosch, was sent on to Durban, so I am afraid the St. Mary's people will have no chance of working together.

Lord Roberts and Lord Kitchener travelling to the front visited our hospital last week. As to ourselves. We live in tents, comfortable enough, though often everything is covered in dust. We mess together in a marquee, and, as we draw our rations and have them cooked, our expenses are slight. What a brotherhood the profession is! although I knew none of the men here, almost all of us have mutual acquaintances. Of work there has scarcely been enough as yet, but possibly there will be plenty soon, and I hope to see some good surgery, although I fear we are in a bit in the background for that. February 11th. No.3 Stationary Hospital, De Aar.

A letter dated March 3rd 1900, from Basil Pares and headed,

18th Brigade Field Hospital, Osfontein,
Just a line to tell you of the St. Mary's men out here, as I have come across most of them, or heard about them.

After a week in Cape Town, at Green Point, I was sent off to Nauuwpoort, where a Stationary Hospital was formed, equipped by the French Aid War Society, a Col. Talvey and two other civilians forming the staff. I was there a month, during which time we got some interesting cases, as fighting was going on at Colesberg, then Rensberg, and ultimately Arundel, so we got the cases generally the same day. After a month at Naauwpoort I came up via De Aar, where Sanders is stationed, and proceeded to Modder. I should mention Brincker and Skevington came to Naauwpoort the day before I left; they are attached to No.6 General Hospital which is to be established there (550 beds). At Modder I met Hatch, who is with a Field Hospital at Jacobsdaal; I stayed the night with Hatch and got to Pardeeberg the same night, and next morning found Low and Wingate in the 18th Brigade Field Hospital, and knowing Major Ford who was in charge, I got attached to this. They had been very busy all the week, and were short handed, as men had been taken from the Field Hospitals, to replace regimental officers wounded. I saw Hewitt at Nauuwpoort when he passed through, he gave me a horse he had commandeered in the Rensburg district; I saw him again up here, he had been to Kimberley with French. We get plenty of work; Low was sent by Lord Roberts with a Captain Malcolm to Kimberley, but we expect him back to-morrow morning. Douglas who was in practice in Grahamstown, is with a colonial regiment and I saw Mantell the morning I arrived at Nauuwpoort, and he was going to take Douglas' practice for him. We had a lot of pseudo-dysentery at Nauuwpoort, and there is a lot of enteric at Orange River. There were a lot of gun shot wounds here, head and spinal cases predominating, but we sent off all our sick before coming here; three days in a bullock wagon to Modder does not improve the prognosis in most cases. It is very hot, but cold at night, and since the last few days heavy rain, the khaki coloured veldt has suddenly become quite green. We expect to move forwards with Lord Roberts in a day or two. Best remembrances from "St. Mary's Field Hospital" to you all – Yours,

Basil Pares.

A letter from J.O. Skevington

March 15th, 1900
6th General Hospital, Nauuwpoort
I utilise the spare time here, which I unluckily have owing to a sharp attack of enteritis, to fulfil my promise to you on leaving. Brincker and I are stationed up here with this hospital, which consists of about 600 fully equipped beds. Our staff comprises two colonels, two majors, and one subaltern of the R.A.M.C., and thirteen civilian surgeons.

After 60 hours journey by single track, we arrived here, a place somewhat aptly described as the last place the Creator ever made; but others say it was only the last but one, De Aar claiming that honour. Sanders is at De Aar and Smith also is there recovering from the effects of influenza. Sanders we saw coming through and he was in fine feather. The first man I came across here was Basil Pares, mounted on a captured Boer pony, and most delightfully got up in aged white canvas suit. To my sorrow he left for the action at Paardeburg the next day, just when we intended hiding the Lancasters at Socker. We have had a busy time here, as we have taken batches of 200 wounded at a time, and we have some 60 or 70 enterics with us always, or as they come down s.c. fever, said denomination being an abbreviation for simple continued fever! We had a big try to save a case which had perforated, but the type is very virulent, and we failed all the way. There is a good deal of surgery here of one kind or another, and Stevenson, a Johaanesburg Gynaecologist, tied the femoral one night by the light of a candle in a tent, for secondary haemorrhage. I shall not forget that night in a hurry, it rained as it only can rain here, and we were wet up to the very armpits. A day later I got a show at a similar case, and tied the anterior tibial just after its exit from the interosseous membrane. Brincker has been doing a good deal too, he is at present very keen on saving the fore-arm in a bad shell wound. At present no limb has been amputated here. Most of the wounds are Mauser wounds, but at Paardeburg the enemy did not play the game at all, the Highlanders being hit with Martini and Express bullets. One man caught a Mauser which had the nose filed off, and a bigger mess of a biceps could not be imagined. We get it blazing hot here by day, but bitterly cold at night. It certainly is a perfect climate, barring the chronic dust storms, but I have not seen a foot of ground yet I would fight my worst enemy for. The civilian surgeons here could not be better treated by the combatant officers, who never fail to express their pleasure at seeing the C.S.'s out here, and really they cannot do enough for one. Low is, I believe, somewhere Bloemfontein way, but I cannot find out his exact whereabouts. Wingate too has gone that way, but before I came up here. As regards the progress of the war, you are far better informed than we are. When we first came here, fighting was going on over the hill around Arundel, and we could hear the big guns hammering some ten miles away, but now the Boers are back to Norvals Point, from which place our next batch will probably come. I understand a good many Civil Surgeons are likely to stay here for a time with the Army of Occupation. With kind regards to all friends at St. Mary's from Brincker and myself –

I am etc.,

J.O. Skevington.

(Basil Pares remained in the Army and served in the First World War, receiving the C.M.G. and D.S.O. He finally retired before the Second World War as a Surgeon Lieutenant Colonel of the 1st Life Guards and Royal Horse Guards. He retired to Woking where he died in 1943.

Basil Wingate qualified at St Mary's Hospital Medical School in 1899 and joined the R.A.M.C. He served in the South African War and took part in the relief of Kimberley and in the operations in the Orange Free State and the Transvaal. He received the Queen's Medal with five clasps and the King's Medal with two clasps. In the First World War he was A.D.M.S. in France and received the D.S.O. as well as being mentioned three times in dispatches. He had a permanent commission in the R.A.M.C. and retired as a full Colonel in 1928. He died in September 1940.

The information about Joseph Skevington was given to us by Mr Ivo Smith, F.R.C.S., who qualified at St Mary's Hospital Medical School, worked at St. Mary's Hospital in his early surgical days and was renowned as an eminent London surgeon. His father and Joseph Skevington were cousins.

Joseph Skevington was born in Rothley, Leicestershire in 1875. His basic education was at Oakham School in Rutland, and he proceeded to study medicine at St Mary's Hospital Medical School. He qualified in 1898, and what seems remarkable in today's medical climate, obtained his F.R.C.S. the following year in 1899. While serving as a civil surgeon in the Boer War, this remarkably enlightened man performed some of the early radiological investigations in military service – X-rays were only discovered in 1895.

In 1903 he was appointed to the staff of the infirmary in Windsor and subsequently had a rapidly growing surgical practice in Staines, Maidenhead and the Royal Northern Hospitals among others. He served in the 1914–18 war as a Captain in the R.A.M.C. He was knighted in 1919 for his work during the war and for his services to the Royal Family. On his retirement in 1936 from the King Edward VII Hospital Windsor, the operating theatre was named 'The Joseph Skevington Theatre', and a new operating table was also presented bearing his name. It was typical of the man that following retirement as a surgeon he continued to work in the hospital as a radiologist until 1942. He died in 1952.)

CHAPTER 6

Letters April to May 1900

J.A.H. Brincker mentioned by J.O.Skevington wrote on 2 April 1900,

Nauuwpoort Cape Colony.

Previous to the outbreak of this war Nauuwpoort could not have been called anything else but a railway station; there certainly were a few houses then, but these were mostly occupied by people who had immediate employ on the railway, and they were nothing more than tin shanties, small houses built of galvanised iron. Nauuwport is an important railway junction, bringing together the railway from Cape Town and Kimberley on the one side, and Port Elizabeth and East London on the other, and taking these up to Bloemfontein, Johannesburg, and Pretoria.

Nauuwpoort means a narrow gate or pass, and takes its name from a farm belonging to a Dutch loyalist of the name of Klass Glasberg; this farm is about three miles from Nauuwpoort, and lies in a narrow pass through which the railway passes on its way to Port Elizabeth. Nauuwpoort lies in the centre of a large plain surrounded by a circle of curiously flat shaped mountains, surrounded by steep wall-like walls. These mountains are of common occurrence in this part of the country, and the name Tafelberg (or Table Mountain) is as common here as blackberries are in autumn. They one and all have the same peculiarities; they are all about the same height as that of Table Mountain, 3,500 feet above sea level. Sloping up gradually at first, they become terraced, and finally they become as vertical as a wall.

Vegetation is very scanty, and consists mostly of short scrubby bush, known as the Karoo bush; water is scarce superficially, but there is plenty underneath, and can be got up with the greatest ease. The rainy season is summer; it then comes down in torrents, flooding the surrounding country, and in a few hours transforming the deep water channels found here (and known as a spruit here, and a donga in Natal) into roaring rivers.

These mountains are about four miles from Nauuwpoort, though to the unexperienced eye they may appear about two thousand yards off; the air in these parts is so pure and clear that distance becomes very deceptive to the eye. Nauuwpoort stands on a slightly elevated piece of ground – that is, ground sloping downwards from the place in the direction of these mountains; it is thus well situated for defence against an advancing army, which will for about five thousand yards be exposed to a deadly fire from behind the earthworks which have been thrown up all round.

Nauuwpoort has grown to tremendous proportions since the beginning of hostilities; it is an important base now for all kinds of military stores, rations and ammunitions. It is said that they have here stores worth much; for instance, there are millions of rounds of rations here. They have here also a very important remount depot; thousands of horses arrive here from South America; these undergo thorough training here, and are then passed into the different regiments.

We have stationed here about four thousand men, mostly Militia, to protect the place; but in addition to them we have recruiting depots here of almost every regiment of the empire, from the 1st Life Guards downwards, so that altogether we have about ten thousand men here. The latter, however, are not permanencies, but go away from day to day. Especially now, things look very busy. Troops pass through here in thousands – these are all bound for the front; they are all going to Bloemfontein, where Lord Roberts is said to be concentrating a force of at least a hundred thousand men before he means to advance. These troops are taken as far as Norval's Pont, where they have to cross the river on ponts, or pontoons and then march on foot to Bloemfontein.

The railway here is very busy, and on average about twenty trainloads, of enormous size, go up to the front daily. These trains are of enormous lengths, never less than twenty wagons, and often drawn by two or three powerful engines; these are loaded with rations, ammunition, heavy guns – naval and garrison guns which have been transformed into field guns, or rather moveable guns, by the genius of Captain Scott R.N., C.B, of H.M.S. Terrible, and up to lately Commandant of Pietermaritzburg. It will therefore be obvious of what great importance a place like Nauuwpoort must be from a point of strategy; and it appears inconceivable how it was that immediately after hostilities began the Boers did not rush to capture this place, for it must have been known to them of what value such a place must be to us.

It is then, in Nauuwpoort that No. 6 General Hospital was founded, on February 21st 1900. This hospital was to be one of 540 beds, but this number has been greatly increased – so much so, that we have 800 beds; and of these 200 are filled with enteric patients, and there is a great likelihood of the number being greatly increased. Dysentery also is very common, and takes up about a third of our beds. Tonsillitis and other inflammatory affections of the throat are also very common. We had a very large number of surgical cases immediately after the fight at Paardeberg; we had them sent to us in two batches of 200 cases each. At the time we had no operating theatre, and what we did in the way of operations had to be done in the ward.

This Hospital is made up of about a hundred large marquees, each holding eight patients; each of these marquees is well fitted out, considering

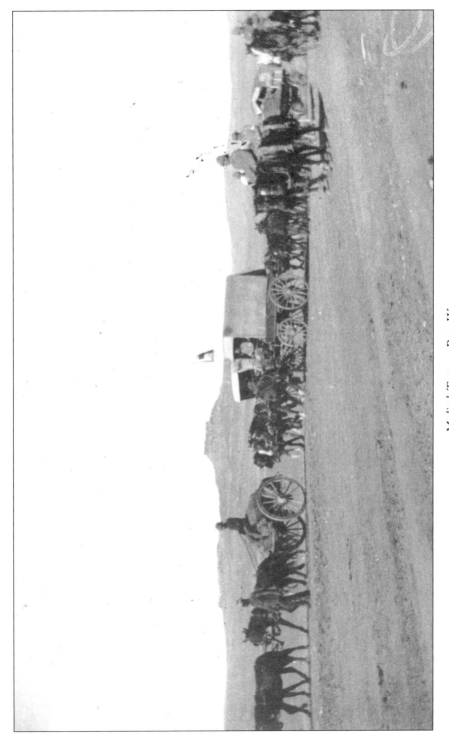

Medical Team – Boer War

Photograph courtesy of the Imperial War Museum, London. Negative no. Q77306

the difficulties of transport. It has a wooden floor, raised a few inches above the ground. Each patient has a brand new spring bed, horse hair mattress, bolster and pillows, sheets, three blankets, and white counterpane; by the side of each bed is a small table with two shelves, the table for mess utensils, the shelves for clothing etc. In addition to these, each marquee is furnished with a large deal table, a deal bench, an easy and camp chair, a dressing table for medicines, table cloth, salt cellar, mustard pot, looking glass, washing basins, brushes, and other necessities for a ward with patients confined to bed.

The hospital is divided into a medical and a surgical division, each with its staff and assistants; each surgeon has a row of tents to himself, usually eight. At first the surgical division was the largest, now it is the smallest. Each surgeon has a nursing sister attached exclusively to his tents, and also a corporal; and to each tent there is an orderly, either of the R.A.M.C. or the St. John's Ambulance.

As to dressings, I have found it safest to have one large dressing tray, which is carried for me from ward to ward, and which I leave in the care of the sister. The sisters, with the exception of one or two, are Army Reserves, and come from the different London or provincial hospitals, but we have none here from St. Mary's.

Night duty is performed by an orderly medical officer, who take it in turn, four sisters who do duty for a fortnight, a sergeant, and a detachment of orderlies. Special orderlies are allowed to each enteric ward, and to such other wards as have bad cases – but the latter is rather the exception.

We now have an excellent X ray apparatus, dark room, and developing room, under the direct supervision of Lieut. Hine R.A.M.C. An excellent operating theatre, with skylights, wooden floor, etc; it is made of galvanised iron, and, but for the heat, serves its purpose well.

We have large sterilisers, a beautiful set of surgical instruments, containing all the instruments one could wish for, beautiful irrigators on stands, and everything else.

The Royal Engineers have laid on an excellent system of water supply. The water is obtained from the ground by pumping; there are two pumping-stations. The pumps can be worked by steam or by wind. The water supply is excellent, and ample for the whole place.

We have also a kind of sewage system; although very simple, it acts well. All soiled dressings, excreta of typhoid patients, and other refuse, are destroyed in an incinerator which we have put up outside the camp. The sanitary arrangements are under the care of our sanitary surgeon, who is a civilian.

I forgot to mention that the typhoid wards are separated from the rest of the camp.

They stand on the gentle slopes of a hill, whilst the general hospital is situated on the other. The surgical and medical divisions are separated by the railway running to Bloemfontein.

Your readers will therefore see that the arrangements of No.6 General Hospital are not only excellent, but beyond the hopes of even the best hospital experts. Sir William Thomson, of Dublin, in charge of Lord Iveagh's Hospital, and other experts, have expressed themselves as highly satisfied with these arrangements.

Facts also prove it, for up to date we have passed over 2,000 patients through No.6 General Hospital, and, further, there is not a case of enteric fever to be traced to the surroundings of the Hospital.

J.A.H. Brincker

(*Author's note*: This is an extraordinary letter to have been written from a battle zone, and then published. It details the numbers of troops in the garrison, the layout of the garrison, the ammunitions held, the rations available, and indeed the movements of the troops with even their destinations. Lord Roberts' plans to advance with the number of troops he would have are revealed. All this information would be valuable to any enemy, yet there was no censorship. Such a letter could not have been sent in World Wars I and II.)

"London to Bloemfoentein"

Towards the end of last year the War Office asked for help from the Volunteer Medical Staff Corps to supplement the services of the Royal Army Medical Corps in South Africa. A large number of members from the Volunteer Medical Staff Corps in London, Scotland and the Provinces volunteered for active service, and after being medically examined the majority were accepted. The London contingent were first of all medically examined by their own officers, and then by the Regimental Medical Officers of the Guards at Rochester Row. Those that passed him were then, on February 19th, attested into the Royal Army Medical Corps for a period of one year as short service soldiers, and proceeded the next day to Aldershot, where we were joined by some of our comrades from Edinburgh, for mobilisation and equipment. We stayed at Aldershot until the personnel of officers and men were completed from various sources, and then left, on February 27th, christened by the rain, as No. 9 General Hospital, for Woolwich. We stayed at Woolwich a few days longer than expected owing to the boat not being ready, but on March 8th, we embarked on the P&O S.S. Sunda, at the Royal Albert Docks, and glided merrily, at about 4 p.m., amidst general cheering into the Thames. We were a mixed cargo consisting of Rifles, Mounted Infantry, Horses, and

No.9, General. The men were told off into various messes, and soon settled down making themselves comfortable in their hammocks when bedtime arrived. We had an easy run down Channel, and early on the 10th entered the Bay of Biscay, where the sea was comparatively calm. On the 12th we passed Gibraltar in the distance, and on the next day sighted Madeira. In the afternoon of this day, twenty-five of the officers on board were each inoculated above the groin with one c.c. of Ante-Typhoid serum, and owing to the preparation being too recent or too strong, the reaction was very great, for within two hours all of them were in various stages of collapse; some fainting, others had attacks of faintness, one or two were seized with violent vomiting, whilst all had more or less severe rigors and pyrexia ranging from 101 to 103 degrees. The following day the inguinal glands, and the lymphatics running from them were enlarged swollen and painful. These symptoms lasted for about three days, and then gradually subsided, so that by the sixth or seventh day after inoculation we were beginning to feel ourselves again. Most of the men on board were afterwards inoculated, but only with ½c.c., and were sent immediately to bed, by which they suffered much less reaction, and the symptoms were less marked.

On the 14th we steamed by the Canary Islands, and about here we unfortunately lost by death from pneumonia, one of the Edinburgh Medical Students. On the 17th we reached St. Vincent, Cape Verde Islands; here we stayed the day to get coal, and some of us took the opportunity to stretch our legs on shore. From here we made a straight run to Capetown, a journey of 14 days without sight of land, where we arrived on April 1st. The passage had been very delightful, the sea calm and the weather lovely, although it was sometimes very hot, especially around the equator. We passed away the time very well on board, with drills in the morning, and afternoon, cricket, quoits, and sports such as obstacle, egg and spoon races etc.

At Capetown we stayed one day, and were then ordered to proceed to Port Elizabeth, where we disembarked with part of our equipment, by tender. At this place we entrained direct for Bloemfontein. The railway journey, taking two-and-a-half days, was at first rather tedious, but it gave us our first experience of the roughness of active service, as there were little facilities for washing, except under a tap at a railway station, whilst there was none for changing our clothes or shaving, and we had to feed on the proverbial Bully Beef and Biscuits. At Nauuwpoort, when we stopped for our breakfast on the 6th, we met Brincker on the platform. He was attached to No.6 General Hospital there, as also was Skevington, whom we did not see. As we neared the borders of the Free State the journey became much more exciting; as we passed through Rensburgh, Arundel, etc., the scenes of late engagements, of which evidence was in view by the broken-down fences and blown-up railway bridges. This was especially seen at Norval's Pont, where the fine girder bridge over the Orange River had been rendered useless. At these places we had to cross very carefully over temporary structures. At Springfontein we were warned that between there and here the train might be held up by the Boers; so the infantry were served out with 100 rounds of ammunition each and we proceeded, without lights in the carriages, but nothing happened, and we reached here safely. We proceeded to the Rest Camp until the site of our hospital ground on the veldt on the outskirts of the town had been fixed upon, when we started to work to pitch tents for ourselves and marquees for the patients. We have now nearly finished, and are preparing to receive the patients. Nos 8 and 10 General Hospitals are also here, and amongst the staff are several St. Mary's men – Corfe, Knapp, Leon, and Walton.

The country is very hilly, with large valleys between; the soil is mostly sandy, of a brown, or reddish, hue. The land seems to be but little cultivated, but allowed, on its own account, to grow grass and other herbage, upon which the herds of cattle and sheep are turned out. Arable land we have not yet seen. The kopjes are not such little hills as we at home seem to have imagined. Most of them are fairly high, and none of them are so very easily climbed.

E.W. Herrington
Lieut., R.A.M.C.
No. 9 General Hospital Bloemfontein, April 18th 1900

Some of the St Mary's students volunteered for service before qualifying as the following letter reveals.

May 4th 1900.
Yeomanry Field Hospital, Bloemfontein.
Seeing that some letters had been written to the Gazette from St. Mary's men in South Africa, may I take a few spare moments to let you know how the St. Mary's men in the Imperial Yeomanry Field Hospital and Bearer Company have fared. We left the Albert Docks in the transport Winkfield; but I will not give details of the voyage except of one night which might have been our last on board. About 1 a.m. in the morning, I was sleeping in the bows of our boat, and was awakened by hearing our whistle going. I then heard the watch call out, and the next thing that occurred was to hear a terrible tearing of iron and wood, and to find myself lying on the floor, having tumbled out of my hammock. The order was then given to stand to our boats and get our life-belts on. On reaching the deck I found there had been a collision with another steamer, the Mexican, which, as

you must know, foundered. The next half-hour was a terrible one as we thought we might sink at any moment. However, we were informed that all was safe. And so we helped the other boat. Our C.O. Major Hale, was one of the first to go into our boats and help the other ship; I too volunteered, but as my rowing powers were not great, I was ordered on duty to the Hospital, where I attended the passengers and crew as they were brought down. It was an experience never to be forgotten. However, we reached Cape Town safely, although very much damaged. We encamped at Green Point, Cape Town, for nearly three weeks, and then left for Bloemfontein, where we are encamped just outside the town. We have to rough it a great deal, but are getting used to it. We expect to go up to the firing line, in three days time. On our way to Bloemfontein we pulled up at Deelfontein, and saw Surgeon Ashdowne, and were treated by him and the Yeomanry Base Hospital with great hospitality. I am a Sergeant in charge of a section in the Bearer Company, under Major Hale, D.S.O., R.A.M.C., who commands us. The St. Mary's men are Major Hale, Corporal Preston, Privates Collins and Wood, and myself.

Ainslie B. Tytheridge

A letter dated 15 May 1900 was sent by 'A Civilian Surgeon', with no other identification. A previous letter signed thus gave an account of the effect of the typhoid vaccination on the writer. We presume this is from the same author.

With the Cavalry Brigade

May 15th 1900

We had fourteen days wait at Cape Town with nothing to do, and then moved on the De Aar, Nauuwpoort, Norval's Pont, and Bloemfontein, each in turn. We waited a couple of days in the latter place, and then marched 10 miles out here due north to a place called Darkee's Hoek. Our Hospital was immediately opened for the sick, but after two days we were told it was to be divided, and that the right half was to return to Bloemfontein. Instead of keeping us as Field Hospitals to the fourth Cavalry Brigade, they made us act as a Stationary Hospital, so we had to treat all our cases on the spot, and send some to the base. A Field Hospital is supposed to be capable of treating 50 cases in 10 tents, but we very soon found our sick increasing, and finally had to treat 104 cases in the space meant for 50. Needless to say, it was very hard to do much good in such overcrowded dwellings, and with only a limited supply of medicines, and very few of those which we really wanted. Our sick were mainly dysentery, a very acute form; enteric, a rather mild form; and diarrhoea. The latter I attributed largely to inactivity of the liver at this high altitude, 4,500 feet above the sea level. This form of diarrrhoea is seldom seen when troops are marching and taking lots of exercise to work off the excess of food which everybody gets in a stationary camp. It very closely resembles the diarrhoea which one sees in the hill stations in India. The enteric we had to treat in the usual way, that is with diet, and treat any untoward symptoms that arose. The dysentery we treated with,

R-OL   Ricini
Tr.   Opii

and got fairly good results. Ipecacuanha and opium alone proved valueless. Towards the end we got some magnesium sulphate, and got most excellent results, but there was much vexation of spirit before we were allowed this drug. It was given in drachm doses every two hours. Had we had this drug sooner we might possibly have saved some more lives; as it is we lost only three from dysentery and one from enteric. When speaking of enteric I forgot to mention that the disease occurred in both inoculated and uninoculated cases. The death was in a case that had been inoculated. In addition to these we had several cases of tertiary specific (called secondary in the army where everything is either primary or secondary), several cases of hernia from riding, and a few minor complaints. We were told to evacuate our hospital five days ago, as we were to move anytime at a moment's notice. The order arrived at 8.30 a.m., and the transport provided for the removal of the sick was eight bullock wagons. As there is a great deal of red tape to be played with on these occasions we did not get away from camp until 4.30 p.m. I landed 82 sick in No. 8 General Hospital at Bloemfontein at 11 p.m., having lost none on the way. How much better for the patients if red tape were put aside, and they had been removed during daylight and warmth. I stayed the night at Bloemfontein, sleeping on the ground with a couple of blankets that had been lent me; they were full of pediculi as I have since found out. I was up at 6 a.m. and did my official business in Bloemfontein, and returned to take in the remaining cases by train, as they were too bad to travel by wagon. Special compartments were to be provided for them. I had them carried from the camp to the siding on stretchers.; when the train arrived I found that the special preparations consisted of open cattle trucks which had not been thoroughly cleaned out. However, they were put in and we started for Bloemfontein, where we arrived in an hour's time. Fortunately there was a medical officer to take charge at once, so I handed my papers in and left. I doubt if they all reached their destination alive, as some were very bad cases of enteric that had had haemorrhages. All the hospitals in Bloemfontein are now overcrowded, whilst a fortnight ago they hardly had a case of sickness in any of them. There are far too many P.M.O. people about, and they love red tape, even at the expense of the life of a patient. The last thing that the R.A.M.C. man has to consider is the life of the patient; the first the filling in of documents etc., I heard that one of our men lost six patients whilst moving from Thabanchu to Bloemfontein.

A Civilian Surgeon

An editorial appeared in the *Gazette* dated 21 May 1900.

St. Mary's at the War

Three more R.A.M.C. officers, Capt. J.H. Campbell, J. Grech, and Lieut. H.E.G. Wafton, have been lately transferred to S. Africa, and with Mr. R.C. Leaning going as a Civilian Surgeon, bring up the total of St. Mary's men serving in various capacities to fifty-two, with four of the Hospital Sisters attached to the General Hospitals. We have received several most descriptive letters of their journeys out and experiences, notably one describing the effects of the inoculation against typhoid, and J.H. Brincker's from Nauuwpoort, one of the letters saved from the ill fated "Mexican". In the former letter it is very interesting to note that of some 200 injected with the antityphoid serum, all suffered from symptoms of malaise, pyrexia, vomiting etc., commencing within two hours of the injection, with the exception of one who had had typhoid four years previously. Judging from published accounts and from private letters, the type of enteric being met with in South Africa is a severe one, and very definite results may be confidently expected from Dr. Dodgson's work on the antityphoid inoculation. Lieut. Wingate, who was present at the battle of Paardeberg, writes "I was giving chloroform to a wounded officer, and Low was operating upon him, when the Boers started shelling us, or at least the shells began to pitch into our camp, and very unpleasant it was. Two bullets whistled through the operating tent over our heads, and the surgery tent, about twenty paces distant, was pierced by four bullets. We had to quickly fill our wagons, and remove all our wounded under fire, and we left our hospital tents standing and trekked away to the west for about two miles, and there, dead beat, with all our wounded except two poor fellows who died en route, we camped, or rather laid down on the veldt and slept. It was an awful night, and I shall never forget it. Several of the patients were groaning, and the want of water was terrible, for the enemy held the river, and our water-carts, which had been sent to obtain water, were captured by the Boers." Speaking of the state of the laager at Paardeberg, he says, "The wagons, of which there must have been over 200, were smashed up and the ironwork twisted into shapeless knots like piece of wire round a soda-water bottle, and in many cases one could see mules, horses, and oxen, which had been struck by a shell, contorted into fearful shapes and presenting a sickening sight. How on earth the Boers managed to live in that awful atmosphere is more than I can imagine". Writing from Natal, another says: "Spion Kop battle was a terrible blunder, there is no doubt if we had only gone on we should have got through the next day, as the Ladysmith people say the Boers were going away in all directions".

We are glad to note Mr. J.O. Skevington's testimony to the excellent and cordial relations existing between the R.A.M.C. and the Civilian surgeons, which from some rumours we had heard, we were afraid were not altogether satisfactory. Hints had been suggested that the Civilian surgeons were not being treated fairly by their official confreres, and that petty bullying and unnecessary slights were the lot of the civilian without official status. That this should be so, would be a slur upon a gallant corps, which we are glad to be able to deny.

(John August Hermann Brincker obtained his D.P.H. from Cambridge and the Royal College of Physicians and Surgeons in 1902. He worked for a time at the Borough Fever Hospital, Croydon and resided in London and in Kensington Park Road, London from 1939 until 1964. He was a Lecturer in Hygiene and Public Health at Bedford College, London and St Mary's Hospital Medical School and a Principal Medical Officer with the London County Council from 1929 until 1939.

Edmund William Herrington became a Divisional Surgeon in the St. John Ambulance Brigade and was a Commander of the Order of St John of Jerusalem. He was awarded a service medal with three bars. He also obtained a Coronation medal, King Edward VII & King George VI. He was Clinical Ophthalmic Assistant at St. Mary's Hospital and Assistant Medical Officer Metropolitan Asylums Board. From 1930 to 1947 he resided at 9 North Side, Clapham Common, London SW4.

Ainslie B. Tytheridge. There is no record of his having qualified in medicine.)

CHAPTER 7

Letters May to June 1900

An editorial comment appeared in the *Gazette*,

A member of the Staff has sent us the following letter from Mr. Jenkins, a Dresser in the Welsh Hospital.

May 27th 1900
Government House, Bloemfontein

You will, I dare say, be surprised to note the above address, and will wonder how I came to drop in here. But to explain, all our staff were sent up to this town until the Welsh Hospital should be established. On arrival here, after a tedious three days railway journey from the Cape, we were ordered by the P.M.O. to remain at different hospitals in this town, pending further instructions. Five of our staff were sent to No. 8 General Hospital, another five to No. 9, while I had the good fortune to be located here at Lady Roberts' private ward, which was opened two days after our arrival here. Lady Roberts with both her daughters is now residing at Government House here, which is the late residence of President Steyn. She has utilised the ball-room as a hospital ward. It contains 36 beds and is entirely for wounded Tommies. Everything is going on most wonderfully well. Major McMunn (of blood pigment fame) is in charge while all the dressings are intrusted to me. Our Sister looking after the ward, is a Miss Smith from Bart's., while Miss Ramsey, a personal friend of the Roberts', also assists. The patients here are quite luxuriously accommodated, and simply get anything which they may desire. Any amount of smoking is permitted inside, while music and concerts are the order of the day. So great an influence does Lady Roberts evince in these men, that she almost daily comes in to see and interview them. In addition to inside comforts, Tommy is also allowed to wander at large in the grounds, in fact, he is altogether a personage to be envied. Most of the cases are those of wounded, the majority being of a slight nature. Twenty-eight cases are those of bullet wounds, the most remarkable feature of these being, the very curious course which some of the bullets have taken. In one case the bullet has transversely pierced the neck, passing behind the larynx, and making its exit in very close relation to the carotid artery. In spite of all this, the wounds are now perfectly healed, and from the day when this man was injured, there has not been a single symptom which would even indicate the presence of an injury. Fortunately in almost every case in our ward, the wounds have been caused by the Mauser bullet, which is undoubtedly the most humane of all the bullets. In every case which I have as yet seen, the wound is a very small one, edges mostly quite clean, and heals very rapidly. There is however one case here where a man's elbow has been hit by an explosive bullet which entering in the back of the elbow makes an exit in front of the joint, causing the tissues there to be simply blown out in marked disorder. There is a large cavity, around which redundant granulations are heaped up. In the first place, both the brachial artery and the ulnar nerve were distinctly exposed. In addition, the surrounding tissues were also so much lacerated, that an amputation was under consideration. It was finally decided to give the arm a chance, a very wise decision as later events have proved, for during the last ten days the wound has made most phenomenal progress towards recovery. The treatment which has been adopted in this case is: The wound is daily well syringed with carbolic lotion (1 in 20) carefully dried and then well peppered over with boric powder. The cavity is plugged with wet cyanide gauze, over which dry dressing is put, the whole being protected with wool, then fairly loosely bandaged, the arm being kept at rest by being attached to an internal angular splint, and kept in a sling.

Another case seems equally remarkable, in that the bullet having penetrated the left breast above the second rib, and about 2½ inches from the middle line, makes its exit just above the anterior superior spine of the same side. For a couple of days after the injury, the patient spat up a little blood, and suffered from shortness of breath. These inconveniences, however, very quickly subsided, while the patient now is as well as ever, and ready to travel down to Cape Town. Before concluding, I must not forget to remark, what excellent patients these Tommies make. They are full of spirit, and always most grateful for anything done for them. They have been good enough to present me with some very valuable relics of this war, not the least of them being a bodice of Mrs. Cronje, taken from her trunk at Paardeberg, by one of our patients here. I have also been given the whole series of Boer pom poms, some dum-dum bullets, in fact, I am hoping to have quite a famous collection to bring back with me.

I had the pleasure of meeting two other St. Mary's men yesterday, viz., Wood and Preston, who are attached to the Imperial Yeomanry Hospital, and to-day are commencing their march on foot to Kroonstad.

E. Lynn Jenkins.

"Transporting of Sick and Wounded from the Front to the Base"
No. 6 General Hospital Nauuwpoort.

There are four fully-equipped hospital trains in use in South Africa for the conveyance of the sick and wounded from one hospital to another. Of these

No. 2 and No. 3 are in use on the Cape Government lines, and No. 1 and No. 4 on the Natal Government lines. The luxurious Princess Christian Ambulance Train has also been in use on the Natal lines for some time, but whether that is the same as No. 4, or an additional hospital train, I cannot say.

I have seen both No. 2 and No. 3, and so in my account I am referring to these in particular. No. 2 has accommodation for 94 lying-down patients, of which about 20 beds are for officers. No. 3 has 96 beds. Each train is made up of eight corridor saloons; of these, the six foremost contain the beds, the seventh is the pharmacy and kitchen, the eighth the private apartments of the two surgeons and two sisters, and their dining-room.

The beds are arranged on each side of the saloon; the first five are for the men, and are arranged end to end in two tiers. The sixth carriage, next the pharmacy, are for officers, and the beds for this are arranged in exactly the same way.

These two ambulance trains run between the large hospitals and the base. For the conveyance of the wounded from the fighting line to the large hospitals trucks are in use. These are so arranged to take stretchers; as the wounded are brought up in stretchers they are lifted into the truck, the stretchers fixed end to end and one on top of the other in slots made for the purpose. These arrive here at all times of the day, and with us they usually arrived in from one to three batches at the dead of night, which means all of us getting up to detrain the patients, sort them, see them into their respective wards, feed them, and see to their bodily wants.

With the tremendous number of sick and wounded now under treatment the two ambulance trains are not sufficient to cope with the traffic of invalids, so that something else has had to be instituted. The ambulance train only takes such cases as are considered serious, cases that are helpless, lying down, or want frequent dressing or attendance on the journey. The others (and by far the large majority) are taken down in the way I am going to recount to you; having had the pleasure of being in charge of such a train from Nauuwpoort to Capetown, I think I can justly claim to say something. To keep to the very truth, I shall give you my own experiences on this journey to Capetown.

We left here on Saturday night at 6 p.m. My ambulance train consisted of four saloons; I had with me in one carriage a lieutenant of the Life Guards, who had returned from the front convalescent from simple continued fever (a term in the army to hide ignorance); in the other compartments I had 100 convalescents from enteric fever. I had a corporal and orderly of the R.A.M.C. to assist me. Rations were found for the men consisting of 100 lbs. bully beef, 120 lbs. biscuits, 30 tins Ideal milk, 13 tins Bovril, 4 lbs. sugar, 4 lbs. tea, 2 lbs. coffee, 2 lbs. butter, 15 tins jam, brandy

4 bottles, whisky 1 bottle. I must remind you that this was the diet for convalescent enterics, most of whom had only been up a week.

The arrangement was that I should telegraph down the line when I wanted hot water for the mess. I may at this stage mention that at all or most stations they have a station staff officer (military), who usually commands a small detachment of militia who are engaged to watch the line and bridges.

Well, we reached De Aar at 11 p.m., taking four hours to do forty miles – and no wonder too, as we were attached to a goods train. To my horror on arrival there I found that we could find no engine to take us on, and had to wait there until 6.40 a.m. next morning; so I arranged for hot water next morning at 6.a.m., and retired to bed. At that hour breakfast was served to the men (prepared by ourselves); at 6.40.a.m. we set forth – once more as goods. The next station was Victoria West Road, which we reached at midday; here the men were served with hot Bovril, biscuits, and beef. It struck me that at this rate of travelling and consumption of food my patients would have to starve the last day. I therefore thought of this plan of action; I knew that there were many patriotic people left in this country; a good many of these happen to be refugees from Johannesburg. A good many of these people have combined to form the Cape Red Cross Society, whose object is to supply the sick wounded with clothing and necessities. So when I wired for hot water at the next stoppage, which happened to be Beaufort West, I requested the station staff officer to communicate with the benevolent ladies of the place to tell them that I was bringing down a batch of sick from the front, and that any delicacies that could be supplied to them would be gratefully received. This telegram acted like a charm, so that when we arrived there I found a lot of ladies and gentlemen awaiting us on the Beaufort West platform, armed with hot tea, hot milk, custards, jellies, eggs, and bread. So much did they bring with them that after all we were fed we had a large supply to take away with us. We reached Beaufort West on Sunday night at 7 p.m., and for want of an engine to take us on, were delayed until 9.30 p.m. Our next watering place was Matjesfontein, which we were to reach next morning at 7 a.m. I got out to arrange about breakfast, but found the train going off without me; Cape Government trains fortunately don't go fast – more especially goods trains, so I managed just to catch hold of the last carriage, and to get myself into the guard's van, where I sat until the next station was reached. There had been some misunderstandings about the hot water at Matjesfontein – which, by the way, is a beautiful little place founded by Mr. J.D. Logos, U.S.A. Olive Shreiner lived here for some years, and wrote her books from here.

I arranged to have hot water at Towers River, and had a row with the guard for nearly leaving me behind. At Towers River, Worcester, Wellington, and Wynberg, the ladies were again to the fore, and we had no difficulties about food. At Wellington I was very nearly left behind again, but I made the guard understand that he was not to leave the station until I gave him leave, as I was in charge of the train, and not he. We reached Salt River Junction (two miles from Capetown) on Monday night, then we were shunted until 5.40 a.m. next morning, when we were taken to Wynberg, there to give my patients over to No.2 General Hospital. It was 8 a.m. before I was clear of my patients, and I had then to go back to Capetown without an invitation to breakfast. The journey of 569 miles thus took us sixty-two hours to complete. The last day of our journey some of the men got into trouble; by some means or other they managed to smuggle beer and spirits into their carriages, with the result that one man was so bad that I thought he would or had developed a perforation. Fortunately that did not happen; by means of a few simple appliances I managed to pull him round. No. 6 General Hospital after being stationed at Nauuwpoort since February, is on Tuesday going up to Johannesburg. I expect we shall have difficulties to overcome, and travelling by bullock-wagon from Kroonstadt will probably be the order of the day. We might then be fortunate enough to see some active service.

J.H. Brincker

No. 10 General Hospital
23rd June, 1900
Bloemfontein, O.R.C.

We have just received a copy of the "Gazette", and, not to be out of fashion, we are writing that friends may know of our whereabouts.

We form part of No. 10 General Hospital, and came out all together in the hospital ship, "Avoca", with a great send-off. H.B.G. Walton was one of our staff, while H. H. Jackson was ship's surgeon. We did not land at Cape Town but went on to East London. At this place unfortunate passengers are transferred from the ship to the tender in a sort of gigantic clothes-basket. The bump one gets in the process is distinctly disconcerting to the victims. We entrained at once for Bloemfontein. At Bethulie, just over the Orange River the railway bridge was destroyed, and we had to get out and walk over the waggon bridge. Here we ran across R.A. Draper, in charge of the 3rd Norfolks. His name is not among the 52 given by the Editor. The country round here was thick with Boers, and an attack on Bethulie was thought to be imminent. From thence to Bloemfontein the country was alive with our troops, who had however only just cleared the enemy out. The Reddersburg disaster occurred only about two days before.

In Bloemfontein No. 10 took over all the different public buildings as hospitals. By a stroke of luck we four were all detailed to the same place.

Walton exchanged into the Inniskillings, and went on with French's division.

In our hospital there are three medical officers, five or six sisters, and an X-ray expert. We found no place to live in, and so commandeered a row of Dutch cottages for ourselves and orderlies. If we have not the luxuries and "social life" of Wynberg, yet we are comfortable enough, in spite of a certain solution of continuity about the windows, and the immediate neighbourhood of many noisy mules and horses.

Sister Joscelyne is just recovering from a severe attack of typhoid and with some subacute rheumatism as a complication to retard convalescence, which is now, however, assured. The rest of us shared the care of her. Typhoid is terribly rife among the medical, nursing, and orderly staff of all the hospitals here. There have been 6,000 sick here at one time, and like Mr. Skevington we find very many sent in from Paardeberg, Vet River, Sand River etc., labelled "S.C.F." Dysentery is common, and often fatal. Not many wounded. There were 64 deaths in one day. Inoculation is not in high favour, but we await the results of Dodgson's investigations. He has written to say he hopes to be here shortly.

We have had much to interest us here. When we arrived fighting was going on at Thaba'Nchu and Bushman's Kop (which looks quite near), and even nearer. A vivid imagination enabled us to hear the sound of big guns more than once. Bloemfontein, now empty nearly, was then full, and Roberts, Kitchener, French, etc., might be seen any day at the Club, listening to the band in Market Square, or at the Cathedral on Sunday. The great march took place right past our little cottages, and we have seen the annexation of the O.R.C.

The climate is grand. Perfect days and frosty nights. Our chief recreation is riding. All the civil surgeons here have horses, and very good ones too. We hope to go to Johannesburg or Pretoria before the show is over, which isn't yet awhile. Kitchener came down the other day, and went off eastwards with a considerable force. They are busy throwing out entrenchments all round the place, in anticipation of an attack which was hoped for, but has not yet come off.

We have seen many St. Mary's men. J.T. Leon is with No. 8; Herrington at No. 9; Atwood Thorne, looking very fit, has just left for Kroonstadt with his Vickers-Maxim battery. We have Mr. Thorne's own authority for stating that these guns are not "pom-poms". We have also seen Low, Basil Pares, Basil Wingate, B.C. Taylor (who lost his unit, wandered off to Winburg, and has not been heard of since that day). Leaning, has just joined No. 9, and we see him often. Whitehead turned up in his ambulance train, looking very fit indeed. J.W. Summerhayes is convalescent from typhoid at No. 9. Sister Tippets, formerly at St. Mary's, is also at No. 9. At this hospital the students are represented by Speirs and Jones, while Jenkins is with the Welsh hospital, now at Springfontein. Kind remembrances to all at home from "St. Mary's Base Hospital".

Sister Lewis Loyd,
Sister Boynton,
R. Corfe,
Herbert H.G. Knapp.

(Dr R. Corfe qualified at St Mary's in 1894. He was a Civil Surgeon in South Africa in the Boer War and after this settled as a general practitioner in Greenwich, where he continued to practise until his death at the age of fifty-seven in 1927. He served in the 1914–18 war in both France and Salonika, retiring as a Lieutenant Colonel.

Dr H.H.G. Knapp D.S.O. came to St Mary's from Oxford and qualified in 1896. He went to South Africa a year later and served first as a Plague Officer and then as a Civil Surgeon with the R.A.M.C. After the Boer War he entered the Indian Medical Service and became a Lieutenant Colonel in 1921. He entered the Civil Department in the Bombay Presidency serving first in the Jail Department and, later, promoted to Inspector General of Prisons in Burma. He retired to Bournemouth where he died in 1944 at the age of seventy-five.)

CHAPTER 8

Letters July to September 1900

July 6th 1900
Pretoria,

Sir, – Having read some of Mary's men's late experiences in South Africa, I feel that a few words of ours will be of interest to your readers. I had the pleasure of sending an account of our doings as far as Bloemfontein before, and will therefore give our movements from there.

On May 27th we left Bloemfontein and marched up to Kroonstad, meeting with nothing of interest except what the country and the inhabitants afforded us. We halted one day at Kroonstad, and marched on for Johannesburg.

On June 6th we halted for the night about three miles from Serfontein. The following morning, while at breakfast, we heard distant firing, and having packed up we went forth to offer any assistance we could. After about two and a half miles march we came close to guns, and found they were Boer guns, and that they had surrounded Roodewal railway station. While deciding what had best be done, we were suddenly alarmed to see some English scouts dash through our ambulance column and call out that the Boers were following. Major Hall then gave the order to "retire", which we had to do. The waggons carried out the order with such good effect that several of us were left behind. The Boers then appeared over the hill, and to our great astonishment fired at us. Major Hall called the fellows together round a waggon that had broken down, but as the bullets still continued to flow he ordered the men to lie down in a drift, at the same time Sergeant Jefferies stood on the wagon and waved a red cross flag, and the Boers ceased firing. The Boers then came up and expressed their regret at firing at us, but explained that they thought we were an ammunition column. The bearer company were then marched back to the wagons. In about half-an-hour the fighting ceased and we were allowed to go up to the station, where we (most of us) experienced the first horrors of war. The station was a perfect wreck, railway trucks with their contents thrown all over the ground, railway buildings one mass of broken tin and wood, pierced through and through by shell and bullet. Amongst all this we found our dead and wounded.

In the meantime the Field Hospital went on about one mile and a half to the unfortunate Perly's camp at Rhenoster River, where fellows had been shot in their tents in the early morning, the remainder of them had then surrendered. We buried eight at the station, and took away about eighteen wounded, and we marched up to Rhenoster Camp and joined the Field Hospital, and every man worked until late that night. Altogether we had about 96 wounded and 25 killed – about nine died afterwards.

The following Sunday we were ordered by the Boers to move about two miles east, which we did (we were then under their orders, to all purposes prisoners). On the 11th Lord Methuen's column attacked the Boers, and they retreated, leaving us on our ground, from which we had watched the battle, seeing English shells bursting on our latecamp. We brought in one killed and about 12 wounded, and after a few days took the wounded down to Kroonstad, and from thence we were marched to Johannesburg, and then on to Pretoria, where we now lie.

This evening we have received orders to go and join a column to-morrow, and we expect to see the final fight of the Boers.

I hope my letter will be of interest, and I would give many details but feel I should take too much space. Perhaps I may have another opportunity of writing later on.

Ainslie B. Tytheridge,

Sergeant,

Imperial Yeomanry Field Hospital Bearer Company,

Pretoria.

A letter from Alfred W. Sanders

The few words last sent by me to the Gazette were addressed from De Aar. Four months of dust, flies, and enteric there, made one very glad when orders came to proceed to Prieska and take charge there. It was on Whit-Sunday morning that having packed my valise and two panniers on a cart drawn by four Cape ponies, I left De Aar, accompanied by an orderly of the St. John's Ambulance Brigade – the men of which have given valuable help out here – a little black dog and a white pony. The former was mounted on the pannier, the latter was tied behind the cart. By mid-day we reached Britstown, outspanned, and made free with a Machonachie ration, and some coffee sent to us by a kindly disposed person. That night we spent at a farm belonging to a Dutchman, who gave us supper, bed, and breakfast. Starting at sunrise, by mid-day we had reached Hanwater, a large farm belonging to Dr. Smartt. Here one saw what money, thought, and hard work can do. A great dam had been made to convert a valley into a fine lake. The waters of this allowed to flow in miniature canals over a plain many square miles in extent – being really a vast alluvial deposit – permitted fine crops to grow where formerly nothing but Karoo shrub would live. Spending the next night at a Dutch farm, on the third day we reached Prieska. The country round is mountainous, and the broad Orange River with its banks clothed with willow and many other kinds of small trees was a very pleasant change after waterless De Aar. Most of the houses are small square little places built of sun dried brick, no stairs, iron roofed, and often mud floored. S.M. Smith of "ours" has been here, but was now away with Col. Adye, and had seen fighting, and done good work at Kheis. The School had been converted into a fairly equipped Enteric Hospital with a sister-in-charge, and besides these two other buildings were in use. One the Kaffir School, a good sized oblong building had a few beds in it. Anticipating more sick and wounded, Smith had sent for beds etc., from De Aar. These having arrived we soon had the Kaffir School fitted out, though in a somewhat rough-and-ready manner. The commandant helped all he could and purchased freely at the local stores. In a few days Civil Surgeon McFadden – a really good fellow from Belfast – arrived with the first convoy, and filled our beds. These were mostly mild cases. For a fourth Hospital we now took over the departed Llandrost's house; by no means a palace. More beds arrived, ordinary iron lath beds, and a gang of "Boers" on parole was told off to put them together. Some windows were put in, and after a general clean down, our fourth Hospital was ready. McFadden had returned to Draghoenda, and soon arrived with the rest of the wounded. These poor fellows had travelled by road from Kheis, and were in a sad plight. Practically all had been struck by soft bullets and all the wounds were suppurating. One had been shot through the knee-joint, one through the elbow, and one through the ankle, while a fourth had a compound fracture of the tibia in the left leg, and most of the calf muscles shot away on the right. Live stock we had in abundance. Part of the journey they had to stand in trek wagons. Seeing a good deal of operating would have to be done, we asked for a third hand, and Richardson from St. Thomas', an old friend from De Aar joined us. We set to work operating, in turn, and in a fortnight's time things looked much better. We had to take off the thigh of the boy who was shot through the knee. The next thing was to get transport to remove our patients to Orange River, a week's trek. One ambulance had arrived from there, and another was now in camp. These and two spring wagons were enough for our eight lying down cases. These, a water cart and a donkey wagon for rations and kit, constituted our convoy. There was not work for all of us now of course, but we had to return to Orange River, so all went with the convoy on our ponies. It was a grand time. Our patients were so far better that they did not find the journey very trying, in fact they benefited from the open-air life. The days were hot and the nights very cold, but sleeping in a valise with a good Karos sheep-skin, it was comfortable enough; though one did wake to find the top blanket white with frost. Up at sunrise we trotted off to get a shot at a buck or anything else we might find, returned to breakfast, then inspanned, and away by eight o'clock. At our midday halt we did such dressings as were needed, and gave our patients an airing, lifting them from the wagons on stretchers. Our guns were always in our hands, not for Boers but buck. None came to my share, though McFadden shot one and a servant another. Bread, butter, and milk were bought when possible, some good friends at Prieska having given money for the purpose. We endeavoured to reach our night outspan before dark, but sometimes an extra long trek prevented. However our camp fires were soon alight, velt-bush and dry cow dung being the stock fuel, and our kettles were soon merrily boiling. It was a good week, – the best I have had yet, and gone too soon. Having reached Orange River, we all three were sent on here, and now I am at Grey's College, running enteric wards again, in one of which I have the privilege of working with Sister Lewis Lloyd.

At present the work is light, there being few acute cases, and there are plenty of chances of out-door sport. Inter-Hospital football is not confined to London Medical Schools, and polo can be played. Having only one pony, and being new to the game, I don't attempt. Several days I have spent hunting the wily buck, it may be his fault or mine, but I've never hit him. The veldt is now dry and brown, but lately it has rained, and they say the grass will soon be growing. War we see little of at present, and news comes slowly and uncertainly. Like all our men out here, I have been delighted to hear of our school's victories, of the Shield, Cup, and honours of all kinds won. Forgive my taking so much of your time, and wish me across the Vaal, –

Yours truly,
Alfred W. Sanders.

Mr Reg. Hughes writing from Pretoria (23 August) to a friend at St Mary's says:

'You will be pleased to hear that I have met Mr. (now Captain) Priddle; he is Medical Officer of the Police here. I went to mess with him on Thursday, 16th August, at the model schools, which building now does duty for Police offices and officers' mess. He is looking very well and has a hospital of his own. He asks to be kindly remembered to you.

Last Friday (17th August) a patrol of thirteen Seaforth Highlanders were fired on about three miles from us. The Boers captured twelve of them, and wounded one in the thigh. They wanted to shoot the wounded man, but a Boer wearing a red cross intervened, and so his (the Boer's) comrades spared the Tommy's life and took him to a farm-house. When the Boers had disappeared with the captured Seaforths, the wounded man sent off a note to his C.O., and he was brought in and came down to our hospital. To-day we are being inspected by Col. Gubbins, P.M.O. of District; he seems very pleased with the hospital

There was some firing this morning at 2 a.m., and the Royal Scots were ordered up. Later on two trains with troops, guns, and transport went in direction of Middleburg, so apparently there is a big fight going on. We often hear rifle shots in the early morning, which usually means a patrol is being fired on. Jenkins and myself send kindest regards,

Yours faithfully,

R.H.St. B. E. Hughes'

By E.W. Herrington, Lieut. R.A.M.C.

Sept. 15th 1900
Orange River Colony,
Bloemfontein
My last communication to you was written soon after my arrival here, and in it I was describing the pitching of the camp, but could only give few details as the work was then proceeding.

I am now sending you a more detailed account, and a brief outline of our work, with the facts of a few interesting cases, thinking that they might be acceptable to your readers.

We arrived in Bloemfontein early in the morning of April 7th, and proceeded to the Rest Camp. We were able on this, and the next two days, having little else to do, to get a look at Bloemfontein and to visit the various Field Hospitals which had been moved, for the better treatment of patients, into various buildings in the town, such as the Raadzaal-Dames Institute, Guy's College, St. Michael's Home, Industrial Home, Landrost House, St. Andrew's Home etc. It seemed peculiar to see the Parliament House filled with patients, who were lying upon stretchers raised upon cross-trees, the majority of them being below the bar, and a few above. In the other places the patients were lying upon beds placed either upon bedsteads or upon the floor. The town, at that time, was very lively, as the "military" were everywhere, owing to Lord Roberts' main army, since its entry on March 13th, being encamped around. The consequence was that large numbers of troops from Lord Roberts and Lord Kitchener and their staffs down to the "lads in Khaki" were to be seen in the streets, but women and children were conspicuous by their absence, as they had mostly fled the town before the arrival of the army.

Bloemfontein is not a large place, and would be very disappointing as the capital of anything. The public buildings are few, but of their kind very good. The Raadzaal is the most imposing, and is a pretty piece of architecture, whilst the Presidency, the Government Offices, and the Post Office, are of themselves striking because of their surroundings. The Cathedral and the Town Hall are very small, and both belie their name. The centre of the town is the Market Square; this is surrounded by shops, and from which lead a few streets, containing a few more shops, all of which are very moderate in character. The houses, excepting those in the Square, are nearly all of one storey, and are roofed with corrugated iron, whilst they are fenced in with barbed wire; this is the universal custom, so that wherever you go you see corrugated iron and barbed wire. The population consists of about 3,000 persons, of whom a large number are English, whilst the remainder are made up of Free Staters and Kaffirs. The water supply is very scarce, and is mostly obtained from wells, and to a less extent, from the Modder River through the waterworks. Sanitation is on the principle of the pail-earth system, whilst the slop-water is allowed to run into the gardens, etc., for irrigation; scavenging seemed to have little attention until the British entry. April 10th. The site of the Hospital ground having been fixed on the western side of the railway below Bloemfontein Mountain, afterwards christened Naval Hill, owing to the Naval Brigade having been stationed there when the army marched into Bloemfontein, we began to set about marking out the position of the camp, and to pitch it. The pitching we were able to do easily enough, and, in a few days, had erected enough cover for our 520 patients. We were then short of the internal equipment, owing to its being at the base, and not able to be sent up, as the needful supplies for feeding such a large army had first to be forwarded. Taking into consideration that the distance from Cape Town by the direct route via De Aar and Nauuwpoort was 749 miles, and that there was only a single line of rail, not in perfect condition the whole way, this was not an easy matter and even then we were not able to be on full rations. However, by degrees the equipment reached us, and on April 20th we received our first patients. The admissions gradually became more numerous, and on April 27th we took in 123 patients, and on the following day 260, so that by then we had 560, which was over and above our complement. On April 30th we were informed that the army was about to move, and that the outlying field hospitals would empty their sick into us, and that we must expect 600 more patients, so as no more marquees were available, we requisitioned for 120 bell tents for their accommodation, and in the first five days of May the admissions were respectively 354 – 170 – 430 – 100 and 180, which was above the estimate, so that to make room we had to transfer some patients to the Convalescent Camp, and to erect 20 more bell tents for the remainder. Our total then was over 1,600, and as we only had the same nursing and medical staff as for the regulation number of 520, the amount of work to be done by that staff may be better imagined than described. Convoys, mostly by ox waggon, came to us at all times of the day and night, and as the majority of the patients were suffering from enteric fever of a severe type, they had to be seen to and made as comfortable as possible upon arrival. Extra assistance in orderlies was at that time imperative, and as trained ones of whatever description were not available, they had to be taken from the convalescent patients of different regiments stationed at the Rest Camp.

Our camp then consisted of over 100 marquees and 150 bell tents for patients, and nearly 50 bell tents for housing the staff, so that it might truly be called a "tented city", even without the addition "of pestilence" used by a critic of the army hospitals. The rule was that the most serious cases should be placed in the marquees, eight patients in each, where they had bedsteads, mattresses, and bedding, whilst the less serious remained in the bell tents upon stretchers and two blankets, and if a case became serious, then room was immediately made for it in a marquee. The strain continued for from six to eight weeks, by which time we had gradually been given more help, and were assuming our normal condition, so that now we have only patients in the marquees, and these reduced to six in each and these are of a much milder type.

Owing to the great strain of work, and to the risk of contagion run by them, a large number of our orderlies, especially the younger one, fell sick, and we unfortunately lost seven of them by death, six being from enteric, whilst a large number were invalided down. We also, I regret to say, lost one of our Nursing Sisters and one of our Civil Surgeons – Civil Surgeon H. Bryant of Guy's – both of enteric, the latter having perforation which was diagnosed and operated upon during life, but without success.

The morning of May 28th was fixed for the reading in the Square of the proclamation announcing the annexation of the Free State, and as this was an unique occasion, which none of us was likely to see again, those of us who could anyhow manage it escaped from our work for an hour in order to witness it.

The Hospital Commission has come and gone, after an exhaustive enquiry into the hospitals here, and from my own personal knowledge, and from report, I do not think the R.A.M.C. will come badly out of the enquiry, but will in the future, have their hands greatly strengthened. They were not able to do impossibilities, and did their best with what materials they could seize upon, whilst no one could foresee that there would be such a terrible outbreak of enteric after Paardeberg or that the disease would be of such a virulent type.

The climate here is perfect, and that is the only advantage one can give the colony, for the country itself is very barren and unpicturesque, when you have said veldt and kopjes you have described all – no trees, no rivers, for the Modder is nothing to speak of, and little vegetation. We have just got over the African winter, which means practically that the very cold nights are gone for the time being, for the days are always more or less hot and sunny.

The weather now is very hot, whilst the rains will soon be upon us. Spring is showing itself by the shrubby trees and patches of grass upon the veldt becoming of a greener hue.

(To be continued)

Editorial comment in the *Gazette*:

A.W. Sanders is now attached to No.3 General Hospital, Kronstadt, and has had a very warm time of it. We give a short extract from a letter of his, describing the affair at Bothaville.

"A few days ago, at Bothaville, we had some hard fighting. On the afternoon of the 5th, our men made a reconnaissance towards the town, and were heavily fired on by some Boer guns which had been placed in a concealed position, and refrained from opening fire until our men were within close range. Fortunately but few of ours were hit. I had not before had any experience of shell fire, and even then was not very close. It was decidedly unpleasant.

That night we crossed the drift in the "Valsch" and camped on the south bank, on the hills where the Boers had had their guns.

Getting but three hours sleep we started at dawn and followed the track of the Boers. About two miles from camp our advanced guard captured a Boer outpost and discovered the Boer laager (a camp formed by a circle of wagons). The enemy being quite unprepared many of them took flight, including Steyn and De Wet. We closed on those that remained and occupied a farmhouse overlooking the laager. The Boers lined the wall of a garden and kept up a very hot rifle fire on our men, but were most fortunately unable, because of the severity of our own shell fire, to work their guns. I spent the morning attending to our wounded commanding officer, lying on the floor of the house. The bullets were coming in fast through the windows and scattering the plaster from the walls over us. We were safe, provided you kept down, and the enemy could not get their big guns to bear on us. It was a most anxious time for us all, but in the end we came off victorious, fortunately having support at hand, but had this failed we should, I fear, have had a bad time. We lost heavily, especially in officers. You will probably have read some account of the fight.

(Alfred William Sanders lived in Pretoria in the Transvaal from 1903 to 1942. He was a surgeon at the Pretoria Hospital.

Reginald Hugh St. Bernard Ellis Hughes served in the Royal Navy from 1904 until 1924. He retired with the rank of Surgeon Captain R.N. He resided at Grove Cottage, Portchester, Fareham from 1925 until 1945.)

CHAPTER 9

Letter March 1902 – Life in a Flying Column

A late member of the staff has forwarded this letter from friend Jenkins, and we have much pleasure in publishing it:

c/o P.M.O. Harrismith,
March 27th 1902.
South Africa.

In writing this, I venture to think that some of the experiences which have fallen to my lot recently, will prove perhaps interesting both to yourself and to the readers of our Hospital Gazette. A somewhat prevailing idea seems to exist in our hospitals at home that the duties of a civil surgeon out here are not over-burdensome, but I earnestly express a hope that this brief narrative of mine will help to throw some light on the question. At the same time I am quite prepared to admit that some of the billets here do not entail more than an average amount of risk, such as being attached to one of the large stationary hospitals: but on the other hand when one is posted to a flying column, or is regimental surgeon to a genuine fighting corps, he is brought thoroughly in contact with actual warfare and its concomitant results. When I became appointed as medical officer in charge of the 1st Battalion Imperial Light Horse, I considered myself very fortunate, and even honoured for if, during this great Anglo-Boer War, any individual corps has covered itself with glory, the 1st I.L.H. have just pretensions to stand foremost. The numerous successes which have been achieved by these men depend on the fact that the majority of them are colonials, who have been born, or have lived out here sufficiently long to know how to appreciate the Boers, and when necessity arises, to fight them in their own particular way. The post of Surgeon to the I.L.H. fell vacant owing to my predecessor, Dr Creau, being severely wounded near Bethlem. I hear since he has been invalided home, is practically recovered, and what perhaps is more, can now boast of the much coveted decoration, the V.C., presented to him for exceptional gallantry in the field. It was on the 15th of January that I rode out to join my regiment at Tigers' Kloof, a place formerly, I have no doubt, which could boast of these ferocious animals, as the name suggests, but now, alas, as the result of increasing civilisation, there is no definite proof that these denizens of the kloof and jungle once upon a time held sway over these parts. When I became properly introduced to this irregular corps, I was much surprised to find men from all parts of the world, and although the greater number were born and bred in South Africa, there were some who came from the States of America, these being mule-drivers from Texas and Kansas, others came from different parts of Europe, while the appearance of some, at any rate, suggested a descent from Jacob and Abraham, the latter hailing from Johannesburg and its vicinity.

The advent of a new doctor to a regiment not infrequently offers a loophole for being placed "off duty", and if there is a particular member who has a weakness for skrimshanking he will generally come to the ambulance tent with a most marvellous tale of the agony, and suffering, sincerely trusting to poach on the tender mercies of a civil surgeon. Such a character interviewed me very soon after my arrival, and endeavoured to impress upon me very forcibly that he was suffering form "Di-sintery", I asked him how he knew he was suffering from Dysentery, to which he replied with a most plausible smile, "Cos I's been passing slime ever since the war begun." The diagnosis was to me obvious, and I ordered him three No. 9 pills to be swallowed in my presence, with the most satisfactory result, for he has never more burdened me with such complaints. From this you will understand that these pills are a most certain cure for "Mauseritis", and if, in addition, you prohibit his usual rations and prescribe "condensed milk" in lieu, then a very speedy recovery is bound to follow. Such cases as these are, however, soon discovered, and very little time elapses before they are weeded out from the regiment. Leaving Tigers' Kloof somewhat suddenly, our trek took us in the direction of Heilbron, where we were to come into touch with the other columns about to participate in one of the "big Boer drives". Generally speaking "Reveille" went about 4.30 a.m., and we would start marching about 5.30–6 a.m., reaching our camping ground for the evening about 6, provided of course that the enemy were not too energetic enough to so harass our movements so as to prevent us camping about this time. Very frequently a rearguard action occurred, so that those squadrons that were engaged might not be able to join the main body until darkness supervened to assist their movements, and as I had to be always present when any fighting was going on my evening meal often became a much delayed luxury. During the day we generally depended on eatables that the country produced, such as mealies and peaches, some very fine specimens of the latter being ripe about this time, especially in the Transvaal. Any poultry which we came across would very soon change hands, our men having long established a most brilliant reputation for looting, and so powerful is the force of habit that ere long I also became somewhat of an adept at fowl-snatching. There are still quite a number of farms which are inhabited by Boer women and children, but in most cases they seem very badly off, and when I made enquiries as to those necessities which they missed mostly, a very average answer was, sugar, salt, and matches.

Although the Dutch women we met appeared very sulky and aggressive, I must speak one good word on their behalf, and that is the very great respect which they entertain for a doctor. In one household where I extracted some teeth for the children, I was prevailed upon to accept a tied-up parcel, which on further investigation proved to be a Bible of no mean proportions. Any empty homestead would be speedily committed to the flames, the idea being to destroy everything likely to prove of material use to the enemy. The Boers were very keen on keeping us always on the qui vive, and few nights were allowed to pass without their sniping into our camp. This usually meant that a few would be wounded on our side, and further, an interrupted night's rest for "yours truly". Our average days' march was about 25 miles, often very trying beneath a relentless sun, and on those occasions when it rained, the situation you will allow was not an enviable one. It is in such cases as this, that rum proves such a valuable part of Tommy's rations, and the medical officer who is not careful to recommend extra quantities during such trying times very soon becomes unpopular. For nearly six weeks the men did night as well as day duty, being compelled to snatch an hour's rest either on the march, or after arriving in camp. My work really only commenced in the evening after pitching camp, when I had to ride round to inspect the different squadrons, some of the latter being about four miles distant from the main body. To ride in the dark and run the gauntlet of pickets, who had orders to shoot at everything after a certain time, was another frequent item on the programme. Again, when any night march took place you can remain assured that the ambulance was not left behind, and if your horse was unlucky enough to step into a hole, and a severe bruise followed, you had to grin and bear it, for a doctor should know how to bear pain as well as to alleviate it. One of these night marches was so very exciting that I will briefly describe it. It was on January 29th, we had arrived in camp about 6 p.m., after an exceptionally long day's march, and in about an hour's time we were quietly told to be in readiness at 9.30 p.m. to march again. How reluctantly we mounted our horses, but a rumour to the effect that there was some fun coming off, helped us to a considerable extent to minimise our vocabulary of nasty remarks. With a little moonlight to assist us, we trekked on solemnly for miles, only halting an hour or so to give our mounts a chance. Just before dawn arrived, our advanced scouts returned with the news that there was a Boer laager three miles ahead. Then indeed excitement ran very high, and after some re-arrangement of the troops the majority of us swept down upon the enemy, who was resting quite peacefully in the valley. They were quite taken by surprise and made no attempt at resistance. It was quite a respectable haul, which included 21 prisoners, 32 cape carts, 15 waggons and nearly 4,000 head of cattle. Among the captured was Commandant De Villiers, who, with his wife and daughter, was riding about the country in a very swagger "spider", which belonged to Steyn. This piece of loot fell to my lot, and with our Colonel's permission I appropriated this for an additional ambulance. Another queer article which I commandeered was a clock, and that same night when two other officers were fast asleep in our tent after our recent exertions (which included riding nearly 60 miles within the 24 hours), we were very suddenly aroused by some sweet strains of music. At first I thought I must be dreaming, and in a cathedral, but soon it dawned upon me that "the old Dutch" was responsible for this entertainment. It seems that my servant, a somewhat curious individual, had wound this clock without my knowledge – hence the music. The hymn it played was "Lead, Kindly Light", which at the time I considered somewhat appropriate, for it was a very dark night, and we were certainly very far from home. The next seven days were most eventful, for we were kept going both day and night without intermission, and it seemed as if there was no rest for the weary. On February 6th matters reached a climax, for, about 11p.m. that night the camp was suddenly the scene of most terrible firing. The Boers had accidentally dropped upon us, and were driving large herds of cattle in front, so as to protect themselves. The night was so dark that it was quite impossible to distinguish between friend and foe. Our tent was perforated in three places, one of the officers sleeping with me being wounded in the elbow. From this you can judge that bullets were not a scarce commodity. It seemed a second Tweefontein, but in this case the enemy met with a reception which they had hardly bargained for. When I cautiously peeped out at the bottom of our tent door, I saw the outline of some Boers not far off, so I took up Adam's revolver and blazed away. I felt quite justified in this, for we were on the defensive, and it was not likely that I should be taken for a red cross man in my pyjamas. That night I was kept extremely busy attending to the wounded, and the cases were far too many for me to deal with properly. When morning light appeared the camp presented a most ghastly spectacle, with dead and wounded men and horses strewn about in different places. Several Boers were found lying dead and those that remained wounded were all very severely hit, for it is the custom of the Boers to take away with them all those only slightly wounded.

It was on this occasion that Commandant Besters fell into our hands. He was very badly hit in the stomach, and expired while I was attending to him. The casualties were so many that we were obliged to heliograph to Colonel Byng's column for assistance. The next night again was a regular panorama, this being the last night of the great Heilbron drive. The enemy was now fairly hemmed in and had to either force through our lines or get captured on the following day. There was not a man of us who attempted to sleep that night, and from 10 p.m. till daybreak there was a regular fusillade of firing, rifles, colt guns, maxims, pom-poms, and 15 pounder guns firing case cartridge, all seemed to vie with one another in creating the most tremendous din. Bennett Burleigh never exaggerated when he described it as a "veritable Hades". Personally, I spent the night in frog fashion beneath the ambulance wagon, and was intensely relieved when dawn arrived. The number of Boers hit was comparatively trifling, when the amount of ammunition expended is taken into consideration. One little Dutch boy was badly wounded in the thigh, and I heard him crying bitterly during the night. When I found him next morning he was in a very bad way. The bullet had entered his hip and could be felt distinctly in front of the thigh. I had little difficulty extracting it, but the little fellow died in about two hours afterwards.

After all this hard work we are actually allowed to rest a couple of days outside Heilbron, after which we must resume operations in pursuit of the ubiquitous Boer.

E. Lynn Jenkins.

(The Boer War ended in 1902 and unfortunately we have no record of letters to the *Gazette* from July 1900 until this last letter of March 1902. It is possible that some were written, but none was found in the archives.

We feel that those letters that are included here covering the early stages of the war give a good account of events, and illustrate the attitudes of medical men, nurses and soldiers serving in South Africa at the time.

There are no letters from Mafeking or Kimberley to record the memorable events at either site, but the letter from Ladysmith gives a detailed insight into the circumstances of a siege.

That chivalry existed during this war was demonstrated in the letter by Ainslie B. Tytheridge when the column was fired upon by the Boers, and the waving of a Red Cross flag caused them to cease. The Boers approached the column and apologised explaining that they thought the column was an ammunition column.

The letter by R.H.St.B.E. Hughes tells of a wounded Seaforth High-lander who was about to be shot by a Boer, but was saved by the intervention of a Boer belonging to the Red Cross.

Another letter tells of a captured British Officer being returned to his unit because he was a Medical Officer.

In World Wars I and II there must have been similar acts of chivalry, but not on any grand scale, and indeed the exhibition of the Red Cross did not protect a building or an individual from attack. It was certainly not the custom for the enemy to return medical officers to their units, on either side.)

An Editorial appeared in the *Gazette* dated November 1902:

"Dulce et Decorum."

Some time ago in these columns it was suggested that some memorial should be raised to commemorate those men who lost their lives in the service of their country in South Africa. There seems to exist a very general consensus of opinion that something of the kind should be done, and already, in numerous other schools and Hospitals, schemes have been initiated and carried out. At Guy's it is proposed to erect, as a memorial, a fountain in the courtyard. Now Guy's is a larger school, and while we would not seek in any way to emulate them, surely we ought to do something at St. Mary's to perpetuate what is certainly an honourable distinction in the History of the School.

During the war seventy-one members of the Hospital served in one or other capacity in the Imperial Forces, and of this number six lost their lives. Lieut-Colonel A. Baird Douglas, Sherwood Foresters, was killed in action: Captain R.H.E.G. Holt, R.A.M.C., died of wounds; Lieut. W. Guy Jones, R.A.M.C., and Civil Surgeons Cecil Courtenay Parsons and Reginald Percy Fort, died from enteric fever; and sixthly, Sec.-Lieut. G.V. Jameson, 1st Border Regiment was killed in action. These are men whose names form an integral part of the history of the School, and yet so short are human memories that in a few years they would probably be forgotten, did not some tablet serve to remind the generations to come that at the call of their country's need men were to be found in numbers to sacrifice everything for their country's sake. The difficulty in the way of the scheme hitherto seems to have been as to who should take the initiative in the matter. If we are right in our opinion that there is a strong feeling in favour of the movement, and we most thoroughly hope that we are right, then surely the people who should make the preliminary arrangements are the authorities. In olden days the question might have arisen as to which authorities, those of the School or those of the Hospital, but in these present days of amalgamation that difficulty will not be an obstacle. On the Committee, when formed, there should be representatives of the Board, of the Staff and of the Students both past and present.

In a matter of this kind it is not a large subscription that is required so much as a wide-spread and general response to the call. It is not necessary to discuss the form that the memorial should take until it is seen how much there is gathered for it. But even a brass of the simplest nature in the

Hospital Chapel would be better than leaving us the stigma of doing nothing to record the names of those men who have served their country even unto death.

We sincerely hope that by the time the next number of the Gazette appears we shall be able to publish the appeal of the Committee for subscriptions, and that the response will be as generous and wide-spread as the nature of the case demands.

(A brass plaque was erected and is on the wall inside the entrance to the hospital. It contains the names of the medical officers and one nursing sister who died from enteric fever, but was not mentioned in the editorial. Four of the seven died from enteric fever.)

CHAPTER 10

World War I (1914–1918)

In 1914 Europe was on the verge of war as the result of rivalries for economical and political reasons between the great powers. At the same time there was an increase in the military strength of the larger nations, supported by strong nationalistic feelings. Europe was waiting for any excuse and this came with the assassination of Archduke Franz Ferdinand of Austria by a Serbian student on 28 June 1914. Austria declared war on Serbia. Russia had a treaty with Serbia and mobilised her forces. Germany declared war on Russia on 1 August 1914. France had a treaty with Russia and mobilised. Germany declared war on France on 3 August 1914 and invaded Belgium. This precipitated Great Britain to enter the war on 4 August 1914.

Germany, Austria, Hungary and Bulgaria faced the Allies, Great Britain and its Empire, France and Russia. Italy joined the Allies in 1915, and the United States of America joined in 1917. Japan supported her ally Britain in 1918.

An Editorial appeared in the St Mary's Hospital *Gazette* in October 1914:

St. Mary's and the War

It is early yet to appreciate the results of the Great War on our Hospital. By its starting during the summer holidays, we have not been disorganised so much as had the first shots been delayed till now. From the administrative point of view, the full effect of the changed conditions cannot be realised for months or years. It is at least probable that our subscriptions will be diminished for a time, partly because the subscribers have gone to the war, partly because they are suffering financially, as we all are, owing to the manifold inhibitions of normal economic functions, within and without our Empire, produced in connexion with the outbreak of communal insanity which we call war. We must each and all do our best to gain new subscribers, since our main function is to succour the sick, at all times and in all conditions. "Business as usual" must go on in a hospital, whatever else goes on in the world around. But it cannot go on unless we all do our extra share, to make up for the inevitable losses due to the war.

For the Forces are doing much: see the lists at the end of this number; note that we are holding over one-third of our hospital beds ready for them here, and that St. Mary's men preside over half the base hospitals of London, and are represented at another. Note also, that Sir Almroth Wright's name and fame are known wherever vaccination is carried out, whether anti-typhoid, or anti-other infection, and that he has been appointed Consulting Physician with H.M. Forces; note the number of units in which we have men; note the by now well known hospital at Paignton, where Mr. Ernest Lane may be found, and where our steward did good work as an expert volunteer; note how almost to a man our Housemen volunteered; read Dr Gosse's article on the work of our Hospital Ship, and then add to all this, the many unpublished names of those connected with St. Mary's who have been helping, by personal service with His Majesty's Forces, or by enabling others to go, or in countless other ways. We may well be proud of our hospital in its National War aspect. But how about its aspect in the matter of war against disease?

Well, we are going to stick to our job, and see it through. We shall, if necessary, do as is often done in America, and get what is necessary to do our duty to the civilian sick, and trust to the great public to foot the bill. We shall continue to train students from start to finish; we shall offer them the chance they shall not get so well in many other and larger hospitals, of doing things with their own hands, which is the only way to learn. We shall probably be able to show them all sorts of war casualties, medical and surgical, and if we cannot show them these last at the first-aid stage, it will be thanks to our good Navy of the sea and air. They will thank Providence that they have this opportunity of testing their constancy to the high ideal of personal service to Humanity, by continuing their medical studies, and qualifying as soon as possible to take their place in the line of fire against disease.

A letter written to the *Gazette* by J. Ernest Lane was published in October 1914:

The American Women's Hospital at Paignton

On the outbreak of war certain American ladies decided to form a hospital for the sick and wounded soldiers, and they accepted an offer from Mr. Paris Singer of the use of his residence.

The entire cost of conversion and maintenance is supported by American money. The hospital is situated at Paignton, S. Devon, overlooking Torbay. It consists of 200 beds and is completely equipped with an operating theatre, X-ray room, etc., and there is a lavatory for every five men and a bathroom for every seven. The first batch of patients were received on September 27th, the War Office having given 24 hours notice. The wounded had sailed from St. Nazaire to Southampton, and had been transferred to an ambulance train, which arrived at Paignton at seven o'clock. The detraining was successfully carried out with the aid of twelve orderlies, and voluntary assistants. Among the 130, 30 were described as "cot" cases, and were removed on stretchers to vans and motor ambulances; the 100 were helped into G.W.R. excursion motor cars.

On arrival they were in fairly good spirits, though naturally tired and worn. The majority came from Mons and Soissons, and had not had their clothes off for two or three weeks, and had had but little to eat, some having had to wait two or three days before being bought in from the trenches. The immediate care was a matter for the sisters, in getting them clean and cutting off their clothes. After the first 24 hours they settled down to sound, restful sleep, though at first they were troubled with dreams, and often awoke with a start to face imaginary Germans. For the first two or three days they mainly required sleep and plenty of food. Of the 130 cases only six were medical. They consisted of dysenteric diarrhoea, rheumatism and pleurisy. The surgical wounds were mostly due to shrapnel, the character of which was dependent on the size and shape of the fragments. The cases were mostly septic, and though discharging pus freely, there was but little tendency to pocketing owing to the free drainage along the open track. Portions of clothing were only occasionally found in the wounds. Typically they presented a small wound of entry with a large wound of exit, frequently of the explosive type. They were situated on those parts which are liable to be exposed when lying face downwards, such as the face, back of the head, shoulder, arm, forearm and hands, buttocks and feet. The severity of the injury varied with the anatomical structures through which the bullet passed, though it is remarkable how the important vessels and nerves so frequently escaped. Contact with bone caused fracture with considerable comminution. The fractures included those of humerus 4, ulna 3, metacarpals and phalanges, femur 1, tibia and fibula 1, spine, jaw, and os calcis. Injuries to nerves included a case of paraplegia from the level of the 2nd lumbar nerve, due to a large shrapnel wound opposite the angle of the 9th rib; this patient had a large bed sore on his arrival, division of the external popliteal, and of the anterior tibial at its origin. Amongst injuries to the blood vessels were a case of division of the femoral vein, the haemorrhage from which was very difficult to control owing to the wound being at the lower end of Hunter's canal, and an aneurysm of the brachial artery. There were two eye cases: one presented a dislocation of the lens, requiring extirpation of the eyeball, the other a wound of the cornea. Rifle bullets cause a small wound of entry and exit with but little damage. Two cases were convalescent 10 days after the passage of bullets through the lung. The treatment adopted was largely conservative, and as

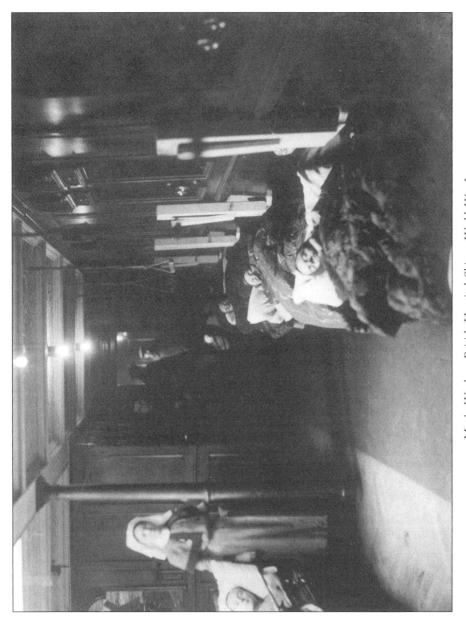

Men's Ward on British Hospital Ship – World War I

Photograph courtesy of the Imperial War Museum, London. Negative no. Q7798

the wounds drain freely plugging is not required. Bullets if superficial or if causing any pain or discomfort were removed. One bullet which I successfully removed had passed beneath the angle of the left jaw and lodged in the right side of the third cervical vertebra; it caused severe dysphagia, occipital neuralgia and oedema of the left half of the tongue. The fractures, though septic and comminuted, united well without necrosis, and without the aid of elaborate splint apparatus. Appropriate treatment was carried out for the cases of special injury. Minor ailments, such as corns and callosities, and toothache are not to be overlooked. A second batch of 29 cases, mostly convalescents, was received from Devonport, on October 5th. Of the 159 cases that have been treated, 70 have already been discharged, which is indicative of the rapid recovery made.

J. Ernest Lane.

P.S – A further batch of 121 patients was received on October 16th.

(J. Ernest Lane, 1857–1926, belonged to a family that played a major role in the development of St Mary's Hospital and its Medical School. He was the son of James R. Lane who was a nephew of Samuel Armstrong Lane. Samuel Armstrong Lane, the son of a tailor studied at St George's Hospital and in Paris and Berlin. He founded an Anatomy School near St George's Hospital and hoped to get on the staff of the hospital. When St George's opened their own school he turned to the prospect of a hospital in Paddington which was completed in 1851. Samuel Lane was a principal in the founding of the Medical School which opened in 1854. He was appointed Lecturer in Anatomy and one of the surgeons to the hospital. He also held an appointment at the Lock Hospital.

His nephew, James R. Lane, was one of the Surgeons to Out-patients at St Mary's Hospital in 1851 and later also Surgeon at the Lock Hospital. He died in 1891, the year his son James Ernest Lane was appointed to St Mary's Hospital.

J. Ernest Lane was educated at Lancing and Magdalen. He qualified from St Mary's Hospital Medical School in 1880. He became Lecturer in Anatomy. In 1891 he was elected surgeon to Out-patients in the hospital and in 1904 took charge of surgical beds. He was also surgeon to the Lock Hospital as were his predecessors. He became a Council Member of the Royal College of Surgeons.

In 1923 he was knocked down by a bus in Regent's Street and fractured his femur. This failed to heal and he spent three years in bed in the Star and Garter Home in Richmond. He died on 4 November 1926.)

A letter published in October 1914 in the *Gazette*:

The Hospital Yacht "Liberty"
By A. Hope Gosse M.D. M.R.C.P.

Until the outbreak of the present war the use of hospital ships in European naval warfare was practically unknown. It may therefore be of some interest to give an account of one of them, the Hospital Yacht "Liberty" No. 10, of 2000 tons, under the command of Lord Tredegar, with a medical and surgical staff of five, all of whom are St. Mary's men. They are:

Principal Medical Officer	Dr H. Gwynne Lawrence
Senior Surgeon	Mr. W.H. Clayton-Greene
Assistant Surgeon	Mr. C.A. Pannett
Assistant Surgeon	Mr. P. Withers Green
Assistant Physician and Anaesthetist	Dr. A. Hope Gosse

Immediately war was declared the owner offered his yacht to the Admiralty and it was accepted. The work of transforming it for use as a hospital was begun at once. Five of the largest rooms in the forward part of the ship were stripped and turned into wards which now contain fifty swing cots. An equal number of cots can be used temporarily elsewhere. A room opening off two of the main wards was turned into an operating theatre. This was fitted with all the requirements of a thoroughly modern theatre, and in its utility would compare very favourably with the theatre of any London general hospital. In a small room opening out of this and previously used as a bathroom a steam steriliser for dressings and an instrument steriliser for instruments was fitted. Each ward also contains a small steriliser for dressing instruments. In another room an X-ray apparatus was installed. The dispensary was already part of the ship's arrangements. All structural alterations and the fitting of beds, sterilisers, steam pipes, lights and the fixing of everything in use and for stock so that it would not move when we encountered bad weather were completed in ten days.

One of the most difficult and important parts of the work of a hospital ship to carry out satisfactorily is the transport of the wounded from ship to ship. It is a difficulty which each ship will have to solve as a result of its own experience. No hard and fast rules can be applied to all. The size and arrangements of a ship will modify its transport. Experience has shewn us that a destroyer can come alongside the "Liberty" when under the lee of the land. Patients can then be passed across on stretchers, and there is in consequence only one move from the deck of the destroyer, where the wounded are placed, to their beds in the hospital ship. The large battle-cruisers and Dreadnoughts have higher decks but the promenade deck of this ship could be used as it is approximately of the same height. When the wounded have to be transported by means of a tender, one with a flat deck will best serve the purpose The canvas cots or stretchers can be laid side by side on the deck in fair weather, as was done when we took in wounded from the Heligoland fight, but in dirty weather they will have to be placed in the hold of the tender. When the tender with its load is alongside, a wooden cradle is swung out by means of a derrick, the cots are placed in this, and the cradle is hoisted up, swung on to the ship, and, on the "Liberty", lowered straight down into the main ward. This work is best done by the sailors, who are, of course, accustomed to the ropes, and very quickly acquire the gentleness necessary for their unaccustomed human freight. In the ward the ten trained orderlies are ready to carry the patients to their beds.

On August 29th we were in Harwich Harbour. Shortly after midnight we were called up and ordered to be in readiness to receive German wounded, who were being brought to Harwich by the destroyer "Lurcher", our first news of a naval action in the North Sea. Three of the surgeons on the ship were sent to meet the destroyer. There was a dense fog, but the launch found her soon after she anchored. First aid had been thoroughly rendered to the wounded while returning from the scene of action.

From the deck of the "Liberty" the outline of a barge was seen through the dense fog in the calm of an early dawn. The intermittent ringing of our fog bell had been its only guide. Silently it came alongside and revealed a deck covered with canvas cots, side by side, each with its wounded man, while some men with less severe wounds were seated or placed below the hatch. Twenty-four in all, saved from the sinking German cruiser "Mainz". There was no restlessness, no groaning, but a careful scrutiny of their faces revealed recent sufferings.

Transhipping was quickly and carefully performed, and then a systematic examination of the injuries was made, immediate operation cases were selected, all others were redressed, and given such treatment as the nature of their injuries demanded. Five major operations were performed before breakfast, some cases needing three surgeons working at different wounds to shorten the anaesthetic and to enable the next case quickly to receive attention. By mid-day all wounds had been treated. They were often dangerous, always multiple, and most contained pieces of shell. There were very few burns.

By this time the cruiser "Fearless" had arrived with some of the English wounded, five of whom were sent to the "Liberty". These received similar treatment to the other wounded, one, an officer, was placed in a separate state room set apart for the purpose. During the afternoon two other patients needed operation; one, for amputation of the leg, was suffering too severely from "shock" in the morning to stand any surgical treatment.

On the following day we left Harwich early in the morning for Chatham, where we were docked. There were two operations in the morning during this short voyage, one of which was necessitated by a recurrence of haemorrhage from the big vessels of the thigh. Without full surgical equipment at hand this case must have proved fatal, for the haemorrhage was from a wound too high to be controlled by a tourniquet. During the morning X-rays were taken of fractures and wounds. It may be of interest to note that in every instance of the latter a piece of shell was demonstrated. Only in gutter wounds was there no shell. There were two or three bullet wounds. At Chatham a row of motor ambulances with a full staff was drawn up to receive the wounded and convey them to a base hospital. As five cases were too ill to move we remained in dock. There have been no fatalities on the ship.

At first our efforts to alleviate their sufferings and make them comfortable were regarded with suspicion by the Germans; some of them refused for several hours to take food or even drink. This was soon replaced by confidence, and when the time came for them to be transferred ashore they were loth to go. It was pathetic to see one man with only a bandaged stump remaining of his left arm, and his right covered with dressings, waving both in protest against leaving us, and asking in German to be allowed to remain. As the last of them was being raised from the ward he shook us warmly by the hand and cried "Three cheers for Nelson".

It was a few days later on September 5th that we arrived at Queensferry, in the Firth of Forth. Within half an hour of dropping anchor we received orders to proceed immediately down the Forth to meet destroyers bringing survivors from H.M.S. "Pathfinder", which had just been sunk. It was dark when we sighted the three destroyers at full steam and line ahead. They were signalled to stop near us, our boats were lowered, and while one destroyer went on to Queensferry we went on board the other two and prepared the wounded for their transport. One destroyer was, as previously described, brought alongside the hospital ship. The other destroyer contained survivors uninjured, but suffering from the exposure to two hours immersion in the sea, and these were brought in boats and were able, most of them, to walk up the gangway. We took on board all the survivors, over fifty, and the destroyers returned immediately to their patrol stations.

When it is remembered how little naval fighting there has been in the first ten weeks of the war, we must consider ourselves very fortunate to have been the nearest hospital ship to the scene of activity on two occasions, and thus been able to render assistance. We are now stationed, temporarily, further south, and our new base will provide far more work.

The utility of the hospital ship has been proved; its existence is essential in that it brings all the aids of modern surgery to the side of the battleship.

Experience has shewn that, apart from temporary treatment at the time of receiving the injury, the cardinal principles in the management of the wounded in a naval engagement are:- The less the wounded are moved in being transported, and the sooner they are warded, the greater are their chances of recovery and the more rapid is their convalescence. These principles must always be subject to the efficiency of the ship as a fighting unit. It is only by means of the hospital ship, which must ever be in readiness, that these principles can be acted upon with justice and humanity to the wounded.

(Dr A. Hope Gosse was born in Australia and went to school in Adelaide. He came to England to read medicine at Cambridge and St Mary's Hospital Medical School. He qualified in 1910. Apart from his time on the hospital ship, he served in Mesopotamia and was mentioned three times in dispatches. Following World War I a staff appointment became available at St Mary's Hospital. Dr Charles Wilson who at the time had obtained a Gold medal in the University of London M.D. examination was the other favoured candidate. Wilson was to become in later years Sir Charles Wilson, the great Dean of St Mary's Hospital Medical School, and later Lord Moran physician to Churchill during World War II and also the President of the Royal College of Physicians. However in 1919 he was aware that Gosse had a panache that he lacked. Gosse was handsome and remarkably self-confident. He had rowed for Cambridge, had an outgoing personality and had published some medical articles, which Wilson had not at the time. The staff at St Mary's was divided but a supernumerary post was created and both men were appointed to the staff. Gosse served St Mary's and the Brompton Hospitals until his retirement in 1947. He died in 1956 at the age of seventy-three.)

William Henry Clayton-Greene was born in 1874 and was educated at Oundle and Cambridge. He obtained a scholarship to St Mary's Hospital Medical School and qualified in 1900. He obtained his F.R.C.S. in 1901. Following his House Surgeon's post he became a Demonstrator in Anatomy at the School. In 1905 he was appointed Surgeon to Out-patients and Lecturer in Anatomy. He was Dean of the Medical School from 1907 to 1910. He served on the hospital ship *Liberty* during World War I and then at King George V Hospital. In 1911 he was appointed Surgeon to In-patients and held that post until he retired in 1924. He served on the examining boards of the Royal College of Surgeons of England and the University of Cambridge. He edited Pye's *Surgical Handicraft* which was largely rewritten by him. In 1919 he was awarded the C.B.E. He was in every sense a great surgical operator and an excellent teacher and popular with the students. Sir Zachary Cope states in his biography of Clayton-

Greene that although he had a charming personality he was forthright in his speech and frank in his dislikes. He retired in 1924 at the early age of fifty and moved to Guernsey, tired from years of a heavy surgical practice. He died two years later in 1926.

Charles Pannett obtained the chair in surgery at St Mary's Hospital Medical School in 1922, and held this Professorship until he retired from St Mary's in 1950. He was primarily a gastro-intestinal surgeon. He published numerous papers, and was respected principally for his surgical skills. E. A. Heaman in her excellent book on the history of St Mary's quotes Dickson Wright saying that he was a splendid professor not side-tracked by obsession with research and foreign travel. He was in addition a good teacher. Following retirement he turned to research in the Pathological Institute which was formed by Almroth Wright.

H. Gwynne Lawrence qualified in 1896 obtaining a Gold medal in his finals. He practised from 59 Green St., Grosvenor Square, London and was a Member of the Harveian Society of London.

P. Withers Green lived and practised in Johore-Bahru in the Malaya Peninsula.

(For information regarding hospital ships we wrote to the Medical Director General (Naval), Surgeon Rear Admiral M. A. Farquharson-Roberts C.B.E. Q.H.S. M.A. (Lond) F.R.C.S., and the following is based on his reply.

Hospital ships have a very long history in the Royal Navy having been used in the seventeenth, eighteenth and nineteenth centuries. The rules governing hospital ships were laid down in the 1866 Articles by the Geneva Convention first held in 1864. These were modified by the Geneva and Hague Conventions of 1897 and 1909. The rules that governed a hospital ship during the First World War required that it be painted white with red crosses and a green band along the hull.

These ships were mainly used as transports with a limited number of medical staff. Most of the treatment in World War I was carried out in France but patients were brought back for further treatment or rehabilitation in the United Kingdom. However there were hospital ships, particularly in the Dardanelles, which had a treatment capability with surgeons on board. Most of the ships were 'taken up from trade' and brought with them their merchant name, hence the yacht *Liberty* actually had the same name as a destroyer.

During the Second World War the United States navy had purpose-built hospital ships to support their island hopping campaign as well as converting land ship tanks for immediate care during amphibious operations. Some of the latter were employed off D-Day until field hospitals were established ashore. Hospital ships again fell into the two types at this time: firstly as transports, but the majority employed by the British again were taken up by trade but provided full hospital facilities (including X-ray).

The present situation is that British capital ships (the aircraft carriers and amphibious assault ships) have a surgical capability and will carry a surgeon and anaesthetist as the situation demands. This is solely to provide Role 2, support, life- and limb-saving surgery. Since the Second World War we have not had a dedicated hospital ship. However the Royal Yacht *Britannia* was available for use as a hospital ship. During the Falklands conflict we had an afloat Role 3 facility in two ships, which equated to a field hospital. There is also a modern Primary Receiving Facility in the Royal Fleet Auxiliary *Argus*. This is a 100-bed Role 3 facility with a 10-bed ITU, 20-bed HDU, capability for four operating tables and full imaging facilities including a spiral CT scanner.

We have chosen now not to go down the road of a hospital ship because of the constraints of the Geneva Convention of 1949. The regulations make the concept of a dedicated hospital ship unworkable, as it must not carry any means of communicating or receiving information in code. Even using GPS navigation is illegal under the rules. Instead we use Primary Casualty Receiving Facilities on board grey ships, which can thus be armed.)

CHAPTER 11

With our Forces in France

A short letter was published in October 1914 from Lt. W.D. Arthur and was headed:

With our Forces in France

Since my departure from England on August 20th, I have covered quite a lot of French ground, and had many interesting experiences. For the first three weeks or so, we had no medical work to do at all, but spent most of our time loading and unloading transport ships, railway trains, and baggage carts, during a course of species of popular tour through the district of France in which we are stationed. A General Hospital carries about 120 tons of luggage (sufficient to fill 33 railway trucks) so you may imagine the amount of work involved in the operations mentioned above. However, we are now settled down in a large institution called a ''Maison de Repos'' about three miles from an important French city, and for the past three weeks have been very busy indeed with the wounded. I have a ward of 36 beds for bad cases, so I have been kept very busy indeed. We receive two classes of wounded: (a) those unfit to travel; and (b) those who will be fit for duty in a month or less. All the others we send over to England in Hospital Ships.

The occurrence of such complications as malignant oedema (horrible!) and tetanus does not add to our peace. However, we are getting plenty of practice. I have done a trephine and many interesting bullet extractions, and hope to get amputations shortly, when the novelty has worn off, and our senior surgeons are getting fed up with them. Many of the wounds are truly appalling, both in extent and septic condition. Bad comminuted compound fractures present most awful problems as to treatment, and amputation is often the only way out. It is possible I may be sent up to the front later on; five of our officers have gone already, and of these two are killed and another ''hors de combat''. These men were from our own hospital staff, civil surgeons like myself, and one of them a married man with three young children. It seems awfully bad luck, especially as so many of us have no people depending on us, and could be more easily spared.

Lt. W.D. Arthur.

The *Gazette* published the following in October 1914:

The Following Extracts from a Letter have reached us from a Late Houseman at The Front

I am now Medical Officer attached to the Middlesex Regiment, and I find my work most congenial –

Will you please send me, as often as possible, the latest newspapers, one or two at a time, and please remind any friends of mine that letters are always welcome – It seems extraordinary that we should be desolating everything, and except for very violent and forcible reminders, at times it is difficult to realise that war is really in progress. The birds sing just the same, though heavy firing and bursting shells surprise them continually. Only yesterday morning I saw a robin singing merrily away in a place where a terrific shell explosion had rent the air only a few seconds before. – The last place I was at, I slept in a billet – on the floor, but now we sleep in "dug-outs", most ingenious little cubby holes in the ground. I have not had a bed to sleep in for weeks, no bath for as long, though I had a bathe a few days ago. I nearly always sleep in my clothes, and washes are very scarce – At present our Brigade has been relieved by other Regiments, and the Middlesex and other Regiments in the Brigade, are having a few days rest in this place, a small French town whose name I may not tell you, some five miles from the firing line. Last week I was up at the front when we were entrenched opposite the Germans. The Middlesex have been through everything starting with Mons. Our Colonel is a splendidly efficient man, reminding me of my old Chief, Clayton-Greene – I have travelled hundreds of miles and had plenty to do. In two places we have been to, the Church was used as a hospital, and in one case we were shelled out. I have slept in all sorts of places – railway station platforms, out in the open, on the floor in houses where we have been billeted, last week in "dug-outs" and now in a hayloft. I am now allowed a horse and a man to act as groom-servant. I met an old school fellow who was in charge of a section of Royal Engineers whose duty was to repair continually a pontoon bridge under shell fire. His party were billeted in a small town which had been looted by the Germans – I am very fit, very brown, eat like a lion, have congenial work and companions, sleep well and have little to complain of.

(It is a pity there is no signature to this splendid letter.)

A publication in the *Gazette* is undated but must have been in the last few months of 1914. It is as follows:

Lieutenant J.F. O'Connell M.B. B.S. London, R.A.M.C.

The *British Medical Journal* writes:

"The death in action at the battle of the Aisne, on September 20th, of John
Forbes O'Connell, was briefly announced a fortnight ago. He was born at
Neemuch, Central India, on February 18th 1889, where his father Lieut.
Colonel D.V. O'Connell R.A.M.C. was then serving. He was the
great-grandson of Dr James Forbes, Inspector-General of the Forces, who
served with distinction in the Peninsular War, and was the founder of the
Army Medical Mess at Fort Pete, Chatham, which was moved to Netley
in 1860.

He was educated at Epsom College, where he gained an entrance
scholarship in 1902. He proceeded to St. Mary's in 1907, and in November
1912 he graduated M.B.B.S. Lond., and in the following January joined the
R.A.M.C., gaining the fifth place at the entrance examination. He left
Aldershot with the 2nd Highland Light Infantry on August 14th."

It is not easy to write of O'Connell. He had no use for superlatives, to us
knowing him they would not fit. The reading of a sentence of panegyric
quickened the corners of his lips, and "the demon of human eulogy" is
quashed by the manner he adopted from instinct and training. He had many
friends who knew the stuff that lay beneath his genial way. Probably no
game appealed to him with the exception of Rugby football, but had he
wished he might have led in all, for he had every gift of the gamesman.
When resident at Hanwell Asylum the cricket XI, a man short, impressed his
services. The missing man kept wicket for the side. O'Connell volunteered
and played his part as to the manner born, then he went to the wicket and
knocked up top score. But to Rugger he was faithful, and the game might
have been made for him. He was twice captain of the Hospital XV, and later
in first-class football he clearly showed his worth. His was the game of the
Irish forward, and when thoroughly roused it was a joy to see him.

The dusty records of textbooks were little to his liking, but when the
thing was to be done and an examination was at hand he became obsessed
of the essential with a singular facility. He did not require to reinforce his
wits with laborious notes, reading medicine as others skim novels, and with
no more effort. He had the gift of concentration, and knew nothing of the
meaning of fatigue of mind or body. O'Connell did not rush into a service
when qualified. The official mind, the dark groping for efficiency of bodies
of men, was for him food for laughter, and the pomp and circumstance he
called the "cinematograph" part of the business. But when he had made up
his mind he was happy in the work that came at once to his hand, that work
in the field for which he was cut out by nature.

Colonel Wolfe Murray, commanding the Highland Light Infantry, sending
the news of his death to his wife, to whom he was married only a few
months, writes:

"He was shot dead in the trenches while attending Lieut. Ferguson H.L.I., who had been very seriously wounded, and who himself died later in the day. We all feel his loss most acutely. He performed his duties as a medical officer most efficiently, and was a general favourite with us all. I have never seen anyone pluckier: he was just as cool under fire as he was at any other time, and the act which cost him his life was characteristic of him."

The words of his Colonel are an introduction to him in person. Nations, like individuals, grow introspective in the evening of their day. O'Connell was of the order of men who, as they stand, are a direct challenge to the common tales of pessimism. He could do nothing badly, and what he undertook might be put out of mind, for that thing would be done, and done well. And when he had gone a willing hand was lost.

C.M.W.

War Correspondence

March 15th, 1915.
Heathfield, Cardigan,
S. Wales.
Dear Mr. Editor,
O'Connell's Father (Lieut-Col. O'Connell) has sent me a copy of the enclosed letter, with the expressed wish that I should send a copy to the Editor of the Gazette. I think you will agree with me that the noble way in which O'Connell did his duty reflects the greatest credit on his old hospital. The letter (of which the enclosure is a copy), was sent by an officer of the Highland Light Infantry to O'Connell's brother.

Yours sincerely,
T.W.W. Powell

December 12th, 1914.
Dear O'Connell,
I am only too pleased to tell you anything I can about your brother, as he was quite one of ours, and in all your life you can never have a prouder boast than that you were his brother.

As I expect you know, we went out on the 13th August, and our first show was at Fanieve, near Mons, where he at once came to notice. He established his dressing station in a little cottage quite in the open, about 200 yards behind my firing line. One of my platoons was not very well dug in and suffered considerably. He personally went into the trench and helped to carry out the wounded, though the Germans had the range to a T, and were raining shells on it. Then they turned on to his cottage, and knocked it to bits, and again he carried everyone out, not losing a single man. When

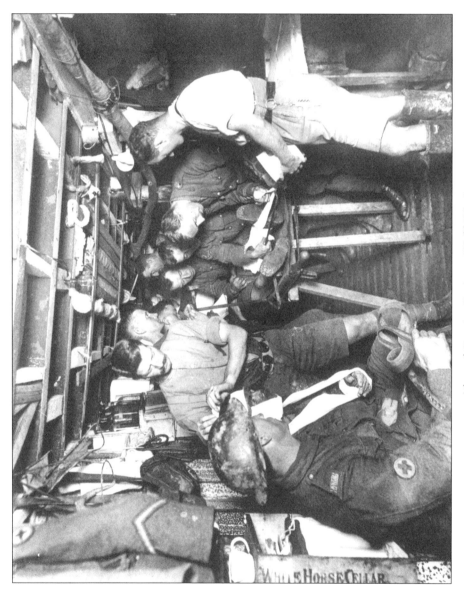

Advanced Dressing Station – World War I

Photograph courtesy of the Imperial War Museum, London. Negative no. E(AUS)672 the order came to retire, he stayed on behind the rearguard, though the Germans were within 600 yards, because he had two men to tie up.

During the retreat we were lucky in that we had no very severe fighting, but your brother had the worst of it, because he had to do with the footsore and sick, who could not keep up. So again he was usually behind the rearguard, but he always kept cheery, when cheerfulness was far more than pluck.

In the advance he was right up with us in the firing line at the Vesle, the Oureq and the Marne. After we crossed the Aisne he again particularly distinguished himself. We crossed on a Sunday. Next morning the 1st Division attacked, but did not get home. We (2nd Division) were launched about 5 p.m., and stormed the enemy's position before dark. We crossed their position and were digging in for all we were worth, when, about 11 p.m. we got word that the 3rd Division on our left had been driven back, and that we must give up what we had won and go back to a little hill above the river, as we were unsupported. I think it was the most appalling sight I saw, or rather felt in the war. Black night, pelting rain and wind, and some 3,000 dead and wounded Germans, lying thick and the wounded begging for help. We could do nothing, as our job was to get back and dig in, in line with the 1st and 3rd Divisions, before dawn. But your brother insisted on staying out there to do what he could for the enemy. It was about certain death to stay out there, but he remained there among them for six hours, and did not rejoin us until 8 a.m. next day. By that time my company was suffering rather badly. We had orders to hold a hill "at all costs", and had not had time to dig in, with the result that I lost 41 men before noon. Your brother, without waiting for food or sleep, came up to look after them, and stayed there for two days while we hung on. The day I was "downed" one of my subalterns was knocked out within 300 yards in a "sort of trench". As I crawled back I saw he was not quite dead, though unconscious, and evidently dying. As I was being tied up I mentioned him to your brother, and he at once insisted on going to see if he could do anything for him, although it was within very close range of a well constructed German trench, and while doing this he was killed by a rifle bullet through the heart. He was buried in the same grave as Fergusson and McKenzie, who also fell that day, and close by Gibson Craig, McDonald and Powell, who had dropped three days before, together with about 50 of our N.C.O.'s and men. I hope I have not over-written about him; but we all felt that his honour was ours and is yours. I also hope that we may meet some day.

(There is no signature reproduced on this extract from the *Gazette*.

John Forbes O'Connell was a remarkably brave and dedicated man who displayed all the qualities of a conscientious doctor. He risked his life repeatedly to care for the wounded, both British and German, and notably spent a whole night under appalling conditions. He also cared for the German wounded in the battlefield returning next morning to his unit, without food or sleep, to attend to the British wounded for two days and nights. Surely his behaviour throughout his service and in the field of battle, ending with the sacrifice of his own It is likely that many gallant men go unheralded!!!)

War Correspondence

November 1914
From Lieutenant R.W. Armstrong, 1st Battalion King's (Liverpool) Regiment, 6th Infantry Brigade, 2nd Division British Expeditionary Force:

I have become a regimental Medical Officer attached to the above battalion. As you know I came out in the middle of August with No. 6 General Hospital, with which were also Bullock, Silcock, Whigham, and Buckell. We were 24 officers in all and had with us 30 sisters and 140 men, with equipment for a hospital of 500 beds. We left Southampton in the "Victorian", and in the fullness of time arrived at Havre, where we received an enthusiastic welcome, chiefly from small children, who pestered us for souvenirs, and pursued us with shouts of "Ami, Mi, Mi". We stayed at Havre some five days sharing with our equipment and bales of rich merchandise – chiefly very smelly hides – some dirty sheds by the side of one of the quais – a French word meaning quays. We then loaded up on to a train and proceeded to Rouen. Here after more delay, we unloaded and set up our hospital on a large patch of heather-covered moor, some distance outside the town. We had just received our first consignment of some 100 wounded, when panic supervened. A German raid in armed motor lorries was apprehended, and we received orders to pack up and quit instanter. We worked like hell and got the whole thing down and packed in less than twelve hours. Got our stuff down to the river and into a ship, and then we ourselves embarking on a second tub amid the frenzied babblings of the pale-faced and much beribboned staff, proceeded leisurely down the Seine, through beautiful scenery and past picturesque villages out to sea and down the Bay to St. Nazaire, at the mouth of the Loire. We lay outside the harbour for a couple of days and in that time the mischief happened. The other ship containing our equipment went in before us and dumped our stuff on the quayside with none of us there to protect it. Two other General Hospitals had got there before us and proceeded to make good their deficiencies at our expense, so that when we at length landed we found more than half of our beds and tents missing. We struggled hard to recover our losses, but the fates were against us, and after about ten days the process of dissolution overtook us, and we were carted off in twos and threes – like sloughs – to go up to the front to join units there. I went up to No. 4 Field Ambulance at Soupir, in the Aisne Valley, midway between Soissons and Rheims. I found them comfortably enconsed for the nonce in a deserted chateau, and working under as nearly ideal conditions as it was possible for a field ambulance to desire. I spent a fortnight there quite pleasantly before I was again shot off this time to relieve A.G.H. Lovell as Medical Officer to the regiment then at Mousay, a little village close to Soupir, Lovell going to No. 4 F.A. in my place. I have now been with the regiment since October 4th. The battle of the Aisne resolving itself into a sort of siege, the little British Army was relieved by French Territorials, and was sent round to the left to do the dirty work there, so that we now find ourselves in Belgium not a hundred miles from Ypres. The regiment has been in action since the 24th October pretty continuously, and has done jolly good work, but has lost very heavily, especially on the two or three days when they have been attacking hostile positions. Once, of course, they get into position and dig themselves in, the casualties are comparatively few, provided the men keep their heads down, for the German snipers are damn good. We have had thirteen officers killed and wounded, during the last fortnight, including our Colonel killed on the first day we attacked, while three have gone sick, so you can imagine we're pretty short of officers. Naturally I've been pretty busy at times, though just now, with the battalion in trenches, things are comparatively slack. Of course, there's not much one can do, separated from most of the small amount of apparatus a regimental M.O. is provided with; in fact, one only has the surgical haversacks and a "monkey box" – a small pannier carried by the medical orderly. One can only get wounded in after dark, and all one can do is to dress them and give morphia – which I do pretty liberally – and keep them at the collecting station, usually a cottage or farmhouse close behind the line, until the ambulance waggons come up and take them away. Some of the wounds are ghastly, especially the shell wounds, while even a rifle bullet makes a horrible hole at times, in spite of what the textbooks tell us. I've seen great gaping wounds as big as your fist made by rifle bullets, either fired at short range or, after ricochetting, though nothing yet which one could say for certain had been caused by dum-dum bullets. Far from the proverbial stories of lives saved by pocket bibles or a threepenny bit carried in the waistcoat pocket, any object of that sort incites a rifle bullet to produce more horrid wounds – in one day I had two such cases, both large holes in the front of the chest, one exposing the trachea and great vessels behind the mamibrium, while through the other the heart could be seen beating, and in both instances the bullet had hit a hard object when passing.

We – that is the Major (now in command), the Adjutant and myself – are living in a fine dug-out at present, in a wood about 100 yards behind the firing line. We have a fine roof which will stop anything short of a direct hit with high explosive, so that we're quite snug so long as we keep in our burrow. We come out after dark and try to feed outside during the day, but the blighted German generally chooses lunch and tea-time to turn shrapnel on to us from a gun we have christened "Little Stinker". We feed excellently – mainly on tinned meats of various brands, bread and jam, all three "rations", and of very good quality, supplemented by eggs and particularly tough fowls, which our mess sergeant catches and cooks at a safe distance away and brings up to us at night. Our staple drinks are tea and rum and water. We haven't had our boots off for a fortnight now, and a bath all over is a dim memory of a happy past, but I generally contrive a daily lick at my collecting station – a cottage behind our wood which has so far escaped being shelled, and sometimes even shave. We get our papers and letters up fairly well, and last night I received the Hospital Gazette for October.

(Dr B.W. Armstrong M.C., O.B.E. qualified at St Mary's Hospital Medical School in 1913. In 1923 he was appointed Medical Superintendent of the Royal Seabathing Hospital in Margate and remained in that post until his retirement in 1954. He was a leading authority on the treatment of surgical tuberculosis. He died in May 1958.)

In November 1914 a short letter from Lieut. Silcock was published:

"I've got a nice job in a way on an ambulance train bringing wounded from the front to base hospitals. We have just arrived here from —— with a full house, including two Dukes, one wounded, one sick. Pattison is the other Lieutenant and a ripping major is in command. There are four sisters, too, who do all the dressings. It's most amusing running this train – one tells the driver which route to take occasionally. I've had two rides on the engine, and one at night was most weird. – We've very little time for writing, it's almost impossible when the train is going, and when it stops anywhere we're always busy – Watermeyer and Buckell I have seen and Bryan and Compton have also been seen."

November 1914
From Temporary Lieutenant C.W.G. Bryan, R.A.M.C., No. 14, General Hospital

We are now settled with a hospital of some 600 beds, and are kept fairly busy. We sleep in a cafe, where we also have our meals, and work starts at

9 a.m. I have surgical supervision of 310 cases, and operate on all that need it of that lot. To take a specimen day's work, yesterday I arrived at 9 and till 9.30 was occupied sorting out the cases fit to go either to a convalescent camp or home to England. From 9.30–10.15 superficial inspection of all cases and transferred those needing it to my operation ward, which consists of about 30 beds. 10.15–11.45 went round the wards and saw all cases the assistant surgeons wanted me to, generally advised re treatment, supervised splinting, gave orders to Sister, etc. During this round the Consulting Surgeon, Mr. Burghard, arrived, and I showed him cases of interest and got advice where I wanted it. We've now been here just over a week and yesterday for the first time the theatre was sufficiently ready for me to use it extensively. Well, from 11.45–12.30, my lunch time, I pottered about with various bits of work, after lunch saw the Daily Mail, which arrives at 1.30, and at 2 began to operate. Compton and another man share the work of H.S. (House Surgeon) at operations with me. First case compound depressed fracture of frontal bone; trephined and found extradural haemorrhage from longitudinal sinus, cleared out clot etc., and drained; next extracted piece of shrapnel from thigh; 3, extracted bullet from region of brachial artery; 4, removed comminuted fragments of shattered olecranon and drained the suppurating elbow; half-hour interval for tea, 5.15; 5, case of bullet entering right cheek, going through right maxilla, cutting tongue in two, fracturing left mandible, and stopped by skin of left cheek. Removed bullet and cleaned up mouth, etc.; 6, extracted bullet from left parotid region; 7, shell or bullet wound right chest, removed two portions of comminuted ribs anteriorly, and drained empyema by rib resection lower and posteriorly – bullet or fragment of shell probably still in lung; 8, explored, cleaned and splinted arm with sloughing wound of two thirds of circumference of elbow region – the lower end of humerus gone, and also musculo-spiral nerve, brachial artery and other nerves intact, and splints (interrupted) and drainage took time, but from the look of things to-day, think we shall save the arm; if so, this is a victory. Meanwhile new cases had arrived and I went over to the ward at 8.45 to help H.S. put up an arm under CHCL3; lacerations and compound fracture of humerus from shell; patient much collapsed. (This patient's arm I have amputated at shoulder joint to-day and have also done 4 other operations) And so dinner at 9.20 and bed at 10.15. Started at 8.45 to-day and had in addition to clinical work, to be orderly officer to whole hospital – on duty indoors 24 hours except 1 hour for lunch and 1 hour for dinner. Shall sleep in my clothes to-night – many bad cases have arrived this evening. I and the other surgeon specialist have alternate mornings and afternoons in theatre, which is going all day long, but he is third in command of his half, and has rather less beds and more assistants, so is rather less rushed than I. Besides theatre

work we do many ward operations, i.e., compound fractures and extractions of bullets in simple cases. I have an appendix and a traumatic cataract
which I am watching and may have to do; on the other hand, if they get
quiet shall send them on to England. I find my ophthalmic experience very
valuable. So you see, we do some work, and miss count almost of days and
dates. I've not had two hours off together except at nights for five days; but,
of course, the Coast Battle won't last for ever, and at present we get our
wounded from that. The patients are very well fed and react marvellously
to treatment, and our results are simply amazingly successful very often.

(T.W.W. Powell was educated at Epsom School. After qualifying from St.
Mary's he obtained his Diploma in Public Health (D.P.H.) and after the
war became a Public Health doctor in South Wales.

  R. Silcock qualified in 1914. Following the war he obtained his Diploma
in Tropical Medicine (D.T.M.). He served for a time as a Surgeon
Lieutenant in the Royal Navy and subsequently gave his address as Maida
Vale Mansions, London W9.

  C.W.G. Bryan as a young Lieutenant had an enormous surgical load as
witnessed in his letter, but he had obtained his Fellowship in Surgery in
1910 and obtained the Middlemore Prize from the British Medical
Association 1911. He was awarded the Military Cross for his work during
the war. Following the war he was Surgeon to Out-patients, Surgical Tutor
and Lecturer in Clinical Surgery at St Mary's Hospital. He was Hunterian
Professor at the Royal College of Surgeons of England 1920–1921. He was
the author of *Diseases of Bones and Joints* and wrote many papers on
orthopaedics and abdominal and thoracic wounds.)

CHAPTER 12

From E.G. Barker, British Red Cross Base, Boulogne

From E.G. Barker,
British Red Cross Society's Base, Boulogne-sur-Mer.
Posted 28 November 1914:

As we have now been out here for just on three weeks, I thought that perhaps a few particulars of the conditions of our existence might be appreciated by your worthy self. The few remaining survivors from our party, viz., myself, Fuller, King, and A.B. Davies are stationed in a large hospital with 400 beds in Boulogne. The building is a large new hotel, and in many ways makes an admirable hospital, for on each of the seven floors there are three bathrooms with accompanying apparatus for cleansing purposes – a feature which is usually conspicuous by its absence in most French hotels. We have one operating theatre, which is on the go most of the day and night, but its equipment is poor, and the table has to be periodically strengthened by bandages and safety pins to prevent it collapsing in the middle of an"op". Just opposite to us is the "Casino", now no longer inhabited by "fortune hunters", but has as its chief occupants the Inoculation Staff of St. Mary's, viz., Sir A.Wright, Capt. Douglas, and Mr. Fleming.

The chief work of these individuals has been in combating the effects due to a hitherto comparatively unknown organism, to wit, the Bacillus Aerogenes Capsulatus, whose presence in wounds manifests itself by an odour which greets you on entering any ward in which an infected person happens to be lying. But we are already on the high road to success, for Sir A. Wright has just recently told us that they have at last prepared a vaccine, and consequently great things are hoped from it; he also advocates the treatment of these wounds with 5 per cent, saline and one half per cent. Potassium nitrate, and from some of the cases I have seen they appear to clear up splendidly with this.

We have been to see Mr. (or rather Lieut.) Bryan, who is stationed at Wimereux – three miles out of Boulogne – at the Casino, which holds 600 beds. He is consulting surgeon (there are four altogether), and is in charge of 150 beds. Compton is also stationed at this place and from what we can see this war seems to be run by St. Mary's men. Silcock, Watermeyer and Armstrong are on an ambulance train which brings the wounded into this town.

103

From H.A. Watermeyer, at the front,
2nd December 1914:

You can tell any of my friends that I am alive and well. Still on No. 7 ambulance train, and enjoying my work thoroughly.

Lieut. R. Silcock writes,
November 6th 1914:

We are still doing our short runs, five or six times a week up country after wounded, our only excitement being certain deficiencies in our rolling stock, or the line, or the driver himself. The other day I drove the train for about 20 miles tout seul and showed the "mechenicien" how the Westinghouse brake should be worked with much success. The other day I saved a catastrophe by spotting at a range of 100 yards that the points were so set as to run us straight into a fully loaded French Red Cross train! I forget whether I told you of our little accident caused by the driver pulling up dead because he suddenly came on a danger signal in the morning mist. Anyhow, we lost all our breakfast, all our crockery, and got on to the line to find our train in three portions, two sets of couplings having carried away! But these little shocks are part of one's everyday life on an ambulance train on a French railway. Those poor devils in the trenches must be having a poor time of it now – hail and rain most of the day and a good hard frost at night. I played bridge with H. last night.

This is first-hand information, for which I can guarantee the accuracy.

G.B. Argles

The following extract from a letter from a late houseman has been sent to us for publication:

I am getting to be quite at home on a horse now, and spend a great part of each day in the saddle; I have got over the initial saddlesoreness. I have a perfectly free hand in all matters medical, and have all the arrangements of attending to sick and wounded and their transference to a field ambulance and so to a hospital. My "staff" consists of a groom, a medical orderly, a personal servant, who assists me with dressings and looks after my kit, a corporal with several men to assist him as a sanitary squad, as I am responsible for the sanitation everywhere we go, a man who looks after the water-cart and filter, and sixteen stretcher bearers. Yesterday I had a medical inspection of the whole battalion – 700 men, and inspected 1,400 feet. At first I found the work quite strange, and it required a considerable effort to get hold of, but now I see my way more clearly.

I have actually been in action since writing the above. From Monday to Thursday last week we had some strenuous fighting. I can only tell you a few details of my part in it. We arrived at a small village on Sunday evening, October 11th, after marching all day, bivouacked for the night, and then went on about four miles early in the morning. I took possession of a farmhouse, from which all the occupants had fled, and converted it into a temporary hospital. It was a beautiful old place, built in the 16th century, but the Germans had been there before us and had left everything in chaos, while the tables were laden with the remains of hurried meals. We are getting accustomed to such sights. There were three rooms in it that I decided to utilise, and had hardly got them ready as receiving room, waiting room and operating room, when a wounded Frenchman was brought in with a very serious abdominal wound. I saw that his only chance of recovering was in operating and decided to do so at once. You can appreciate the difficulty of sterilising things under such circumstances. I started the anaesthetic and handed it over to the orderly, who gave it under my direction, and then proceeded to operate. It took an hour and a half to patch the poor man up, and he recovered well and became quite conscious and comfortable. I heard afterwards that he had died next day, but it was worth the effort, and it was his only chance. That same afternoon the Germans shelled the village, and moving about in the open was rather risky work. One of the shells set the church alight, and the burning tower fell on some houses and set them alight.

Next day we followed the Germans up and I had to move my hospital to a new farmhouse, which this time was quite close to some of our trenches. I found a German helmet, one of those with a spike on the top, and intend to bring it home with me.

Each day for four days we advanced, and now I have converted a barn into a hospital. Heavy firing on both sides has been going on, and with bullets flying one has to be on the qui vive on going outside.

During Wednesday a message was sent from one of our trenches, asking me to go out to one of our officers, who had been badly wounded. I set out with my medical orderly and two stretcher bearers and a stretcher. It was a most exciting journey. By carefully crawling along ditches, and keeping low we arrived at the trench, and after dressing him we succeeded with great difficulty in getting him on the stretcher, for he was very badly wounded though conscious. We then started back with him, but this was extremely difficult, for a shower of bullets greeted one if the smallest piece of one's body was to be seen. However, all went well till we had gone about fifty yards on the way, and were crawling on hands and knees along a ditch, the two bearers in front, then myself and orderly behind, when the orderly got shot in the leg, having by accident got his foot too high while crawling along. It was not serious, but disabled him so that he could not get along. I had to take him on my back for the rest of the way.

That evening there was a night attack by our troops and continued the
next day. The noise was terrific, and a general advance by our troops
followed. I spent some time in searching the field for wounded, and only
stopped because darkness came on. In a village which we captured we found
an old man lying in bed in one of the houses which had escaped destruction.
He seemed quite unconcerned and ignorant of what had been going on.

The Germans seem to have retreated several miles. The inhabitants came
back very quickly to the villages behind us, though when we enter them
they are absolutely deserted, though the big places are full of refugees. The
churches seem to be very attractive to the German artillery.

One of the officers who had been running the officers' mess was slightly
wounded, so the Colonel asked me if I would take on the work of mess
president; now I keep all the men's money and get what forage I can for
the officers on our journeys. Yesterday I got three bottles of milk at a farm
for 50 centimes, 2 fine hares for 5 francs, etc.

Last night we slept a little again, while the Tommies were put into some
barns. After all this time I fully appreciated the bed and being able to undress
after weeks in my clothes.

A Lieutenant, R.A.M.C. writes:

In August I was sent by the War Office – that was last year – to Fort Pitt
Hospital, Chatham. This extraordinary old spot is an old fort on a hill.

I found about fifteen other doctors there. We all lived in the town, and
twice daily panted up the hill to the orderly room, and after that dispersed
to work either in the hospital, save the mark, or else visited the outlying
forts to see the morning sick, carry out typhoid inoculations, or in other
ways air our brand new uniforms.

On our arrival at the A.D.M.S's office for the first time a record of our
appointments was made, and as far as possible our duties were based on this.

For instance, I had spent two or three months in the ophthalmic
department at S.M.H. (St. Mary's Hospital), and was the only individual
there that confessed to any inkling of knowledge pertaining to the eye.
Therefore I was posted to the ophthalmic ward, and for other reasons I was
given any nose, throat or ear case to investigate. This, of course, was
delightful. I visited an old dispensary, really quite an excellent place, and
found a gas lamp for eye and throat work, also a case of lenses and a box
of throat mirrors, and with this got to work.

I had more to do than anyone else. I worked all the morning – and all
the afternoon! Others only worked in the morning, at first. I was at
Chatham until the beginning of October, and long before I left there I had
to give up the special departments and become a house surgeon to attend

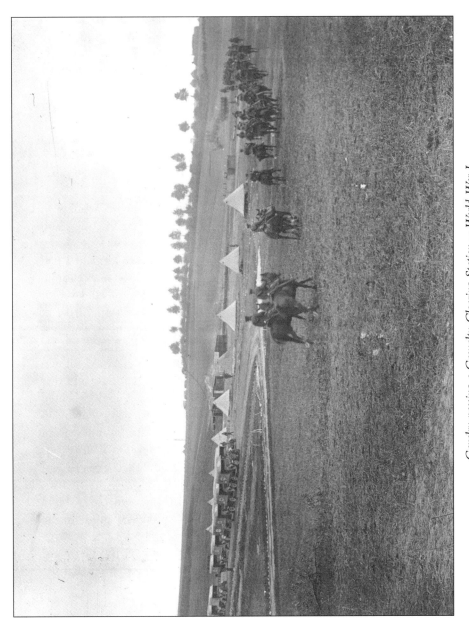

Cavalry passing a Casualty Clearing Station – World War I

Photograph courtesy of the Imperial War Museum, London. Negative no. Q4339

to the wounded, who began to pour into Chatham, from the retreat of Mons, and later.

Our first consignment of wounded were German from the battle of Heligoland, men who were landed for the S.Y. "Liberty". (On August 29th after the outbreak of war there was a naval engagement off Heligoland in which several German light cruisers were sunk.)

Because of the lack of space these men were placed in the old casemates at Fort Pitt – ancient wards, used last at the time of the Crimea, so local history has it. A pocket-case of instruments, carbolic, iodine sometimes, lint, and an occasional meagre allowance of peroxide and lighted by candles – that was the complete equipment of my ward. I forgot to add morphia and chloroform.

With these we did everything, and the men made excellent, though slow, recoveries from almost impossible wounds.

One fellow had a hole in his chest, and a temperature with a bulge in the side. I administered morphia, then chloroform, opened up the bulge and extracted some shell and pus, and in five minutes (this is true) he was talking to his fellow Huns and examining his piece of shell. All the Germans I had under me, who had chloroform, woke up from their anaesthesia as though from sleep, very soon after we had stopped its administration. Well, I've got to the sixth page, and I'm only at the beginning of October. From Chatham I went to Aldershot to join a general hospital mobilising there, and was lucky to meet Bryan, who was for the same unit. We embarked on a boat at midnight from Southampton and steamed away – and steamed for ten days, and at the end of that time we arrived at Boulogne. I should add that on the way we went to Dover, Ostend, Dunkirk, Calais, and executed other manoeuvres at sea, what time the 7th Division was being cut up in Flanders. We fixed up our hospital at Wimereux, three miles from Boulogne, and there I acted in the capacity of dresser for nearly four months. At the end of this time my ambition to hear a shell explode got the better of me, and I applied to be sent to the Front.

At the end of two days I was sent to the 1st Division, to a Field Ambulance, and woke up next morning to hear a few shells explode in the little town we were in – Bethune, by name.

The next day, the 25th January, there was a big attack by the Germans, and we had many wounded passing through the Ambulance. After that life in the Ambulance was domestic.

We bathed and clothed, with clean clothes, Thomas Atkins in his thousands.

The 1st Division had been cut up and was recruiting.

In March I was sent to the 1st Division of the Coldstream Guards, and am with them now.

We have been sitting in breastworks and trenches when we haven't been in billets "resting" – except on May 9th, when we were in reserve at the attack at Richebourg – a very bloody battle, which showed no obvious result as far as we were concerned, but must have been a great help to the French and other parts of our line, where similar attacks were being made.

Life with a regiment is far more amusing than with any other unit I have been to. The medical work except during an attack, is very little.

During an attack, and afterwards, there is no rest, until one is relieved; and the noise is tremendous, until one becomes dulled to it. I have seen men sleeping during a bombardment – snoring. My small knowledge of the throat and ear is always being tried, and I must return to the old out-patient department after things are quiet once more, if you will allow me to sit at the feet of Wisdom to learn. One sometimes gets ear cases, and has to send them on to the Field Ambulances and Hospitals, when if one could only have the means to transport a few extra instruments and bottles about, one could do the treatment oneself and keep the man as out-patient. We are all wondering if there is to be any end to the war. However, here's an end to this letter, at last.

Published in the St Mary's *Gazette* dated December 1914,

St Mary's at War

October 26
From a Lieutenant, 10 Field Ambulance, 4th Division, B.E.F.

It was on Wednesday morning, October 21st, I had just got up after a short night's rest, for I had been attending to wounded until early morning, when a message came from Major Wilding, commanding the Inniskilling Fusiliers, to say that they had a man with his leg off that required attention and would a medical officer be sent a soon as possible. The stretcher squad under Corporal Fremlin was paraded, my horse saddled, and we were all soon on the road. Outside, as we passed along, there was the atmosphere of tension, the civilians showed expressions of anxiety, and there was a good deal of activity round headquarters. Our little band turned the corner and proceeded along the street leading to the place, where, from the message I expected to find my wounded man. On the way we passed our other dressing station, and here I decided to leave my mare, for soldiers whom I met slightly wounded informed me that it was scarcely safe. I sent my stretcher squad on, telling them I would follow, and in the meantime went inside the hospice civil warning them of the possible arrival of wounded and for them to be ready to receive them. When I came out I found an officer with a small transport wagon on two wheels, who said he was willing to do what he could to help the wounded back. So we both went along in the conveyance as far as was safe, passing my squad on the way. About 800 yards up we halted at a spot marked by an old barn at the side of the road, here, lying on a stretcher, I found my man with his leg almost completely severed at the knee except for a flap of skin. I applied a tourniquet, dressed him, and sent him back in the wagon. In the meantime my squad had arrived and several wounded down from the firing line. These we treated and told them to wait for the wagon which was now plying between this spot and the hospice civil. Things here were working in an orderly fashion, but I thought I would investigate further, so on we went, on the road were some slightly wounded straggling along; I instructed these how to proceed, and they no doubt found their way to the hospital. About 50 yards on men were lining the trenches on either side of the road, I was told that it was safe except for an occasional stray bullet, so, in spite of discouragement from my squad, I continued along until I reached a green shuttered estaminet on the right just at the corner of the wood. Here I found the Major of the Inniskillings, who welcomed me at the door: "Just the man I want," said he, "Did you get my message?" "Yes, I said, "and I have seen your wounded man, amongst several others, all of whom are in hospital I hope by now." With this I thought I had completed my job and would have been dismissed, but as it happened the Inniskillings had lost their medical officer and so I fell in for the work. They had had several wounded that morning, none of whom had been attended to. The major pointed out to me where they were. Behind the house was a ploughed field, bounded by a small lane which led up to the farm. This farm was still occupied by the troops. This was the place then that for the moment was the object of my mission. I got my squad together who were very sick when I told them what our little game was, for they considered it the work of the regimental stretcher bearers, and so indeed it was. Still I tried to buck them up and we proceeded across the ploughed field in open order. As it turned out it was safe enough until we got to the lane, and here we literally crept in the ditches and clung to the trees in order to make the most of cover, for the bullets were singing by.

    When within 50 yards of the farm the Captain waved to me the easiest way to approach. Now we were in the farm. Just like the rest of Belgian farms, it was built with three fronts surrounding the yard. These yards seem to be central drainage area of the place, and are on a lower level than the surrounding brick ridge. The house itself was of brick with a thatched roof, the barn, or place where the corn crop was stored was of wood. This, with other outhouses for pigs, hens, and stables for horses, completed the building. Behind stood two small buildings, apparently used merely as sheds to protect implements from the weather. They had no doors and were detached. I walked with the Captain and he showed me where the wounded were. Some of the troops having a rest from the trenches were grouped about the small yard. I investigated the rooms of the house. In the corridor leading to the kitchen I found a man with a wound in his back; I made him comfortable and then attended to one or two in the kitchen and stables. After this I turned my corporal on to fix up the barn, laying it out with straw ready for any more casualties, should there be any.

Having done this my hands were free and I rejoined the Captain to take in the situation. He explained how they had been surprised at dawn before they stood to arms and had lost a little ground in consequence. They had been defending the farm since six o'clock that morning. The trenches were manned about 10 yards in front of the farm and extended out on either side. They had done well but were hard pressed, the fighting being fast and furious. While I stood with him in the yard under cover of a wall, smoking cigarettes and contented, the bullets whizzed through the trees behind us. The branches fell from time to time from the fire. Wounded men crept back to shelter and I treated them in the barn. At one part the wood-work was riddled, and as the barn filled it was necessary to use this corner as far as we dared. On one occasion a bullet hit the wood and fell just a foot from a patient's head as I was dressing him. That there were two sides to this question was evident from a glance at the roof. At the corner of the thatch where two roofs at right angles slope together and where a chimney might stand, lay two of the best shots of the regiment. It was splendid to watch them: they fired, the rifle kicked, they darted down with their guns, the empty cartridges came tumbling down, they reloaded and took aim. "How are you getting on?" cried one of the men below. "I'll tell you, listen – Hear that? well that's one of the grey devils, and that, and that, that makes two, not bad for three shots." This is the way he added to his glory. They were also useful fellows in keeping us aware of movements, for after all the Germans in the trenches were less than 100 yards away. I was watching our snipers then crossed the yard to the Captain who was directing operations. We were leaning against the wall very lazily when a terrific report was heard, dust rose in the air round us, and bits of brick and mortar were flying about. We both looked towards where the sound came from, and we saw men moving from the spot whilst two lay helpless on the ground; obviously a shell had burst in our midst; it dusted up the ground a bit and took a corner off the roof. The men both suffered from severe abdominal wounds. One had a good deal of prolapse, both large and small intestine protruding from the lesion which was about 8 inches in length. It was not possible to return the gut to the abdomen in either case; plenty of gauze was applied with a bandage to hold them in position; a condition of extreme shock immediately followed the infliction of the wound from which they rallied later; for the pain I gave a hypodermic of morphia; they remained where they were until we could return and collect them under cover of night. It was just at this time that things assumed their darkest outlook: it was thought that the farm must fall if we were not reinforced. The next shell was, of course, to finish us; the Germans now had got the range. Well, as it happened, the time that we seemed most to be in danger was the time in reality when we were most safe. The Captain kept a good look-out on the left towards the wood, and there in the direction of Le Gheer between a clump of trees and a house was an interval. In this interval moving objects were to be seen. He passed me the glasses: "Yes," I said, "I see them, are they our men?" He took the glasses again and said "Yes, there go two in Khaki. Pass the word to the trenches, Sergeant, not to fire on those on the left: they are our own men advancing." The previous hour of suspense made this sight most comforting and there was a feeling of relief. Now we were going to do things, we thought, when up came a dispatch rider with a message, which you will see showed us how. It was from the C.O. of the Somersets and ran as follows: "We have come through the Bois de Hoegsteert, and have advanced to Le Gheer. We have taken the village and are ready to open heavy fire on the enemy. Will you be prepared to advance with us and get in touch with us on your left flank." The Captain made his reply, the gist of the whole thing being in the affirmative. Evidently a flanking movement was to take place. I watched developments with great interest. The Somersets kept their word, and the sight of them on the German right was evidently too much for the enemy, for the white flag was soon in evidence in the opposite trenches. Our men, overjoyed, rushed out, led by the Major, and made about 150 prisoners. These they marched back to the farm and then to headquarters. The wounded they handed on to me. I dressed them and then left them with a guard in a convenient place until I could remove them later. Now, of course, came the first lull in the fighting. I took the opportunity of searching the foreground for wounded. I passed dead bodies of men and cattle and finally reached the monastery, which had been the headquarters of the Inniskillings on the previous night. Everywhere things were lying about in great disorder, the remains of a recent meal apparently hurriedly left were upon the table. I found one or two wounded in the stable. Having seen these I returned enquiring for wounded again but there were no more. Satisfied with this I took my squad back to the green shuttered estaminet by the road and reported to the Major. Now for the first time I began to feel hungry. I had had no food that day, and it was now just 2 o'clock: one of the men spared me a small piece of bread and cheese – how I relished it! I felt ready for more work, and it was just as well for the Inniskillings had more wounded up at the cross roads which the Major wanted me to see. My stretcher squad had gone back, so I went out with Sergeant Birch, who happened to be there from a section. In company with the Major, another officer, and a few men, we went through the woods as the road was not safe. This was the direction taken by the Somersets a few hours before. At last we were out of the wood, and on the cross roads, a place well under shell fire. To remove wounded was impossible, but I decided to find out where they were, making collection at night easier. Sergeant Birch took one road and I took the other. Shells were singing through the air. The groans of the wounded led me to the spot and then I found several bad cases lying in rooms which were in a state of utter confusion, with debris all over the place. I treated them and came away. As I left the door I saw across the road in the field opposite two farms blazing away for all they were worth. This, of course, was the work of German shells. I took cover to the cross-roads. Sergeant B. had not returned so I went in search. I ran down in the direction he had taken, and on the way something whistled past me and I felt a warm glow at my left breast pocket. "A near shave, sir," shouted a Tommy, sheltering in a cottage. I looked up and absent-mindedly said, "I suppose so," for I had not realised that a piece of shrapnel was within an ace of putting my light out. After about ten minutes' hunt, during which I treated the Somersets, who had seen my little adventure and had a few wounds for me to dress, I returned. A few minutes through the woods and I was again at the estaminet. Here I met Lieut. Hairsine. We decided things were too hot for stretcher bearing, and as I had given all first aid treatment it was unnecessary to do more until night, so we walked together to the hospice civil, where Stewart had a nice meal ready. It was my breakfast delayed until 4.30 p.m., and how I enjoyed it! Later I rejoined my unit and heard the best bit of news of all: the Inniskillings had found their Medical Officer who had been captured in the monastery by the Germans and then recaptured by the Inniskillings again during their advance. I will write again when I get an opportunity.

(What a pity there is no name attached to this letter but merely the note 'From a Lieutenant, 10 Field Ambulance, 4th Division, B.E.F., October 26'.)

CHAPTER 13

From Lieut. Handfield-Jones, B.E.F.

Published in the *Gazette* in December 1914.

Sunday, November 1st.
From Lieut. Handfield-Jones, No. 6, General Hospital, British Expeditionary Force, France

I went to Southampton last Wednesday week, went on board at night, slept in dock, and then started at about six. A few of us turned out early to see the last of England, for the time being. As soon as we got outside the Solent it was blowing big guns, and for about three hours we had a pretty stiff bit of sea. Fortunately I survived in great style, and enjoyed it thoroughly. We arrived at the English base in time for lunch, and then we found ourselves billeted in the town to await orders. The four of us who had come from Tidworth managed to keep together, and so we had a very cheery time. We got attached to No. 2 General Hospital for lectures for a day or two, and then were ordered to join No. 6 here.

There are several hospitals, and at present all our hospital equipment is still packed, and we have nothing but our mess kit and sleeping tents. As soon as this show on the Belgian coast is decided, up we go some way from here, and then we get what we are all longing for now, viz., work. It is a great life up here – we are all in tents and it is a ripping spot, high up above the town, but it is decidedly chilly, especially at night. At Southampton they bagged our camp kits, and so we are sleeping in our valises on the hard, hard ground. Last night was the first real good night I've had here. However, we are all very fit on it. Yesterday the hospital personnel turned out for a route march in charge of another man and myself. It was a horrid jar, suddenly to have to brush up one's old military knowledge and march these people off. It was a lovely walk: we did about ten miles through absolutely lovely country. We struck a road through the most topping forests. To-day we are turning out to church parade in style. It really is a humorous life so far: our shopping in the best French we can manage is most amusing, and everybody is only too glad to be able to do something for "les Anglais."

Yesterday afternoon three of us went down town and had the luxury of a hot bath, my second in nearly a fortnight. The washing in the early morning is rather a cold and dreadful business. After our bath we went to a cafe for tea, and I ran straight into a Mary's man named Arthur. He has been out here most of the time, and is in one of the General Hospitals, which has been rigged out in great style, and is a fixture here. We have absolutely struck oil in the matter of senior officers, both Colonel Le Quesne and Major Cochrane being of the best.

We had a joyous surprise at breakfast this morning. Two ounce tins of tobacco reposed on our plates. Every man on active service gets it, of course, but we had forgotten that.

English cigarettes and tobacco are obtainable here at absolutely ruinous prices, so we give them a miss. At the moment our mess is not in a very good state, as we are only just starting, of course. We live on rations, and other things we get in, and although we live simply, we live well and cheaply, which suits us all. Our tents are absolutely new, and we are very comfy: two of us share one and have a servant apiece, and they look after us well. This hospital has had a perfectly rotten experience since the show started; it was here originally, had to clear out during the retreat to the Bay of Biscay shores, and has altogether moved 16 times. The Colonel and Quartermaster are about the only two original men now in it. But now we hope to change its luck. One move into things, and then we hope to settle down to work in earnest. We have got quite a cheery crowd here really, mostly Scots and Irishmen.

November 24th
No. 6 General Hospital B.E.F., France

We have been through many changes since I last wrote to you, changing camp and repitching tents, and now we are rapidly closing down, and next week we are going into a very large building in the town, which will take us all, 600 patients and all the staff and personnel. We have had a fair stream of men through No. 6, and now we are sending them all to another hospital preparatory to moving. It has been real roughing it lately: for 8 days we have had thick snow on the ground, with the temperature below freezing night and day, and it still goes on. It has been awfully hard to keep warm, but we are all remarkably fit and still more, happy. Just think in a day or two the Mary's Ball should have come along. How different it all is now. It is great work here, these men are most extraordinary cheerful. Really the soldier type of man is a particularly fine one, when one gets to know him, and we get to know them here well enough; there are only a few grumblers and grousers, and they get sat on rather badly.

November 26th

Our plans are once more changed, and we are moving to a new site about a mile further out from Rouen. The building idea has been knocked on the head, and now we are beginning to strike camp here, and settle down higher up. We are dogged with bad luck: it was a toss up between us and No. 3 General Hospital as to who should go up to the sea coast, and No. 3 got it. The rotten part is that up there they will get so much better cases than we shall. However, I hope I shall get up to the front soon. We get a man here and there sent up. Two are off to-day to join an ammunition column. Wilson, the Casualty Physician, is out here with No. 8 General Hospital, and so is Cuthin. I had news of Vickers lately. One of our Staff Sergeants was in the same Cavalry Field Ambulance at the beginning of the show, and they were in the whole thing from Mons to Aisne. I believe Vickers is still with them. How is Diana? Is she going really strong? Do let me hear all about you all. Letters are coming through well now, and I am kept well supplied from all round. Have Mary's had any wounded yet? It seems just ages since I left London. Just think of Christmas out here; perhaps it will be better out here than at home.

(R.M. Handfield-Jones was related to Charles Handfield-Jones, who was elected F.R.S. in 1848 and appointed Physician to St Mary's Hospital. Charles Montagu Handfield-Jones, the son of Charles, was Senior Obstetrician and Gynaecologist at St Mary's for twenty years.

R.M. Handfield-Jones was Assistant Director of the Surgical Unit of St Mary's Hospital Medical School from 1922–1928. He was Consultant Surgeon to St. Mary's Hospital and along with Arthur Porritt, later Lord Porritt, wrote an excellent surgical text book. His letters to the *Gazette* have a particular value as they illustrate, more than most, the expressions spoken by the upper middle and professional classes at the time. Many of the phrases eg 'we passed through topping forests', 'it is a ripping spot', 'we had a cheery time', 'rigged out in great style', etc, would not be used to-day. The language was that used at home and continued in the prep school.

The attitudes to circumstances was also typical of the times, eg 'when the show began', referring to the onset of hostilities. Such a statement as 'the soldier type of man is a particularly fine one, when one gets to know him', would be considered patronising to-day, but was not meant or thought to be so at the time. It emphasises the strong social and class structures of society that existed, and were to remain unchanged until World War II.

It is remarkable that so many letters give the impression, a real one, that going to war was just another type of sport at which one would try one's best along with 'chums', and remain 'cheery' at all times. One must never let the side down!!!)

An undated letter from R. Leonard Ley described the naval bombardment of Yarmouth:

Although Yarmouth has been put badly in the shade by the bombardment of Hartlepool and Scarborough, I think you might care to have the following account.

At about 7.10 I was awakened by gun-fire, which was distant but continuous. I got up but could see nothing, so thought it was practice and went to bed again. During the next ten minutes the firing got much louder, and then shells began to shriek and explode, apparently in the town, to judge by the noise. I rushed on my clothes and cycled to the pier, which is about 400 yards from my home, and got there just in time to see the last broadside and shell striking the water about three miles out.

All you could see was the flashes of the gun (about thirty at once) and the columns of water. These seemed to keep suspended in the air for a tremendous time. No shells hit the land but several came very close, one within 600 yards of the pier. This one, according to a spectator, threw up columns of water as high as the Nelson Monument (Yarmouth), about 150 feet.

Later we saw British ships manoeuvring about and thought the enemy ships had been sunk; also we saw the submarine go out that was sunk by a mine.

The German ships were right among our fishing fleet, and the fishermen expected to find Yarmouth destroyed.

According to them they had three dreadnought battle cruisers and three smaller cruisers. We owe our escape to the fact, I believe, that the buoys had been shifted further out. The Germans, of course, knew how far from land they should have been, and as it was foggy took their range from the buoys, so all the shells fell short.

They were easily in range with the 11 and 12-inch guns of battle cruisers, as several people from the tops of their houses could see the ships' masts and funnels with glasses, and we all saw the flashes of the guns. The Halcyon, a small fishery protection cruiser, was saved by the destroyers circling round her and covering her with their smoke, plus the rotten shooting of the Germans.

We occasionally get alarms and periods of excitement, but life goes on pretty normally. Still, we shall be glad to hear the German High Seas Fleet (so styled) has been put under.

R. Leonard Ley.

Zeppelins

Count Ferdinand Graf von Zeppelin (1838–1917), a German army officer born in Konstanz, S.W. Germany, constructed his first airship in a factory in Friedrichshafen, between 1897 and 1900. Over 100 Zeppelins were used in World War I.

The first German Zeppelin raid was in January 1915. Three came across the North Sea cruising at a speed less than fifty miles per hour. They could however stay aloft throughout the night and the whole of the next day. As they crossed the English Channel they ran into bad weather but could see the lights below them. They dropped their bombs on Yarmouth and Kings Lynn. During World War I, Zeppelins made about forty raids on Britain and killed 537 people and injured 1,358.

A letter appeared in the *Gazette* from R. Leonard Ley:

27, Nelson Road S., Great Yarmouth.
Dear Sir,
I am sending you a short account of our Zeppelin Raid. We were playing bridge, and about 8.30 we heard an engine.

I said it was an air engine, and my wife also thought it was, but our friends said no. We sat arguing about it, and one lady said Zeppelins always turned to drop their bombs. I said, half jokingly and half in earnest, "Well this one is just hovering for its patch." The words were hardly spoken when there was an awful crash. Our friends fled, and we grabbed the children and retired to the cellar. I have only a confused recollection of events after the first crash, but heard other crashes and saw flashes of light. One of my servants told me our friends had left the door wide open with the hall lights on, so I went up to turn off the light and shut the door. While at the door the road was frequently lit up by flashes of light from their search-light. At that time the noise of the engine gradually passed away. The whole affair from the time we first heard the engine could not have been five minutes. A few minutes later I was called by telephone to see a soldier who had been hit by a bit of bomb. I found him suffering a little from shock and was sweating freely, pupils dilated. He had a wound over the heart, ragged at edges and circular in character. I had him moved to the hospital and saw him again there. The pulse rate was normal on both occasions, and he recovered in a few days without anything being done. There was no suppuration. I also saw at the hospital an old woman. Her clothes were not much damaged, but her abdominal wall was blown away and intestines were protruding. Next day her arm was found at the site of destruction. No one had noticed its absence from the body at the hospital owing to a heavy cape she was wearing, I suppose, which was undamaged. I did not see the body of the other man who was killed. Later I returned home, and after removing the children's cot to the ground floor, my wife and I retired to bed. We were just settling down when we heard the cursed engines again. We again retired to the ground floor, and I reconnoitred from a window. The brute passed over to sea without dropping any more bombs. The damage done was very slight. At least ten bombs were dropped – probably more – only five exploded, one of these incendiary, and two houses were partly wrecked and a lot of windows shattered, two people killed outright, and three or four slightly wounded. The two I have personal knowledge of recovered without suppuration in spite of the presence of a bit of bomb.

I saw the incendiary bomb after it was dug up. It weighed about 40 lbs., and was composed of a cylinder of about 6 inches diameter. The lower end was heavily weighted and was conical, with the object of piercing a roof. At the other end were the wind vanes (so-called propellers) to balance it, and above a handle like a milk can's to attach it to the bomb carrying apparatus. The high explosive bombs were sugar loaf in shape, and weighed up to 100lbs., the explosive was yellow and crystalline, rather like demerera sugar, and was, I believe, tri-nitro-toluene. They had "propellers", which were supposed to act a safety catches. The action was as follows: so many revolutions of the propeller will remove the top of the bomb and so free a detonator which comes into action with the jar of the bomb striking. So if the Zeppelin was 1,000 feet up, they would set the propeller so that it would screw out at say 800 feet, so many known revolutions being produced for each 100 feet it falls. The Zeppelin was probably much nearer the earth than they thought, and thus the safety device was not removed in time. Some such device of course is necessary to prevent accidents in starting and descending. Count Zeppelin's explanation of rendering them harmless before using them as ballast is not widely accepted here.

I might add that the noise of the engine once heard is characteristic and gives plenty of warning, or at least I hope it will if they come again. We have had three or four grand Zeppelin nights lately, and nothing has happened, so we feel more hopeful. I have called the enemy a Zeppelin, but it may have been a Pareseval.

Apologising for length,

I remain,

Yours truly,

R. Leonard Ley.

(Richard Leonard Ley qualified in 1907. He was Assistant Surgeon and Radiologist to the Gt. Yarmouth Hospital and Hon. Medical Officer to the Children's Convalescent Home, Gt. Yarmouth. He was the author of 'Tropical Forms of Adenitis' 1909, 'Case of Spinal Meningocoele' 1910, 'Case of Urethral Calculus' 1920, and 'Irregularity of Pappiloedema in certain cases of Increased Intracranial Pressure'.)

CHAPTER 14

Dear Mr Editor

January 18th, 1915.
France
Dear Mr. Editor,
The Hospital Gazette for November has just reached me via India. I was very glad to get it. I was most pleased to see the order about enteric inoculation, which I had not seen before. In India, as you know, we push inoculation for all it is worth, nearly all the men being protected. I had to examine one battery of R.F.A. and a British Infantry battalion for active service before we left, and made it one of the reasons for rejecting men if they were not inoculated. The battery volunteered to a man, and only two of the infantry formed the depot party left behind for this reason. The result was both units left 100 per cent protected, including officers. Since we arrived in France we have received drafts of over 600 men. Of these about half were already protected, 260 were inoculated a couple of days ago, 23 are waiting to be done, and only 36 in the whole battalion refuse. Thanks to the Army order you have published and to other means, I hope to get hold of these few before long. The publishing of lists of soldiers sent to Mary's for treatment will, I feel sure, prove of the greatest interest to all Mary's men out here on service, as it is always interesting to hear what becomes of men who pass through our aid posts and hospitals. Quite recently over 200 wounded passed through my aid post within 24 hours, from 16 different units, excluding a German, they included British, French and Indian troops. I was able to get along well enough with British and Indian, but regret to state that my French is bad and my German, if possible, worse. I think the worst time I have had out here was when a Sepoy asked me to buy him a watch in a French jeweller's shop. The Indian knew no language other than his own, and the woman in the shop knew only French. Complications ensued when the Indian insisted that rupees, he had no other money, were worth two francs each. Finally the ordeal was over, the native got his watch, the French woman her rupees at one franc sixty centimes each, and I escaped with more or less honour! There is little need to say much, however, to the wounded; the majority do not want to be worried, all they want is there dressings seen to, and what in most cases is more important, is a hot drink of tea or soup. I am glad to say most of them were able to get this except a few abdominal cases. So far I have found that

very few require morphia, and always give it in cases of very severe or abdominal wounds. I am not allowed to say anything about the behaviour of our troops, much as I would like to do so, the way they stand for days in muddy trenches, often with water almost to their knees, is grand; but the class that requires the highest praise is that comprising the stretcher bearers, they are willing to go out anywhere to bring in wounded, quite regardless of all the risks they run.

The question of men giving up their hospital work to come out here as dressers and such like has been raised, and I quite agree with those who consider that students should not do so. We will want many doctors after this war is over, owing to the gaps made by those killed, severely wounded, and those who have to retire through illness. This will affect both the civil and military branches of the profession. My humble advice to students is to stick to their studies and get qualified. I myself left Mary's whilst a student to go to South Africa in 1900, and although I do not regret it for many reasons, I now find myself junior in the service to men who entered Mary's after I did. I fear I have no war news to send you, as the experiences of most medical officers with units are similar out here unless they happen to get into one of the larger engagements. These experiences have already been described by much abler pens than mine. In most cases our work begins after dark, as the wounded cannot be brought in from the trenches during the day, at least that is my experience. I have personally only been in the trenches on one or two occasions, as an order was published stating, "The place for medical officers is not in the trenches, they should remain in their aid posts where their services may be of some use;" but of course in cases of urgency the medical officer would go. It is impossible to be of much use in the trenches, owing to the lack of space and general state of dirt. All men are instructed in the use of the first field dressing, and anyone can apply one, and the medical officer is much more useful at a fixed spot such as his aid post, where he can get things more or less cleaner than he would in the trenches. The aid post should always be under as much cover as possible, and should have a good cellar in which the wounded can be placed in case of shelling by the enemy.

Only the most urgent operations such as tying of arteries and such like should be undertaken in aid posts, owing to the fear of sepsis. Iodine I am glad to say is in almost general use. All my stretcher bearers carry a bottle of the tincture, which they apply at once when a man is wounded. In most cases the first field dressing is not interfered with at the aid post. The man is simply examined, given a hot drink, and then cleared off to a Field Ambulance as soon as possible. Warmth is a most important factor in the treatment of the wounded in the aid post, at least this is my experience, others may have found it otherwise. Coming over from India, as I have done, it has been most interesting to note the gradual falling off of tropical diseases, and the gradual onset of the commoner ailments seen in England. The day we left Ferozepore last August, we had 16 cases of heat stroke with four deaths, the shade temperature was about 120 degrees. Malaria is now almost non-existent, although a few old cases occasionally come in with it still. On the voyage we had 23 cases of neuritis, said by some to be beri-beri, but I do not think this diagnosis altogether satisfactory; now all we get are cases of myalgia, coughs, and a few colitis. So far I have only met one Mary's man, Barker in the I.M.S. is with the 15th Sikhs, and came over with the Indian contingent.

Up to date I have only had a couple of near squeaks. I was hit on the shoulder in November, at the mythical point X, by a piece of a high explosive shell, but luckily only bruised. On the other occasion a five-inch howitzer shell cruised in through the window of my bedroom and tried to make itself comfortable in my valise, greatly to the detriment of my kit and of the house, but luckily I was out at the time. I have not, I fear, given much news, but you asked Mary's men to write, so I have given you what I can. As we are just now in a state of constant readiness to move, I must pack my odd sock and toothbrush, and so will end. With best wishes to all Mary's men, past and present,

Believe me, ever yours sincerely,

J. Errol M. Boyd, Captain R.A.M.C.,

Indian Expeditionary Force, A.

February 4th 1915.
c/o Gordon Highlanders,
Fernhurst,
Haslemere,
Aldershot Command,
Dear Sir, – I am sending some account of my work and experiences in case they may be of interest.

I have worked with Kitchener's Army since I joined on September 1st. Throughout I have taken "sick parade" daily, seeing numbers varying from 30 to 200 per diem. For the first fortnight I helped another man see 400 or so sick – in the open air at first. Then I was attached to the 7th and 8th Seaforths, and from the end of September I have been attached to the 9th Gordons, having the 10th battalion as well at first.

For two months I was under canvas, and now for two and a half months have been billeted.

In camp the men could never dry their clothes and walked in seas of mud; here the village is too small, and we are not much better off in these respects, and being scattered, discipline is difficult.

Apart from seeing sick I have charge of the sanitation, have given a course of lectures, inoculated 2,000 men against typhoid, and 1,000 against smallpox, and now am training the band in first aid and stretcher drill

Latterly I have had a horse, so have learnt to stick on and get exercise on off afternoons.

There are some points in my experience that may be of interest.

Throughout, particularly at first, I have been discharging men as medically unfit.

These men come under three heads:

(1) Cases of hernia, varicose veins, phthisis, chronic heart disease, chronic bronchitis, defective vision, defective teeth, generally unfit, and such like; cases, in fact, which should never have reached us.

(2) Cases of overstrained heart – functional dilatation, due to violent exercise for 8 hours a day 7 days a week, commenced abruptly.

(3) Malingerers

Apropos of the above groups:

1. I hope the profession realises how culpable it is to be careless about the attestation of recruits. In the case of the Seaforths and Gordons alone it meant that, say, 300 men were clothed, fed and paid for 6–8 weeks, sent to the length of Great Britain, sent home again with a suit of clothes, and 20 to 30 shillings in pocket – in the first place. Secondly it meant loss of discipline, because numbers of men were perforce loafing about camp, and slackers loafed with them unnoticed, so making discipline, which anyhow would have been poor, deplorable.

2. I think it undeniable that at the commencement of the war common sense was made to bow before zeal in the manner of quantity of drill.

3. Don't imagine you have to be an old soldier to be a good malingerer.

My experience of Inoculation for Typhoid went to prove that with a little arrangement it could be done quickly, the longest job being the taking of the names. I had helpers. First the arm was painted with iodine, then I pushed in 0.5cc or 1.0cc for the first and second dose respectively, then a man painted with collodion, and finally the name was taken. I used a 10cc Record syringe, and sterilised the needle before each prick by dipping it into hot olive oil. If no hitch occurred with the names I did the men at the rate of 200 per hour, ie, 3 per minute.

Vaccination against smallpox was done in a similar way and at about the same speed. An assistant blew on the vaccine, I scratched, then a square of lint was fixed with Mead's strapping over the place, then the name was taken. Making the squares took longest here. I have had no sepsis. In the case of the smallpox vaccine I at first cleaned the skin with iodine, allowing it to dry, but then only 20 percent or less took. Without the iodine a high percentage took.

Yours truly,

Aubrey W. Venables. Lieut. R.A.M.C.

(Dr Venables was obviously a stickler for discipline and was disturbed considerably by malingerers. We are surprised that he rejected as soldiers those with defective teeth!! During World War I many recruits were rejected for heart murmurs which were physiological and not of significance, but a number of these were so affected by this that they developed into cardiac cripples quite needlessly, spending the remainder of their lives in anxiety.

Sadly, Dr Venables was killed in action in France in 1916.)

German Occupation of Brussels

At the outbreak of war the German First Army attacked Liège. In spite of a brave defence by the Belgian forts and garrisons the invasion of Belgium continued and rapid marching enabled the German troops to cover nearly 200 miles in two weeks and to enter Brussels on 20 August 1914.

The Belgian army retreated to Antwerp where they resisted further German advance for another three weeks and so enabled the French and British Forces to move to a defensive line to protect the Channel ports.

The Germans behaved badly in Brussels at the start of the occupation by burning university libraries and shooting some priests and English nurses.

May, 1915.

From a St. Mary's Nurse in Brussels

The following account of the German occupation of Brussels and the treatment of English nurses and doctors has been most kindly written by Miss Hilda Speak, and we have permission to publish it. We do so in the hope that we may realise something of the dangers, privations and hardships our devoted nurses and doctors are facing and enduring daily in order that they may prove good Samaritans indeed to those in desperate need.

"On August 10th the first contingent of nurses left London, in the charge of a surgeon, for the front, I being one of the twenty. We arrived in Brussels and had a very hearty reception. We were given charge of various ambulances (an ambulance in this context is according to the Concise Oxford Dictionary, "a mobile hospital following an army") in which were Belgian wounded. For some days we kept receiving new wounded, but unfortunately the news arrived that the Germans were approaching Brussels. For a day or two the city was very subdued and quiet, and while taking a walk a day or two later I met a portion of the German Army, which was then pouring into Brussels. This was at 1.30 p.m., and they continued to come into the city until 6.30 p.m. About 80,000 soldiers, with their guns, etc., took up their quarters that night. Ambulances which had not till then received any wounded were invaded and used as quarters for the Germans. From this time the town was very busy and the streets alive, the Germans appropriating everything possible for their own use. Milk became very scarce. The ambulances were chiefly used for German wounded. Fortunately my ambulance was a little way from the main road, and contained only Belgian soldiers, of which together I had fifty-two. In the other ambulances the nurses still remained and attended the Germans, who were continually being brought into Brussels. Later other Red Cross nurses arrived in the city, and were asked by the Germans to go down to the station and feed and dress the wounds of the prisoners and others passing through on their way to Germany. Some of the poor men were in a wretched condition, lying on straw and their wounds greatly needed attention. The nurses were amply repaid by the smiles on the men's faces when they saw the English nurses. For a month the doctors and nurses went daily to the station and attended the soldiers. One day a German officer ordered all there to be locked up in a waiting room, saying they were acting as spies. They were thoroughly searched, and kept there for thirty-six hours, until the American Consul interfered. A few days after an order was issued to the effect that all the English nurses and doctors were to go out of Brussels or they would be taken as spies. As there was no possible chance of our getting out of Brussels without help, the Germans were asked to find some means of seeing us away. After considering for some days, we were told to be ready to leave on October 6th. We arrived at the station with our luggage, and after three hours consultation, we were told we could not leave that day in the train that was being specially run for the American citizens trying to leave Brussels. We were also ordered by an officer to take off our British flags, as we were on German territory. We were also told that if we were at the station at the same time the next day we might possibly be allowed to go. Needless to say, we were there, and after a roll call by a German officer – a list having previously been supplied to the authorities – we were allowed to pass into the station, which was in a filthy condition, through lines of soldiers. We carried our own luggage as best we could, some of the doctors helping us as they could. At last we got into the train. In each compartment there were German soldiers. There were three other nurses in my compartment and two soldiers of the roughest and most objectionable type. They smoked and ate continuously until we reached Cologne, and would insist on having the windows closed. The carriages were the worst I have ever seen – hard wood seats and backs, and very, very dirty. There were also soldiers riding on top of the carriage. It took twenty-eight hours to reach Cologne; in ordinary times it takes four hours. The train crawled, and we seemed to stop every few minutes. During the journey through Belgian territory we noticed the awful devastation all along the line, many towns and villages containing only a roofless lot of ruins. Louvain appeared to be practically wiped out. Imagination can never picture the terrible ruin done to Belgium. At Stolberg, a small station just before Cologne, we were very roughly told to get out of the train. There I saw a young German officer take two of our doctors by the shoulder and throw them across the platform. At this point I was more alarmed than I had been since entering Brussels. Our luggage was all turned out on the platform and the soldiers searched it. All knives and forks were taken, surgical instruments, and even a nurse's fountain pen. After looking through our papers and a great deal of consultation, we were told to get into the train again by the soldiers, and we started for Cologne. I think if some of our young men in England had witnessed the treatment of the British Red Cross at this station it would help them to make up their minds as to where their duty to their country lies. There were twenty doctors; they could not retaliate, their only thought and care being for the hundred and twenty-four nurses who were in their charge in the country of the enemy. At Cologne we got our first meal and were treated quite reasonably, but at the last moment bundles of magazines were placed on each table with very objectionable cartoons. After our meal we entered the train again for a place unknown. We still had a guard with us, and arrived at Munster at 7 a.m. on October 8th, where we were evidently expected, and given breakfast at the station. It appeared to be a camp station: there were a great many soldiers round about. They gave us basins of coffee, sausage and bread. We washed our hands and faces under a pump, and felt much better for the food and wash. After an hour's wait we entered the train again, and as far as we knew we appeared to be going towards Denmark. At 4 p.m. we stopped, and were given basins of soup in the train. We continued the journey and that night had no light in the carriages. We arrived at Hamburg at 1 a.m. on October 9th, but were not well treated there. We left the train for ten minutes, guarded by soldiers each side to a refreshment room, but we were waited on very badly, the food being practically thrown at us. In fact, some of us were unable to get any at all. From Hamburg the train was well guarded, the blinds being drawn and windows closed. We guessed we were passing the Kiel Canal, and were disappointed at not getting a glimpse of the German fleet. After travelling four days and three nights, we arrived on the Danish frontier, and there we stopped for the German guard to leave the train. No one except those who have experienced it can imagine our feelings as we left the Germans behind and knew we were prisoners no longer. Then our destination was Copenhagen, where we were kindly received by the British Consul there. The people were exceedingly kind to us. This was shown by the words written in English in the Danish paper on the morning following our arrival:

To the British surgeons and nurses passing through Copenhagen on their way from Belgium.

Silent we bid you welcome,
In silence you answered our greeting –
Because our lips must be closed
And your teeth set against the gale,
Our mouths are mute,
Our minds are open –
We shall greet you farewell in silence,
Sowers of good will
On fields where hate is sown,
Fare ye well!

After six days in Copenhagen, we left for Christiana, thence to Bergen, where we took the boat to Newcastle"

(Miss Hilda Speak writes of the harsh treatment they were subjected to by the Germans and quotes the display of newspapers with inappropriate cartoons!!! At that time *circa* 1914–1918, nurses and doctors expected good treatment as prisoners, especially as they were non-combatants. By and large this was respected. This group were returned to England. The treatment quoted in this letter was quite good as compared to modern times. They were fed and watered and there is no evidence in this letter of any abuse of the nurses, which in terms of modern warfare was a blessing. This was not always so, and it is horrific to think of the fate of nurses in the hands of the Japanese in World War II.)

(J. Errol Boyd qualified in 1906. He was in the 1st Field Hospital, Rhodesian Field Force, and gained the Queen's Medal with five clasps, 1900–1. He was a major in World War I, and was mentioned in dispatches. He gained the War Medal and Victory Medal. He was the author of 'Suggestions for arrangement and Marking of Microscopic Slides in a Cabinet' and 'The Philatelic Zoo-Stamp Lover'.)

CHAPTER 15

Rawal Pindi British General Hospital

Sunday, May 30th 1915.
Boulogne Base, France
Dear Mr. Editor,
I have spent a most enjoyable and somewhat instructive afternoon, and it suddenly occurred to me that details might interest some of your readers. After lunch a friend and I walked out to the Boulogne Golf Links, the home of the Australian Hospital, borrowed clubs and balls, played 18 holes in far too many strokes, and returned to the Club House (the officers' mess) tired but happy. Our hosts invited us to attend a discussion, just started, on "Gas Asphyxia", of which we have had a great deal lately. The Medical Officers of the Australian Hospital have a "talk" on a selected subject every Sunday after tea, and invite two members from each of the numerous hospitals and convalescent camps of the Boulogne Base, and, of course, all the consultants. We were in time for all the big guns, starting with Sir William Herringham, who gave his experiences of gas cases seen at the front; Sir John Rose Bradford followed with a description of those seen at the base, with details of post mortems; then Sir Bertrand Dawson gave his observations. The surgeons took no part; Makins looked interested. Burghard slept most of the time. One would have thought everything had been said till Barcroft, the only man not in khaki, gave his "facts". He was sent for from Cambridge to investigate gas poisoning. He returned home and experimented on cats. Result: he found that the blood after inhalation of chlorine contained an excess of acid, both fixed and Carbon Dioxide, and its coagulability was lessened. The excess of Carbon Dioxide was the chief cause of the intense cyanosis, not the deficiency of Oxygen. Lastly Sir Almroth Wright at about 7 p.m. brushes the talk of two hours aside, and in a few pregnant words says what amounts to, "You have heard what the chemist says, now you know the cause, find and apply the remedy." Up rises Sir J. Rose Bradford, who had sent for Barcroft, and had a last word – lest there should be any misunderstanding.

However, Sir Almroth Wright made some suggestive observations. He said he had made his "urine alkaline in 8 minutes by taking lactate of calcium," and again, "Sir Wilmot Herringham's observation that ammonium carbonate was the one drug that all the Medical Officers at the front were emphatic in saying was of real benefit, might be explained by the fact that it was an alkali."

An interesting fact we heard for the first time was pointed out by Sir Bertrand Dawson; our atropine treatment of these gas asphyxiated patients had been worked out by the Germans in preparation for its use. A small but significant instance of Teutonic thoroughness.

I am etc.,

H.L. Hatch, Lieut. R.A.M.C. (tempy.)

(Dr H.L. Hatch qualified from St Mary's Hospital Medical School in 1894, with Honours in the Intermediate and Final M.B., and went to live in South Africa. He served as a Civilian Surgeon with the South African Field Force and in the Boer War. He served in World War I in the R.A.M.C. and reached the rank of Captain. He returned to the United Kingdom and settled in practice in Pinner where he remained until his death in 1963 at the age of eighty-four. He was the author of 'The X-Rays', and 'Chloroform: its Action and Administration' and 'The present Position of the Roentgen Rays in Surgery and Medicine'.)

July 19th 1915.
A.P.O.S. 11,
25 General Hospital,
B.E.F., France.

A chiel's amang ye takin' notes,
An' faith he'll prent it.

Dear Sir, – I do not know who edits the Gazette at present, but there is, I presume, still an editorial demand for copy. This letter from "somewhere in France" will tell you of the happenings of some old Mary's men. The mobilisation and getting off of this hospital is no doubt typical of many.

We mobilised at Aldershot about five weeks ago, waited there for a day or two, and left for Southampton early in the morning. Escorted by two destroyers, which nosed round us like two playful terriers, sometimes ahead and sometimes astern, we reached the pleasant land of France in the early morning. We landed and soon got into a camp of canvas tents which was waiting for us. At Aldershot there came up to me one Robbs, and said he was from St. Mary's, and was now a member of 25. We have been together since. I had never been in a tent before, except to buy lemonade at county cricket matches. I now found I was expected to sleep in one. Robbs explained many things to me. He fixed up his tent bed, and mine, tightened the tent pegs, and generally got busy, as the Americans say. We slept in the same tent, and in the morning, as Robbs was shaking the earwigs out of his socks, he told me that sometimes tents blow over. I now noticed that his bed was on the side from which the wind was blowing. Robbs said, "Yes, it is safer on that side, as the pole may fall on you in the night and break your back." I said: "Thank you for those kind words. Let me fix the tent to-night." Robbs has been a very present help in trouble, however. We moved on, however, down the coast, and took up our regular quarters that day.

Our camping ground for this hospital is well chosen. About four miles from the sea are the Sussex Downs (or Downs exactly like them). Under them our tents are pitched in what were once cornfields; then comes a railway, which is hooting day and night and carrying all the paraphernalia of war to the front. This runs parallel to the Downs. Then come sand dunes, and finally the sea.

It is interesting to think of how this town, in which we live, sprang into being, think of the cornfields and poppies, and then, I suppose, the first little tent. This was followed by other tents, and pathways arose, and then roads, and the roads were made better and tarred. Then came the Post Office telephone, Y.M.C.A. concert hut, signposts with the names of the roads, and finally a town, which will shortly have a population of 5,000 inhabitants, possibly more. And all because Kaiser Bill is a megalomaniac; and, after all, this is such a small item in what is going on here. The other night a concert was given in the Hall, and the first performer was Milner Moore, who obliged with the "Whistling Coon." This, of course, brought the house down, and incidentally made the writer think of how much had happened since he first heard that same coon whistle in the O.P. Department at St. Mary's in happy days gone by. Milner Moore was in great form and the star performer of the evening. An excursion on the railway brought us to the seaport in which is 13 General Hospital. There we found Kelly, who has done great work during the past winter, and after congratulating him on having become a father, and interrupting him in an account of how surgery had been revolutionised by the War, we were taken to the top of the building and brought face to face with the Professor. The Professor was as kindly and untutored, in the Prussian sense, as ever. A happy band of Maryans were performing their usual evolutions with test-tubes and various glass tubes drawn to a point.

After this a tramway took us to what had once been the Hotel Splendide at Wimereux. I must say, in passing, that we are supposed not to mention names out here. In playing this great game of make-belief, the Huns, by all the local rules, should not know that English people are labouring in the Northern ports of France. If the war has at long last brought a dim sense of humour to the Hun, he must be smiling some. The wily fellow probably knows more about Wimereux, and the number of Goddams there, than Baedeker himself.

On reaching the second floor at the Hotel Splendide, one was confronted by Carmalt Jones. Carmalt occupied a pleasant room looking sheer down to the sea. He quoted Keats:

"Our open casements facing desolate seas,
Our magic window fronting on the sea," and so on.

In his student days it was Browning he quoted. Otherwise Carmalt was the same. He has been at the Front with a Territorial Battery, and is very pleased with them, and will never, he says, take "T" off his tunic. He scoffed at my suggestion of danger, although in very modest terms, and seems to have developed an absolute taste for high explosive. He was at the time, however, making a cardiographic recording apparatus out of a blackened cigarette box and a piece of hat elastic. On the other side of the road Bryan is doing good work, but we had no time left to look in on him. An excursion to Montreuil, a beautiful old walled city inland from here, revealed the fact that Corbett, a clerk of Dr Luffs, too many years ago, was orderly officer for the day to the Indian Hospital there. He showed us round, and said he found the life interesting. There were to be seen Sikhs, Gurkhas and Pathans in various stages of convalescence. We saw their cooking arrangements, and smelt that smell that comes from East of Suez, and is indescribable, but pathognomic to those who have been there.

In a tea-shop at Le Touquet (I will mention names) was sitting John Pooley. Everyone knows that Pooley was a forward, that time Cowey scored a try in the final, and Mary's successfully sat on it. Pooley had a grievance. After working hard and establishing their hospital out here, his lot had been turned out for a bevy of Americans from Middle West. He had my sympathy, but the ways of the War Office are inscrutable, and I could offer no explanation. Otherwise Pooley was well, and cheered up in a neighbouring Estaminet.

So far the work out here has not been too strenuous, but when and if the Bosches make their big offensive, or we make ours, or both of us kick off together, then we expect to be "for it", as Tommy says. Well, if we can do anything to help Tommy after what he has done for us, we ought to feel grateful for the chance. In the meantime the life is healthy if a little monotonous, and we are doing our little best to cement the Entente Cordiale. We are fortunate in our C.O., a quiet man, possessed of charm and tact, and our surgical and medical specialists. The former Major Alexis Thomson, adds greatly to the gaiety of nations, besides making it unnecessary to carry a Rose and Carless (always cumbersome in the tunic pocket) for is he not half of Thomson and Miles, always on top as it were? Of the latter, Major Melville Dunlop, I can only say that Edinburgh's loss is our gain. Yes, Scotland stands where she did with this outfit.

Our ambulance driver is a sporting parson who goes to the Old Testament for inspiration, but Jehu is left standing. This sportsman had driven at the front, and seems to think he is still dodging Jack Johnsons.

He is shortly going home to be married, and, by this simple act, probably saves many lives.

Did I tell you that our radiographer is only with us by the grace of God, in the manner of speaking?

We were told to foregather at Southampton at 5 p.m., and the X-ray expert was on the scene at 5.2 p.m., watching the gangway caught up by a crane and dangling overhead. He shouted, "Can you take me Captain?" but the man on the bridge muttered the nautical equivalent of "nothing doing", and a following transport had to meet the case.

Well, Mr. Editor, this is a sketchy piece of copy, but if you can decipher it, and it has any interest for Gazette readers, there you are.

Hoping that all of us, now serving abroad, may be spared to go on paying our subscriptions to the Gazette,

I am, yours,etc.,

SCRUTATOR.

November, 1915
A Year with the Army in France
By A.G.H. Lovell F.R.C.S. Late Temp.-Lieut. R.A.M.C.

Through the columns of the Gazette news is asked for from Mary's men at the front. That is my excuse for this, in which I will try to tell you something of my experiences and impressions during these last eventful twelve months. I received a temporary commission from August 7th for twelve months, and in a few days found myself in Amiens with a General Hospital. We received our first train load of wounded and sick within 24 hours of arrival there, before we had properly established our hospital. I was very impressed then by the huge preponderance of incapacitating trivial ailments among the sick – boils, sore feet, varicose veins, and the like.

Then came a week of rumours of victories and defeats, and all the time trainload after trainload of troops passed through the station – cheering men packed into cattle trucks going up and trains with empty trucks or wounded going down.

Personally, I had charge of wounded officers in a girls school, which we were converting into a very excellent hospital of 100 beds. The engineers were putting in a lift, gas burners, an autoclave, and other conveniences when the D.D.M.S (Deputy Director of Medical Services) of the L. of C. told me that the English were leaving Amiens, and we were to remain and hand over everything to the Germans if they arrived! All the English, including the D.D.M.S. and R.T.O. (in charge of travel), except our hospital left within 24 hours. We waited for two more days while stragglers came in telling us they were the survivors of their battalions. It became remarkable how many sole survivors there were from one battalion. On the second day we left hurriedly with our personnel and our remaining 50 bad lying cases – the latter were laid on stretchers and mattresses in cattle trucks. The Germans arrived next day. I think that jolting journey to Havre, which took about 20 hours, was one of the worst times I have spent, for I was with five very badly wounded officers and could do so little for them; their pluck was stoical. To add to our troubles, one of our orderlies fell out of the train in the night and had his leg run over, necessitating the use of my first field dressing and my puttee as a tourniquet.

Having handed over our wounded at Havre we went to a camp near the town, only to be turned out that night (again wild rumours of Germans approaching), and eventually I was sent off with 150 R.A.M.C. details, St. John's Ambulance men from all walks of life, and five other officers in a train. All we knew was we were reinforcements, but our destination was vague, and even our engine driver did not know it. When we got to Paris we found that the truck with all the officers' luggage had been slipped and lost. I then learn the hard and fast rule, "Never part from your valise." We spent the next ten days living in trains travelling round Paris, down to Tours and Le Mans, and back to the environs of Paris. At Le Mans we bought some essential articles to replace our lost kit, and eventually we reached Coulommiers, three days after the Germans had started their retreat from there. Here we saw our first signs of German "Hate" – shops and houses broken into, mattresses ripped up, chairs and beds broken, and in every house and farm the inevitable bottle with cherries at the bottom and all the brandy gone! We also met a number of German prisoners, one of whom asked us if he would be shot or have his throat cut. At this point I was told off suddenly one evening to go to Rebais, five kilometres off, with 70 men and another civil surgeon as reinforcements for the first army. At this spot I was to have directions given me. Well, we arrived there with no kit, transport, maps or detailed orders, and only half a day's rations. We found no English troops there and no orders waiting for us. I never felt quite so out of my element before, being totally ignorant of usual army procedure, so I took the men into a field and slept there until 3 a.m. Then I discovered a field ambulance that had been left behind when the other troops advanced. They were moving off, so we had a hurried meal and marched off northwards with them. That day we did 28 miles, reaching the Army Headquarters at midday and getting to Hautes Vesnes that night. There had been a very successful fight that day there. We slept in a field next to a large enclosure containing some 500 German prisoners. Next day we were off again at 7.a.m. to reach the divisional headquarters, at which we had to report. It was said to be four miles ahead, but it moved too, and remained four miles ahead, and we marched 22 miles that day, eventually reaching our destination, Ouchy le Chateau, at 8.p.m., soaking wet and very tired. Next morning we were told off to No.4 Field Ambulance. This Ambulance had lost half its transport and personnel, and all its officers except two, at Landrecies, so we were warmly greeted. We at once started again on a long, slow, wet trek, crossing the Marne and ending in very poor billets at Courcelles. Next morning, September 13 th, we watched the Guards and the Artillery move out to the opening of the Battle of the Aisne. We followed them, and that day from the heights on the Southern side of the Valley I saw a battle for the first time: a marvellous sight it was, and one I shall never forget.

It was the following morning, when we were waiting by a bridge to cross the river that our ambulance came in for our first dose of "Johnsons." For myself I had not realised we were in range of the Huns – at that time I was innocent and had no fear of shells, though by the evening the wholesome dread was instilled. We were just making tea for lunch while we awaited orders, when some artillery came across the bridge, retiring as fast as they could, and aimed at them came a series of "Johnsons." The first fell 50 yards short of us, the next 40 yards, and we all moved off; a moment later and a shell had fallen where we had been standing, and then we scattered, each choosing his own way back to our collecting post, 400 yards behind us. Meanwhile shells were coming among us faster. On getting back I heard my civil surgeon friend had been hit. I went back and found the artillery had got by unhurt, but my friend had pluckily stopped to dress a R.A.M.C. man who had been hit beside him, and the next shell had taken off his big toe. He had said the day before he wished he could cut it off to get rid of a painful ingrowing toe nail! We took them to a cottage close by and I dressed them both and brought them back to the collecting post. No sooner had we done this than more artillery came down the road and were shelled badly. When they had passed my Major, eight bearers and I went down to help where we could. We found a horrible mess – disembowelled horses, several dead men, including a medical officer, and some 15 wounded; the cottage was now a pile of bricks. We did the first field dressings there and then. One man had his arm almost off at the neck of the humerus, and another his leg almost off at the knee. In both the main artery could be seen divided and closed by retraction, a feature of many shell wounds of arteries I have seen since. I put Spencer Wells on them and left them on, and finished the amputation by dividing the remaining skin with my pocket scalpel. The next evening we crossed the river, but by another bridge – a pontoon – and arrived at 11 p.m., very tired at the Chateau de Soupir. Here we were badly wanted, for in caves at the top of the hill to the north of the Chateau were some 80 English wounded, and outside the caves as many wounded Germans, the latter in a huddled, gory, soaking, shivering mass. I was sent up to bring these down. We got the English down that night and the Germans the next. The Chateau and Church already contained many wounded, and we were only three medical officers. Most of the wounded had received their wounds 36 hours before, and were consequently now in a most smelly condition. I never shall forget, though words cannot fully describe, the interior of those caves, lighted here and there by the stump of a candle, while a farm close by burned merrily. We evacuated most of the wounded at once on motor lorries without attempting to re-dress them. Then each M.O. had two hours sleep in turns and set to work to dress the remainder, starting with the English. We then established a dressing station in the chateau, which was about 1,500 yards from the German trenches. The library became the operating room and the drawing-room the chief ward. We had no beds here, but collected all the mattresses from the huge double beds upstairs.

From here I was sent to the 1st King's Liverpool Regiment as M.O. It was at Moussy, two miles off. As I received the order I looked at Moussy and saw it was in a cloud of shrapnel bursts and had a series of Johnson explosions going on in it − truly, a cheery spot. I waited till dark before going there, and found it a small village with two good cellars and not one house intact, most of them being completely ruined. That night the regiment moved out to so-called rest I know I tried to sleep on a very hard billiard table and spent five days inspecting feet and treating an epidemic of enteritis. Then we went back to Moussy for a fortnight, and I lived in the H.Q. in one of the aforesaid cellars most of the time. We always had an hour's shelling each morning and evening, and often it lasted all day. The "evening hate" was a very regular performance. However, our men were pretty good at finding funk-holes, and we had very few casualties. My great difficulty was to keep the sanitation of the village anything approaching good. Then I was relieved by Armstrong and sent back to the Field Ambulance. By this time things had settled down a bit, and, thanks to our A.D.M.S., I did most of the surgery from this time onwards. This was an early stage of the war, and we were learning by bitter experience the importance of several of the cardinal points of surgery. Gas production was the outstanding feature of the wounds at this time. I consider the following are the cardinal points, and if they seem obvious now, they certainly were not being acted upon at the beginning of the war:

(1) All shell wounds and large (explosive) bullet wounds are septic, and good drainage should be established at the earliest moment;

(2) All cases should have Tetanus Antitoxin at the Field Ambulance;

(3) No wounds should be stitched − especially no amputations or scalp wounds;

(4) Amputations should, for the most part, be circular, or done by a mere trimming up through the site of fracture;

(5) Peroxide of Hydrogen is the most useful lotion we have for use at a first dressing.

Beyond this the mechanical effect of any irrigation of wounds is the most effective part of the using of a lotion, and saline is probably as good as any antiseptic.

At this time we had no supply of peroxide with the Ambulance. While at the chateau we did some surgery. It included amputations and ligature of bleeding points, but was chiefly the making of counter openings for drainage and incisions for gas infections. I drained the pelvis in one intra-abdominal wound with peritonitis, and I know the patient was alive six months later. We next moved up to take part in the first battle of Ypres. I spent Oct 21st with the bearers at St. Julien, returning with the wounded that night to the Tent Section, who had established themselves in a school at Ypres. We were three M.O.s, beside the C.O. and each worked 43 hours on end and then got two hours sleep in turns. I could have slept on top of spiked railings by this time. The wounded poured in, and evacuation at first was slow. We only had one portable light, and no conveniences. Our work consisted chiefly of changing the first field dressings, many of which became very tight, making splints, putting up innumerable awful compound fractures of thighs, arms, and legs, tying arteries, deciding which cases were abdominal and which could be allowed food, passing catheters, and giving morphia. The quarter grain dose of civil practice seems quite ineffective on these occasions. It was an awful ten days, in which one lost count of night and day. We fixed up a theatre in a scullery, and there I did the most imperative anaesthetic cases when we could spare an hour from the "wards." We were seeing at this time truly appalling shell wounds, gas infections, and gangrenes in large numbers. I have seen definite and marked gas formation one and a half hours' after a wound was received, and have amputated an arm black and stinking from a small wound on the forearm 36 hours previously. In this case the emphysema could be felt even over the breast, and the amputation was done through the shoulder, the patient recovering. One felt that more M.O.s and better accommodation would indeed have been a boon. The chaplains and interpreter were willing helpers. Then we moved out of Ypres just as the heavy shelling started and took up our quarters and had a "breather" about one kilometre outside, only to start similar work there next day while the shelling and burning of Ypres went on. At this so called chateau the available water was all muddy, owing to the heavy rains, and we had to use the hall which was nothing more than a narrow draughty passage to do our dressings in. Here the surgery was even more reduced to a minimum, but one found oneself from time to time dead tired, and, with a very bad light, wrestling with such things as wounds of the popliteal artery, a most elusive vessel at the best of times, but especially when the tissues are part of a large haematoma. We hear these last three dressing stations of ours are now all razed to the ground.

Christmas Day found us installed in a big French Civil Hospital, with proper wards, sterilising apparatus, etc., at Bethune – probably the best dressing station any Field Ambulance could have had on the front. We also established an officers' hospital in a building previously so arranged by the French Red Cross. In this town the French were more than kind and helpful in every way. It is impossible to express how much the English, Indian and French wounded owe to the Mother and Sisters of the Order of St. Francis who staffed the hospital. During the winter months were had many minor cases of sickness and very few wounds. The latter were very largely bullet wounds of the head. I did a lot of surgery while at this hospital. Many of my head cases have given most pleasing results, and I know nothing more gratifying than seeing an aphasic, hemianopia or palsy recover after operation, unless it be seeing the patients in the ranks again some months later. At this point, perhaps, I may refer to the abdominal wounds I saw at this hospital. In the four months following Christmas there were 23 deaths out of 49 cases entered as "abdominal."

In this period the total deaths were 106. Of the remaining 26 cases entered by the Clerk as abdominal and subsequently evacuated, 11 were kept from three to eight days, and probably were definitely intra peritoneal. As regards operative treatment, I made it my rule only to operate immediately on bowel wounds when I was convinced the patient would die if not operated upon. Hence my results were heart-breaking. I have only notes of twelve abdominal operation cases (excluding bladder wounds). Of these nine, admitted 4 to 20 hours after being wounded, were operated upon at once and died. In all these cases there was much free fluid, blood and faeces in the peritoneum, and in most cases there was a hernia of bowel or omentum. I was struck by the frequency with which the small gut was completely divided as if by a knife. In only one case did I resect bowel. In the others I drained the pelvis and stitched the divided bowel to the wound. It was remarkable that draining the peritoneum in these dreadful cases always relieved the great pain they were in. This is certainly an argument in favour of putting a drain in even obviously fatal cases. The other three cases were for drainage of localised peritonitis after three to seven days, and have recovered. Of these, two were of ascending colon wounds. I have notes of four remarkable abdominal wounds which have recovered without operation, one being from a shrapnel bullet which I removed from under the skin below the left costal margin. It had entered the right loin, and the patient developed some localised peritonitis, which cleared up. The Mother Superior gave most of my anaesthetics, and the French civil surgeon, Dr. Fleury, would often help when we were busy. He also showed me many interesting civil cases, among them a Hydatid of the liver and an Ectopia vesicae. Though he had had a shell through his bedroom and consulting room he never seemed disturbed, but continued to take his X Rays and to operate daily. He was, indeed, a man to admire. Four of the nuns later received the Croix de Guerre for their splendid work during the war. We stayed in this town five months, and during this time we had three particularly busy periods; the first a few days during the Neuve Chapelle battle, then a furiously busy week following May 9th and another following May 16th. This period culminated in shells falling near enough to the hospital to wound several of our men and kill a wounded man in an ambulance, and to break our mess room windows, so we removed our remaining wounded out at once and were ourselves shortly moved to a fresh area. Here we had a quiet time with only sick to deal with, and even had time to play cricket in the evening. We moved none too soon, for when we had gone a shell came through the orderly Officer's bed and another into our mess room.

After a few weeks here I went out to the bearer section. The headquarters of this was about one and a half miles behind two advanced collecting posts where we worked One of the latter was a truly war-worn spot, having been blown to pieces by the French when they recaptured it at Christmas. Now a few cellars remained, and the rest was little more than a pile of bricks, among which were graves (mostly German) and remnants of trenches. The whole was overgrown with cornflowers, poppies, garden flowers, and corn, and was curiously picturesque. Shortly after this I was transferred to one of the officers' hospitals at the base, where I am now spending a quiet time, for, mercifully, the wounded arriving are few at present. It is a joy once more to be among perfect surgical surroundings and to see patients in pyjamas instead of in khaki and mud plaster. As I send this to press I have just read a "Surgeon in Khaki". It is a wonderfully written, accurate, interesting and humorous account of an M.O.'s life at the front. Let me recommend it to all.

(The First Battle of Ypres took place between mid-October and mid-November 1914 and was where the Allies finally prevented the Germans from breaking through and occupying the Channel ports. The penalty the British paid was the decimation of the British Expeditionary Force. The final German assault came on the 11 November 1914 and with its failure the war of the trenches took over the Western Front for the next three years.

The Second Battle of Ypres took place in April 1915 and was the first occasion the Germans used chlorine gas.

The Battle of Neuve Chapelle commenced on 1 March 1915. The village of Neuve Chapelle had been captured by the Germans in October 1914 and behind it was the Aubers Ridge, which although only forty feet high had a commanding view over the surrounding flat lands and meadows where the Allied front line was entrenched. It was a much-wanted prize. This was the first time detailed planning and preparation occurred and the initial attack by the Allies was successful and Neuve Chapelle was captured almost within the first hour. The battle continued for another three days but there was little further advance. There were 13,000 British casualties.)

(This is a long letter from Lieut. Lovell, with many technical points, but it illustrates the life of a surgeon at the front. Lovell was called upon, even as a surgeon, to oversee the sanitation of a village. One wonders what equipped him for this task, but presume that common sense and his general medical training helped.

His many moves, apart from being disruptive, may have helped him avoid becoming battle weary. He recorded periods of work without sleep for forty-three hours.

What would to-day's doctors think of this?

Especially interesting is the variety of surgical operations he was called upon to do. Other letters from other surgeons paint the same picture. Lovell's conclusions on the immediate treatment of wounds at the front are in line with the conclusions of Sir Almroth Wright and Sir Alexander Fleming which they reached from their work in Boulogne, but Lovell made no mention of the need to remove dead and devitalised tissue from the wound in addition to foreign bodies. He recognised the value of wound irrigation. The lack of antibiotics influenced the results of his surgery, but his work, with the knowledge available at the time, was of a high quality and must not be compared with surgery in the Second World War.

Arthur Gordon Haynes Lovell qualified at St Mary's in 1909 with the Gold Medal and Honours in Surgery, Medicine and Midwifery. He obtained his F.R.C.S. in 1912. He became a Clinical Assistant in the E.N.T. Department of St Mary's and was Surgical Registrar at the London Temperance Hospital. He was the author of 'Synovial membranes, with special reference to those to the tendons of the foot and ankle' 1908, 'Vaccine Treatment of Hay Fever' published in *The Lancet* in 1912, 'Hay Fever' in *The Practitioner* in 1914, 'Actinomycoses of Bone primarily involving the Inf. Maxilla' in 1913.)

CHAPTER 16

The Dardanelles

In October 1914, the Turkish navy under German command bombarded the Russians at Sebastopol and as a result Britain declared war on Turkey. Turkey in 1914 was still in the Ottoman Empire which comprised Asia Minor, Syria, Palestine, Mesopotamia and the western flank of the Arabian peninsula. The Dardanelles was strategically very important as a route from the Mediterranean to the Black Sea, and crucial to the defence of Constantinople. The strait was forty miles long and up to four miles wide. Winston Churchill, First Lord of the Admiralty in 1914 adopted a strategy for a Naval forcing of the Dardanelles and a military seizing of Gallipoli. This was supported by the War Council, Asquith the Prime Minister, and by Lord Fisher the First Sea Lord. Fisher subsequently changed his mind and resigned. He was persuaded later by Churchill to undertake the plan. The total operation was a disaster from the beginning. An attempt to free the passage with Naval craft on 18 March 1915 failed. Even transport ships were incorrectly loaded and had to return to port. Surprise was lost. A combined French and British fleet was met by heavy shelling from the Turkish guns on the Gallipoli peninsula and many hundreds of mines had been laid in the sea at the entrance to the Dardanelles. Of the sixteen battleships engaged three were sunk and three severely damaged by mines. The fleet withdrew and severe storms prevented them returning. HMS *Ocean* and HMS *Irresistible* were struck by mines. A French battleship *Bouvet* was hit by a shell and her magazine exploded. She sank in three minutes and 639 men drowned. On 23 March Lord Kitchener sent the Mediterranean Force from Egypt to land on the peninsula. These were mainly Australian and New Zealand troops – Anzacs. Landings were made in the wrong places. The 29th Army division landed at five separate points on various cliff-backed beaches at Cape Helles, the tip of the peninsula. The Australian and New Zealand forces were to be landed nine miles further north to take the highest ridges. Unfortunately they were landed one mile further north than intended and found themselves up against a lunar landscape of dry gullies, ridges and precipices at Anzac Cove. Both at Cape Helles and Anzac Cove the Turks held the heights overlooking the Allied troops and the frontal attacks of the latter proved costly with little or no ground gained.

In August 1915 allied reinforcements were landed at Sulva Bay but failed to break out of the beachheads. This led to trench warfare, complicated by dysentery, and in late November floods, snow and frostbite.

The British Government realised the situation was hopeless and moved towards withdrawal. Finally the Army was evacuated from Gallipoli. By the end of the campaign 410,000 British and Allied troops and 70,000 French had served in Gallipoli. The British casualties were 43,000 killed including 7,500 Australians and 2,500 New Zealanders. The French lost 5,000 and the Turkish army *circa* 60,000 men.

A Surgeon of the Royal Navy writes:

April 30th, 1915.

Dardanelles

I have had one or two adventures since I came out here nearly two months ago. How and why I came is a matter which, for the present, is to be shrouded in secrecy. It seemed quaint that the first shot I was to see fired by an enemy should come from the Plains of Troy. Nothing much happened for a fortnight or so – we got an occasional glimpse at the "curtain raiser" from the back row of the pit. A lot of the fellows in the ship I was in were growling because we had not taken, nor were ever likely to take, an active part in the show – at any rate, directly.

Well, I had been saving up a little collection of cases for hospital and daily expected a boat or destroyer off. On the morning of 17th March a t.b.d. (torpedo boat destroyer) was reported coming our way. She came alongside, and I pushed the sick into her. One being an officer it was my duty, if I could be spared, to accompany him in, but I hesitated, as it was a longish run in, at the thought that I might not get back that night. Anyway, having asked the Captain, I went aboard. I turned over my patients, and went aboard the hospital ship, an old friend in other waters. I was told that I would be taken back later in the day. In the afternoon I went aboard the "Inflexible" about one or two things, and then I heard whispers about the first instalment of the big show coming off the next day. I went back to the hospital ship, and in the end had to stay all night. Early in the morning the t.b.d. (torpedo boat destroyer) came for me, with several errands to perform before putting me back. These were carried out, and we were just setting out when the flagship "Queen Elizabeth" called us up.

I can't say that I was at all surprised when we received orders to close and accompany her into action up the Dardanelles.

I saw practically the whole of the day's action from the upper deck. The ward-room hatch, and the "band stand" (i.e. the circular mounting for the after 12-pounder) offered a certain amount of protection from splinters, and one is no better off, if as well off, below.

We got a very good view of the battered forts and earthworks at Sidi-el Bahr and Kum Kale. In one earthworks we saw four big guns pointing skywards at different angles, the result of a previous effort.

As we passed the line AB we came under an irritating fire from a battery at B. We were going very slowly, and each shot dropped closer and closer on either side of our stern. I got wet twice from falling spray, and several bits dropped on deck by my feet.

"Triumph," I think it was, closed and let go with half-a-dozen, and he piped down. It was a perfect day – wind just perceptible from S.S.E. We had the advantage of the light just behind us, glaring strongly into the eyes of the enemy's gunners.

11.30 a.m. About now the big ships passed up to their stations, and practically stopped, opened up a deliberate fire at long range at the forts around Chanak and Kilid Bahr. The volume of fire increased as time went on, after the range had been found. The enemy's replies were not long coming; they were dotted about all over the place, and seemed at first ineffective and wild, but in reality it probably was far from it. It takes trained observers from elevated positions to judge really what is the accuracy of fire. And we soon saw our ships getting hit, chiefly in the upper works, and doing little vital damage. An officer of the "Ocean" told me that during the action proper she was hit 28 times, yet the only casualty all told was one man missing. About noon, as we were lying stopped near "Queen Elizabeth," whose tender we were, a shore battery about "C" in diagram opened a heavy fire on us, only missing us time after time by feet, even inches. We moved astern and did not get any more. That is why I think it was a howitzer battery, because they simply fire when a ship comes in line with a mark on the opposite bank. A naval gun mounting allows not only for elevation and depression, but for side to side training. So you can put on "deflection" allowing for the speed of your opponent's ship.

Lying where we were it was quite impossible to gauge the amount of damage we were doing. I saw a magazine go up – there was a sheet of flame about 200 feet high and dense clouds of black and white smoke.

It was when an oil tank caught fire that we saw the most obvious damage. The dense black smoke must have been 3,000 or 4,000 feet high.

12.30. The action by this time was brisk. The remaining divisions by this time had entered, "Ocean" leading our ships, preceded by "Suffren" flying the flag of the French Admiral. I hope to be able to give you a diagram later of how these ships engaged. They passed us at some speed and went up close, each taking on some definite objective, and in a short time they were so far up that it was impossible to make out what they were actually doing.

When I came up from lunch and a smoke I looked around, and about four miles off I caught sight of what appeared to be the bows of a ship

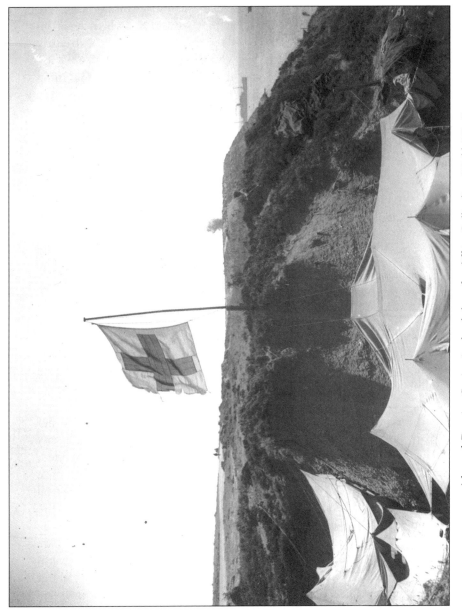

Advanced Dressing Station in the shelter of a cliff in Gallipoli – World War I
Photograph courtesy of the Imperial War Museum, London. Negative no. Q3314

disappearing rapidly. It was the "Bouvet." Q.E. called us up, and a moment later we were racing to the spot. We got the whaler and skiff away and they went searching among the debris. There was very little except wooden wreckage, spars, a few hammocks and the like. Such survivors as there were had already been taken into the three or four steamboats which were on the spot (they had been down all day in the thick of it and did extremely well, so we heard.) There were five Frenchmen sculling around in a whaler which looked like one of theirs; in fact it must have been. The only thing we salved was a chronometer which had floated up. As soon as we were sure that there were no more to be picked up we shoved off (to use a naval vulgarism) as there were a few "proggies" dropping around.

From what I have since heard, I understand that the French Division came in very shortly after our big ships, and that our older ones, "Ocean" etc., came in after them. However, that is a matter of detail and you will see it in the full official report, whenever that comes out.

At 4.10, or thereabouts, we were called up again, and a few moments later we went off at full tilt to somewhere near the same spot, and it was only a very short space of time before we saw what was up – the poor old "Irresistible" in trouble. She had a big list to starboard, and was slowly sinking. She was getting hit every now and again from batteries on either side of the Straits. Her crew were on the quarter-deck, after shelter deck, in the battery, and on the port torpedo net shelf. As we came up they gave us a cheer. There was no panic – it might have been "abandon ship" drill almost, except for the very real shells bursting short or inboard and taking their toll from the crowded ship's company – a very small toll considering the number of rounds that hit. We were quickly alongside; our Captain handled his destroyer with all the skill of the expert, and they simply poured in, the nearest way. Some swam the small gap between our stern and her after-part, and were hauled in. We must have taken in about 700; at any rate, including our crowd, there were 750 on board in all when we left, crammed into every possible spot – engine room, ward room, cabins, mess deck, upper deck, and you know that there is little room to spare in a small destroyer. We were alongside twenty-five minutes, under a poisonous fire from both sides, only just being missed, and when we did get off it was only just in time, because another minute would have seen us hit fair and square by a big one which got home (so I was told by an officer who was forward) on the "Irresistible's" waterline, just where we had been. A few, about twenty in all, remained on board in an effort to save the ship, but they had to be taken off later.

I was kept busy of course. We soon got under the lee of the Flagship; the "Irresistible" started a cheer and the inevitable "Tipperary." Then we got them out as soon quickly as possible once alongside.

Then we went back to have another look. There was no sign of anyone on board, and she was still sinking.

We put back, and then suddenly turned – we saw the "Ocean" in a similar plight – the destroyer division that had been at the entrance all day arriving simultaneously lay themselves alongside and took the crew off. It was only prompt action that saved a heavy casualty list – only one man was missing from that ship – because the fire was overwhelming. It was the Turcos' last chance, as it had already gone sunset, and they seemed to have brought every gun to bear.

I was not at all sorry when I got on board the Flagship at 7.30 p.m.

In the wardroom all the survivors and the ship's officers were comparing notes. I found several fellows I knew, some in the "Queen Elizabeth", and some in the "Irresistible". Two of the latter I had met some time previously at a boarding-house on Christmas Day last, where we three, with our respective wives, dined together.

The S.M.O. of the "Irresistible" was an old Mary's man, Fleet Surgeon Facey. We also had brought off the two other doctors, one surgeon R.N. and one surgeon R.N.V.R. Well, since then I have had several changes. There is no further incident to record.

We are at present playing a subsidiary (although of importance strategically) in the general operations.

As to previous experiences, well, very little. Plenty of pestiferous weather in the North Sea, an occasional chase after submarines was about the only excitement, bar participating in one or two big moves that might have been "It" – only it takes two to make a battle. Many dreary days on patrol. I had three weeks of duty in a hospital ship just before I came to these parts. I got the medical side, and some jolly good cases. I left her with regret.

The Captain I was with the whole of the first part of the time got mentioned in dispatches, in addition to being promoted for the good work he did mine-sweeping. Mine-sweeping is "nervy" work, much more so than being under gunfire.

I have met a few Mary's men since the war started. I had a pleasant afternoon, going with F.H. Stephens to tea on board steam yacht "Liberty" where, as you know, were Clayton Greene, Gwynne Lawrence (whom I had not met before), Pannett, Gosse and Withers Green. Stephens was then in the mine-sweeping flotilla with me. I also met Williamson at one of the home ports, Hobbs (the elder, who is a temporary surgeon), and Shaw. Also Silcock's brother, a King's man, Surgeon Probationer R.N.V.R. I once heard the Surgeon Probationer described as "Medicinal Midshipman." I don't know which way they take it.

Apropos of getting qualified before serving, everyone I have talked to about it agrees that a qualified man is worth ten times an unqualified to either Service.

I don't know whether you know that Fergusson, the Gunnery Lieutenant of the "Bulwark" was a brother of our Fergusson – I knew him at school, and after. He was a topping fellow. He got all "ones" in passing for Lieutenant, gaining something like two and a-half years' time, and he was a jolly good half at Rugger, playing for the United Services a good many times. He was sporting enough, I remember, on one or two occasions when some of our own people had failed us, to turn out for our "A" team That was about 1906 or 1907. I expect that you must have met him.

(Yet another letter with no name attached. What a pity!!)

Surgeon F.H. Facey, R.N. writes:

I will give you a short account of our escape from poor old Irresistible on Thursday, March 18.

When we went into the Dardanelles that afternoon we had no idea we were to be in special danger of being mined. On that morning the Queen Elizabeth, Lord Nelson, and Inflexible went in and fired at long range: later the four French ships went in to closer range. At this time we were off the entrance, and saw (but not for certain) the Bouvet meet with disaster and sink in 2 minutes 45 seconds. I went down below at 2.p.m., when the Irresistible, Majestic, Ocean and Albion went up to close range to relieve the French ships. You can understand that I did not think anything very dangerous was on, as I went to sleep down below from 2 p.m. to 3 p.m. At 4 o'clock I had a nibble of biscuit and a few chocolates. At 4.30 p.m. the explosion occurred. Everyone seemed to realise it was a knock-out blow, the whole ship being lifted up, and when she settled down she had a distinct list to starboard. I think I must have been dozing at the time, as the explosion did not seem so terrific to me.

A shipmate said, "Come along," meaning up through the turret – a somewhat intricate way out – and after a moment's hesitation I followed him. When we got up the first ladder all the lights went out. Fortunately he had his electric torch, and found the way up quite easily. We climbed out on the quarterdeck and found the men mustering there. There were no destroyers visible, so the prospects were rather dismal for getting away. In the hurry for getting up the turret I left my cork lifebelt at the bottom of the turret. The inner tube of my "bike" tyre was in my cabin, so I nipped down below to get it. My first effort was a failure, as the watertight door near my cabin was closed. Meantime the ship kept floating very well, so I thought we should be all right.

On coming to the quarterdeck again, I found someone had opened the wardroom skylight, so I climbed down there, got to my cabin in the dark and brought up the tyre and pump, which I blew up, together with the

swimming collar. All this time we had been drifting towards the beach –
our engines being disabled – and about this time the Turks began to shell
us with 6in. howitzers and other big guns. We were trying to take cover
behind the turret, and I noticed two shells explode about 10 to 15 yards off.
A destroyer came up alongside us. I then turned round to look for our
engineer lieutenant, but he had disappeared. Afterwards we heard he had
taken to the water and was picked up by a steamboat. I now thought it was
about time to clear out myself, as the shells were exploding all round us,
and the combination of that and the possibility of the ship sinking, was
somewhat alarming.

The destroyer's stern was some way from the stern of the Irresistible, and
only her bows were touching us right forward. I did not fancy going
through the battery where the shells came from, so I decided to climb over
the side and walk along the net shelf and get on the destroyer. There were
a number of men there and progress forward was very slow. Lots of them
jumped overboard and were hauled on board the destroyer by rope-ends.
I caught a line that was thrown from the destroyer, and the R.N.R.
lieutenant in her beckoned me to jump, which I did, and was hauled on
board.

There were 610 of our men in the destroyer – it would have been a
calamity had a shell dropped in the middle of them. They shoved off soon
after I got on board, and slowly we were all put on board the Queen
Elizabeth. We had 16 wounded and 13 killed; among the latter were a
lieutenant, a midshipman, the warrant officer, and the assistant clerk
missing. The last named was killed or drowned, we fear. Poor boy, he only
joined the ship about four weeks before. We spent two nights in the Queen
Elizabeth off Tenedos and one night in the Phaeton. I hardly had a wink
of sleep these three nights. However, I am now sleeping like a log, and feel
none the worse. The Captain, Commander, and several lieutenants
remained on board the Irresistible with the idea that she would be taken in
tow, but they went to the Ocean about an hour after we left and were soon
again mined and eventually got off in a destroyer. The Ocean was not
shelled as we were, and did not lose any killed or wounded. Of course, I
lost all my belongings.

May 15th 1915
Anzac Cove, Gallipoli
Dear Sir,
The sight of the St. Mary's Hospital Gazette which suddenly appeared in
my "dug out", apparently from nowhere (really the result of the fine mail
service maintained by the Navy) as I "carried on" my daily round of duties
in the battalion to which I am attached, and which is the right flank, at

present of our bite into the somewhat tough old bird we propose to make a meal of, brought back to me with quite startling suddenness (as the appearance of a mail did to most of us) the fact that there is a world outside the little patch where we have obtained, and are maintaining by some little strenuousness, a foothole on this interesting, picturesque, and damnable part of the globe. I could hardly have conceived it possible that the affairs of the moment could have so entirely have engrossed one's whole consciousness; but for the last ten days since we landed it is no exaggeration to say that fighting, working, eating, noise, and wonder what will be doing next, have been our world. You will know before you get this (if you do), more of the circumstances of our little affair than I am permitted to tell you here. But your quite touching appeal for copy – real hot stuff from "The Front" – impels me to send, not, I am sorry to say, what you really want, but what little I can give. The life of a regimental Medical Officer is no sinecure under the circumstances. My "dug-out" and my aid post are 15 yards from the firing trenches: a shell burst in the latter (before we were able to get in deep enough) and killed my orderly, two stretcher bearers, and wounded four others (I was the only one not hit!). But the evacuation of the wounded and the maintenance of the water supply and sanitation have required all one's efforts to carry out in a way not satisfactory indeed, but sufficient to save one from a feeling of abject incompetence. And here I would ask your permission to put in my comment on the discussion of the supply of medical men in the Army, letters on which from Drs Nangle, Cope and Raven appear in the number I have (January). I most emphatically agree in protesting against the medical profession putting itself on a pedestal of importance, above others of the community, and claiming some exemption therefrom from the call to serve the Empire at the front. There are many ways in which the medical profession can come to infamy; but the most despicable and permanent will be if we do not supply our due and necessary proportion of properly trained medical men. And by trained I mean men who have made equal effort with combatant officers to fit themselves by training and study for the special work they are going out to do. The self-complacency of medical men has often been the source of grave errors arising; but there is no excuse now for us to allow ourselves the delusion that our medical training has fitted us for all the duties which we are called upon to perform in our positions, whatever they may be, in the Army or Navy. I feel sure that this will be agreed with by men who are in the Service. The regimental Medical Officer certainly has to know quite a lot that even the training given at St. Mary's Hospital does not afford; though I need hardly say that it is some special application only of knowledge already present that is needed, an a long training is quite unnecessary.

This comment, which will, I fear, be belated, is unpleasantly dogmatic and unsatisfactory, I can see, but I have not time to re-write it, and, after all, it may "provoke discussion", if the subject is not by now worn out, or better, rendered unnecessary. If so, will you please delete it.

To continue, we get our wounded down the steep hills and gullies to the beach by night to avoid the shrapnel, which is very unpleasantly persistent and searching. On the first three days getting men away was a hell of a job – there is no other word for it; but now it is well organised, efficient and rapid, and they get on to the well equipped hospital ship and to good care and attention promptly and easily. The regimental Medical Officer has really only first-aid and casualty work to do; no surgery falls within our scope here except, perhaps an occasional insertion of a few sutures or ligatures of an exposed vessel. The training of one's stretcher bearers and water duty men seems to me one of the most important functions of the regimental Medical Officer, and next the art of keeping up his supply of medical stores and of looking forward, the art of digging rapidly, and to the point, to escape and assist one's patients to escape injury, is a very important duty. The only books I have with me are R.A.M.C. Training Manual of Field Fortifications. The first three days quite a large part of my time was occupied in providing shelter from shrapnel for the injured in the aid posts till they could be evacuated. Water supply! The horrible difficulty of preventing pollution and the hideous possibilities of its becoming unavailable, and the difficulty of preventing indiscriminate use are always present. We are, thank God, inoculated against typhoid, and in the eight months since I have been at the job, I have not seen a case. One simply forgets that there is such a thing! I expect a rude awakening as summer advances, but I hope and with confidence great exemption from this pest. Lice! there only redeeming feature is that, like David Harum's idea of the dog and the flea, they keep us so occupied that we forget we are harassed soldiers. Food. We feed like fighting cocks. We drink, by the way, Tea, which is the quite effective solution of the water contamination question at present, and as long as the wood lasts and men not too thirsty to wait for it.

Sickness almost nil at present. Shipley's Lectures are very useful; I have put my bit on kerosene and manual labour, and supply kerosene whenever I can to the men. It is a lovely spot here. On afternoons when things are quiet one sits on the cliff and gazes as Old Prometheus did, and from a spot not so distant, and by the Gods I have never, even in sunny Australia, seen the like. It is a lovely spot. I hope I shall get out of it. There are, indeed, quite a few places greatly inferior to it in beauty where I would rather be at the present time. At present, however, one's concern is to do one's job, and pray one will not funk any call on one, however difficult, and that to

my mind is the one all-engrossing anxiety to many of us – will I do my
job? As a Johnian, I murmur, "Si je puis" – as a St. Mary's man I send this,
hoping to do so, and with the signature only (in case I fall short)"

OLD STUDENT

(This letter from a nameless graduate is written with long sentences often
used at the time, immaculate punctuation but difficult syntax. It illustrates
again the unusual life and duties that the regimental Medical Officer had to
cope with, not covered by his medical training. Here too is mentioned the
value of anti-typhoid inoculation and also the fear that one might fail one's
colleagues and patients in the hour of need.)

A letter from W.D. Arthur, who had written also in October 1914:

I left England in September in a huge transport carrying several thousands
of troops to the Mediterranean. I was one of 90 unattached R.A.M.C.
officers aboard, and we none of us had the least idea where we were going
to be stationed, though many rumours were circulated. Save for an exciting
episode with an enemy submarine in the Aegean Sea, the voyage was
uneventful, and we arrived in Mudros Harbour a week after we left
England. Here, after a few days delay, we received orders to go, some to
the Gallipoli peninsula, and some to hospitals ashore. I was sent to the most
recent sphere of activity – Sulva Bay, where I was attached to a service
battalion of the South Wales Borderers in the trenches facing Scimitar Hill.
The battalion was very much under strength when I joined, and the men
remaining were most of them in a bad state of health after a long and
arduous campaign carried on under very trying conditions.

  A sick parade in the morning of about 20 per cent, of the strength was
the usual thing, most of the cases being dysentery and jaundice. Practically
every officer or man who had spent a week or so at Sulva developed
dysentery in a more or less severe form: it was impossible to escape
infection, for flies infested all our lines in immense numbers, contaminating
all our food and cooking utensils. The equipment of a field medical pannier
does not permit of any great variety of treatment, the difficulties of which
were much increased by the shortage of many important drugs. In the early
days of dysentery emetine in one third gr. doses was sometimes successful,
but a recurrence of symptoms nearly always occurred as soon as the
treatment was stopped, and the patient ultimately had to be sent off to
hospital. On the whole the treatment of dysentery and jaundice in the
trenches was very unsatisfactory. Proper rest was, of course, impossible, and
the food supplied, though of good quality, was sometimes rather unpalat-
able. Shortly before I left the Peninsula orders were circulated that such
cases were to be sent as early as possible to a hospital, where the facilities

for treatment were much greater than in the firing line, and where there was a reasonable prospect of recovery after a period of rest.

There were comparatively few casualties while I was with the regiment, and though we were shelled daily from every direction, we lost more men hit by "snipers" than by shell fire. The treatment of wounds consisted in putting on a dressing and sending the man back to the dressing station, where he was detained until dark, before being sent to a Field Ambulance on the beach.

An attack of appendicitis, following on a mild bout of dysentery, cut short my sojourn in this land of flies and dust (to say nothing of the aromas) and I was sent back to a base hospital for operation.

Since I left the Peninsula, I hear that the positions of Sulva and Anzac have been evacuated. It is difficult to imagine how such a manoeuvre could have been effected without enormous casualties, but by some means it was done without loss of life. Everyone who knows the conditions of life out there will rejoice to think that our troops have been removed from what has proved to be a veritable plague spot.

W.D. Arthur.

(No account of the Dardanelles campaign would be complete without consideration of the effect it had on Winston Churchill. Much has been written about this and there is none better than that written by Martin Gilbert in his biography of Churchill. Much of what is written here is based on his writings.

Churchill was held responsible then and subsequently for the failure by the military and naval forces of the Dardanelles offensive. He was criticised for an ill-conceived and ill-thought out plan. Failure of the Naval and military chiefs was not considered and errors made in the execution of the offensive were not considered. Churchill found little support from political colleagues of either his own party or of the opposition. He was devastated. He felt sure that he was the victim of political intrigue in the light of subsequent events. Asquith invited the Conservative Party to join his administration and to be part of the War Council. They had one condition – that Churchill should be removed as First Lord of the Admiralty. Churchill consulted many of his colleagues including Bonar Law, Leader of the Conservative Party, with the hope of remaining in the Admiralty. All efforts failed and it was decided Churchill must go. Many thought that not only was his time as First Lord over, but that his career was also at an end. Churchill himself thought he was finished, and Clementine, his wife, thought he might 'die of grief'. Following his removal he was subjected to repeated criticism in the newspapers, which publicly held him totally responsible for the complete failure of the Dardanelles campaign. Thus nationwide the people of the United Kingdom were led to the same view.

Churchill next resigned his parliamentary duties and on 18 November joined the Queen's Own Oxfordshire Hussars and sailed for the Western Front, with the rank of Major. Even the military chiefs wished him not to have any leading part in the conduct of the war. His many letters and plans to politicians were ignored. It is a measure of Churchill's character and ability that he bore and overcame what was indeed a devastating assault on him and his leadership qualities in time of war. That he was a man of destiny the nation found out in World War II.)

(There is no record of an F.H. Facey in the Medical Register between 1905 and 1945, but there is an S.H. Facey who was registered between 1897 and 1942. He gives his address as Royal Navy throughout his career.

William Daniel Arthur qualified M.R.C.S., L.R.C.P. in 1914 and his various addresses were: 1914 North Glam.; 1923–1924 c/o Holt and Co., 3 Whitehall Place, London, and 1925–1953 c/o Glyn, Mills & Co., 3 Whitehall Place, London. From the entry of 1927 he is referred to as M.B.E. He provided no details for the *Medical Directory* and there was no obituary for him in the *British Medical Journal*.)

CHAPTER 17

Salonica

Bulgaria joined the German side in September 1915 following the Gallipoli and Italian failures which altered the balance in the Balkans.

Austrian and German forces attacked Serbia in the north and the Bulgarians attacked it from the east. Serbia was overrun and what remained of the Serbian army was taken off by Allied shipping from the coast of Albania and brought to Corfu.

It was decided to land an Anglo-French force at Salonica to help the Serbs. This took place in October 1915 and a force of 600,000 men including Italian, Russian and Serbian forces was gradually built up. This large army made several attempts to break out from their bridgehead but failed. One of the major catastrophes was the sickness of 480,000 men in the campaign. It was not until 1918 that the Allied forces succeeded in advancing through Salonica to the Balkans to defeat the Bulgarians.

Capt. D.H. Anthony writes from Salonika:

"For a congenial life I commend you to a Field Ambulance – in this country at all events – and when one is in the best Field Ambulance in the best Division in this (or perhaps any) Army. Well! I ask you.

You see there is no war here relatively speaking, except now and again and then one experiences a little discomfort, but it is transient and one soon settles down to quite a pleasant life. What do you think? Our Ambulance boasts of a golf course, rather small, but as Mr. Robey says: "What is there, is good." One plays football, hockey occasionally, and there is plenty of shooting – I mean wild geese, duck, hare, pheasant, partridge, etc., not Bulgar, though he comes in for it too. A horse to ride, and would you believe it, one could follow the hounds on three days a week in winter.

Some War, isn't it?

"I hear Major Langmead is in one of the Hospitals at the Base, and next time I am down I shall try to call to see him. Mary's men must be very rare in Macedonia. I have met three only, and they were years my senior."

"Leave, or the lack of it, is the great drawback here, otherwise this is not at all a bad spot in which to spend a war. A few diseases are rather annoying, but hitherto I have been fortunate and have escaped with only two attacks of Sand Fly Fever (the books say you can't have two attacks, but I've managed it, and I suppose the Books must be wrong. I was taught that they were of no use, and this seems to be more evidence of a damning nature!)."

(Douglas Harris Anthony qualified in 1916. He became Medical Referee Australia House and Medical Referee to the Ministry of Pensions. Following qualification he was a House Surgeon at St Mary's Hospital.)

This next letter was published in the *Gazette* in January 1918 but was dated:-

December 15th? 1915
Dr Langmead writes:

I promised to write you and am over-long in keeping my promise. My Army life started with the usual period of inactivity three weeks at Blackpool, three en route, not unenlivened by experiences, and about six weeks out of work here. I was first attached as officer in charge of No. 68 General Hospital, and on arriving here we were told that our equipment, which was coming all the way by the sea, had been sunk in the Atlantic shortly after leaving Liverpool. Consequently we were all sensible of having made a faux pas in the eyes of the brass hats out here, and awaited and suffered gradual but persistent disintegration. As one of the disintegrated elements I was next attached to No. 60 General Hospital in the same capacity as I should have been with the other, and have continued with them since. I cannot complain that I remained inactive after being attached to No. 60. It was in process of expansion, with frequent shuffling and re-shuffling, until we arrived at the respectable size of 1,540 beds, of which about 1,000 came into my division, and we did not keep them empty, I can assure you.

The enemy was chiefly malaria; without it about 200 beds would have sufficed, for the surgical side was chiefly filled by malaria also, much to the chagrin of the surgeons, especially of Captain Bromley, the O.C. of the Surgical Division, and in happier times Assistant Surgeon and Dean of Guy's. I suppose he has done altogether about as much surgery as he gets in 24 hours at home. The other chief foe has been bacillary dysentery, but numerically it has been a very bad second worst. A few P.U.O.'s (pyrexia of unknown origin), and a very few civilian medical diseases practically complete the roll. No definite sand-fly fever, epidemic jaundice, dengue, cholera, beri-beri, or the hundred and one tropical diseases which in one's ignorance, after a perusal of the literature, one expected to find. Only three of the enterica group all told.

The malaria has been a thing to remember, though they say it has been much better than last year. We drained the worst source of cases the Struma front, which probably accounts for the severe type I met with. About our own site, there were no great numbers of mosquitoes, perhaps 3–10 in a marquee in the morning, but each seemed capable of doing a good night's work, judging by the incidence of malaria among officers, sisters and personnel.

We met with malaria as an infection able to produce every sort of manifestation – cerebral, algide, enteric, colonic, gastric pneumonic, nephritic, etc. 30–40 grains of quinine daily failed to touch many cases, and a large proportion required either intramuscular injections (12–18) b.d. or intravenous injections of similar dosage instead, or in addition to, orally, before the temperature and other symptoms made any sign of diminishing.

This all refers to the season, during which time we were up on the hills about 12 miles out of Salonika. As we were part of a summer arrangement we have now come down to another site about 2 miles out of the town, and are just setting up house again and expanding to our former dimensions, and during the growth I am temporarily having a much easier time. By about three weeks we shall be a 1,540 bedded hospital again and have sick prisoners in addition.

Prisoners of war are now our only patients – Bulgars, Turks and local suspects, and one Hun airman, who, true to his race, is the only troublesome inmate, but a hole the size of the inevitable tangerine orange, in his tibia, caused by a machine gun bullet, provides a recompense. The Bulgars and Turks are Orientally resigned, anxious to be of help, easy to deal with, and bear no ill-will. Naturally they dislike each other, but they unite in hating the German and apparently Germans generally. So much about one's work. About Salonique its magnificent situation, its ancient glory, its cosmopolitan inhabitants, its sanitation (lucus non lucendo), and its fire, which ends an era, you have read descriptions from abler pens than mine.

Without the mosquito and the fly, and with a Western nation in possession, Macedonia might be a veritable promised land, running with milk and honey. Mile upon mile of country need only the plough to yield two crops a year of practically anything you like. The Struma valley alone could grow enough corn to feed the whole of the Balkans. Minerals, too, I hear, are plentiful. But there seems to have been no enterprise and little change since about the time when Father Abraham wandered out with his herds from Ur in the Chaldees.

I have met a few old Mary's men out here, Easton, who is D.A.D.M.S. for eastern half of base area, Clarke, who is on a travelling medical board, Rickman, now invalided home, Moorish now home on expiration of contract among them. They all seemed in the best of spirits bar Rickman when I last ran against them. Clarke lent me a S.M. Gazette a short time ago, and by it I find that you still have a very definite opinion of our masters for the time. Please remember me to Spilsbury, and

Believe me, yours ever,

Frederick Langmead.

(In the book on *St. Mary's Medical School* by Zachary Cope published in 1954, Cope says, 'the report of the Royal Commission on University Education published in 1913, was not very complimentary to the consultants of that time.' The consultants were more interested in pursuing their private practice than taking up academic posts, which would require their attention full-time. It was recommended that full-time posts in the medical schools should be encouraged, devoted to teaching and research, and suitable candidates should be found. In 1919 four medical schools appointed Professors of Medicine and Surgery. At St Mary's at the time the money was not available to appoint full-time professors to the Medical School, but the dean, Dr Wilson was greatly in favour of these academic posts. As a step toward this Dr Wilfrid Harris was appointed Director of the Medical Unit and Clayton-Greene of the Surgical Unit. Private practice was not excluded. Some time later the necessary moneys were found and in 1921 Dr Langmead was appointed the first Professor of Medicine and Mr Pannett the first Professor of Surgery. Academic clinical units thus began with full time professors. Professor Langmead held this post until his retirement in 1939. He died thirty years later at the age of ninety and a ward at the hospital was named after him.

Spilsbury whom Langmead mentions at the end of his letter, went on to become the best known Forensic Pathologist in the United Kingdom, famous for his court appearances for the prosecution for many years, and whose medical evidence was rarely if ever questioned.)

A letter was written by Capt. L.B.Clarke dated 1.11.1916:

I have been with a Battalion for some time, the 2/17 London Regiment. I have been with them since the middle of August, and as they have been in the trenches ever since, I have now had some interesting experiences.

Regimental work is quite different from field ambulance work. You have quite a good time if you are with a decent crowd of officers, which I am glad to say has been my lot.

The M.O. is the one person in the battalion whose opinion is asked for on all varieties of subjects which have any bearing, however remote, on matters scientific or hygienic. My headquarters was in the Regimental Aid Post situated about 400 yards, as the crow flies, from the Bosch line. There I saw the wounded, and such as were sick.

The Aid Post consists of three large dug-outs in a small trench, close to the Headquarters of the Battalion.

The three dug-outs were side by side and were used, as a surgery, where all cases were brought, and where I had my bunk; as a sleeping and general living room for the medical orderlies, sanitary and water orderlies, and

R.A.M.C. bearers attached to the Battalion, and as a small hospital, where a dozen cases can be accommodated.

There were about ten or a dozen orderlies in the 2nd, and owing to the irregularity of the floor and ceiling, the general congestion inside, this dug-out went by the name of the "Rabbit Warren."

In the third dug-out we used to put cases that required minor treatment and would probably be well in a couple of days.

In this way we saved many men to the Battalion who would otherwise have become enmeshed in the numerous tentacles of the R.A.M.C.

A number of early cases we had were mild cases of shell shock, which were successfully treated by being given plenty of digging to do in the day time and a mild sedative at night. We found it much better to keep these people employed close up to the front line, where they were under intermittent shell fire, than to send them down the line for a time, only to get a relapse directly they return to the danger zone.

Just at the back, we had an old disused French trench dug to a good depth and laid with rails. We had an enthusiastic A.D.M.S. and an equally keen field ambulance behind us, and they succeeded in completing a fine new trench, along which we could send trolleys, holding a couple of stretcher cases. There is no harm in my mentioning these details as we have since left that half of the world.

The completion of the trolley line was a greater acquisition to the Battalion, as there was considerable difficulty in getting cases down to the field ambulance. In many cases the main communication trenches were very narrow, and frequently anything from an hour to an hour and a half would be required to get a stretcher case from the sap head to the Aid Post.

If we were to sit down and think of all the adverse conditions one could devise for bad cases, you had every one of them as a patient was carried from sap head to Aid Post.

Frequently one would have to scrape off with a knife thick mud from the region of a large wound. Portions of clothing, boots and socks, for example, would frequently have to be removed from the wound.

You can quite realise that asepsis is entirely out of the question, and one is not surprised at the enormous number of septic wounds which are seen in the base hospitals.

During our stay in the trenches, the Bosch opposite to us were relieved, Saxons taking the place of Bavarians. We found the Saxons much less aggressive and not nearly so bent on things as the Bavarians.

The casualties became fewer, and one had less excitement all round.

It is not, perhaps, advisable to indicate the number of casualties we had, but one outstanding fact is this – that the Bosch sends a lot of stuff over without inflicting any casualties.

It is quite extraordinary hearing intermittent shellfire all day, and in the end nothing happens.

For some few nights we were kept on the go for about ten hours at a time, and one had to snatch sleep when one could.

We are now in another part of the country, and our ultimate destination in unknown.

A further letter was published in February 1917 written from Salonica but not dated:

Dear Mr. Editor,

A few sentences from a letter I addressed to you in your private capacity from France were published in a recent number of the Gazette.

As the letter was not intended directly for publication, being a matter of fact, written during the rush of a big move, it appeared, I am afraid, very scrappy and disconnected, and I therefore hasten to apologise to all concerned, including even the printer, who apparently was unable to master the intricacies of my writing.

I trust that this present letter will atone in some measure for past defects.

At the time I wrote our destination was unknown, and conjecture was the order of the day. Since then all doubt has been removed, and we now find ourselves in a country whose people are rent in two factions by the World War.

We came out on His Majesty's Transport "——", and as ship's medical officer I had a full time of it with sickness (sea and other varieties), inoculations, inspections and so on. The rough weather of the first few days gave place to tropical heat in more southerly parts.

I was then unfortunately taken ill, and after four days in my bunk was somewhat ignominiously carried ashore on a stretcher and removed to hospital, where I spent the whole of the first month. A severe attack of 'flu resulting in a dilated heart has changed the scene of my activity from a battalion to a general hospital. The intermediate step of field ambulance work was condemned by the powers that be owing to the mountainous character of the country, and I was only with the 2/5 for a week.

A note by the way may be of interest to readers of the Gazette. The 2/5 London Field Ambulance, which I was in France before joining the battalion, contained four St. Mary's men: Lt. Col. Corfe (O/C), Capt. Hardcastle, Lt. Marshall (returned from the Soloman Islands, I believe), and myself. Marshall has taken my place as M.O. to the 2/17 London Regiment, and is, according to all accounts, having a fairly heavy time of it.

The change from France is a considerable one, from trench life to hospital life, from the desolation of ruined villages to the increasing activity of a great town.

Salonica is a strange place in many ways. I suppose it would be impossible to find in any other town in the world, certainly at the present time, a greater variety of people than one does in the Macedonian capital.

Situated at the head of an enormous arm of the Aegean Sea, with the mountains surrounding it, the town has one of the most wonderful sites imaginable. Both on account of its people and its locality it takes a place apart from other towns, and one wonders at times which is the more interesting of the two. The inhabitants or the place itself; which the more extraordinary, which the more varied, for both people and place are quite unlike anything which the average man has seen before.

To see Salonica at its best you go to Floca's (pronounced Flocker). You will probably wonder what that may be. Well, in England it would be best described as a public house, in America as a saloon, in France as a cafe, and in Greece – well it's Floca's, and that's all there is about it. A large square room, plainly furnished and not overclean, and filled with a number of small tables overflowing into the street outside, it serves as a rendezvous of Thessalonian society. Here you sit at tea and watch the nations of the earth parade in front of you.

Civilians of all sorts pass in and out, and you see the Greek of the educated classes, dark and olive skinned; the Turk, with frock coat and fez; the Spanish Jew, driven here in the 15th century to seek sanctuary with a tolerant race, and now the wealthiest and most powerful of all; and crowding round the door and loafing at the corner a motley crowd composed of the scum of Macedonia.

Hospital sisters and nurses are here in all sorts of uniforms – English, French, and Scottish women from the Serbian hospital – perhaps escorted by a male friend or else forming a party by themselves.

But I suppose the most interesting of all is to watch the Allied officers as they come in, their various uniforms adding to the general colour scheme, and forming such a picture as you will see in no other country, neutral or belligerent.

First the Greeks themselves, newly dressed in smart looking uniforms, fussy and hesitating in manner as though not yet at ease in the presence of officers of other nations. Greek Naval officers and middies, too, looking for all the world like their English confreres and often difficult to distinguish.

Then you see Italians of all ranks, but not in such large numbers, as they prefer the macaroni of the "Hotel Rome" on the next floor.

French are everywhere, passing in and out and appearing very much at their ease, as theirs is the language of the educated classes.

Serbs, too, in great numbers, recognised by their long grey coats and their dented felt hats, similar in many ways to the Greeks, only with more strength of character.

But the finest looking of all – a sort of race apart – are the Russians; tall, well built every one of them, with fair hair and blue eyes, their fawn coloured tunics decorated by the ribbons and medals of various orders.

I will say nothing of the British officer, except that here at Floca's one meets nearly everybody one ever knew, and here and there a passing face recalls memories of Town or Cambridge.

Tea is served and the man who brings it can talk to you in Greek, Spanish, French or English, the latter being acquired in Ohio, U.S.A.

The pedlars from the street come through and ply their trade in cigarettes, post-cards, boot laces and so on, for which you are asked to pay exorbitant prices. Perhaps the most honest of all is the little girl with dirty hands and tear-stained face, who comes and weeps alongside your table, mutely asking for alms. She has no wares to sell, and you feel you are not being done when you give her a copper or so. But even she is playing her part, and the smile of triumph on her face when she has reached the safety of the street with some ill-gotten morsel is a sight worth seeing.

One passes out into the crowded square, and turning up the hill on the left one enters the Rue Venizelos. This is the principal shopping thorough-fare.

Running from the front up into the old Turkish quarter, narrow and ill-paved, it appeals, however, to the Thessalonian as the Rue de la Canniebiere does to the Marseilleaise, or the Rue de la Paix does to the Parisian, and as Regent Street does to the Londoner.

Here you see every kind of shop you can conceive – a jewellers, resplendent with electric light and brightly burnished silver, and alongside a lock-up shanty with an unsavoury looking gentleman clothed in a motley assortment of coloured rags selling winkles and other varieties of shell fish.

Presently this curious mixture of Burlington Arcade and Whitechapel is crossed by an equally dirty, ill-paved and evil smelling thoroughfare. This is the celebrated Via Ignatia, leading from Rome to Constantinople. There is not much glamour attached to it now, and save for a Roman arch, which has survived the vicissitudes of time, it is little more than a slum street and a tram route.

The trams are wonderful creations of a Philadelphia firm, worked on the trailer system, and replete with every modern convenience for hanging on, a method of travelling rendered necessary by the fact that no one ever walks anywhere and fares are cheap. The result is that there are always crowds hanging on all round the cars, and when they pass one another gymnastic efforts are required to maintain one's position. You can hang on to a first-class car all the way for a halfpenny.

Trams are the only things which are cheap in this country, everything else being of high price and inferior quality. Now and then shops are put "out of bounds" for a time and then prices are lowered.

The currency is a mixed one of paper and metal. The former are printed in Greek on one side and French on the other, and are made in New York. The coins are of silver or nickel, the latter variety being perforated by a hole in the middle. You can use any coin you like, from Turkish to Italian.

On leaving the tram route you pass through streets which are comparatively clean and wide, but even here in the West End houses have the appearance of being dumped down regardless of symmetry or order.

At the upper end of this part of the town you turn a corner and suddenly recognise on a large building the familiar Red Cross and Union Jack. This is the principal Military Hospital, worthy of note as being the only one in this country actually housed in a building.

Rumour divides its origin between a Greek orphanage and a princely harem. An imposing entrance of white marble stairs and columns lead into a lofty hall traversed by a long corridor.

Medical and surgical floors and a basement for special departments and stores completely occupy an enormous building.

Huts and tents outside bring the accommodation up to the standard Army hospital of 1,500 beds.

This then is the hospital in which I find myself at the present time. The work just now is not heavy. Medical cases always predominate, marshes, mosquitoes, and malaria playing their part, and causing the greater number.

The transport of the sick and wounded is a difficult matter owing to the non-existence of roads. Mules fitted with cacolets, travoirs and litters form the only means of transport in many parts.

The weather so far has been fine and warm but cold at nights, more like early summer in England, with an occasional storm of wind or rain.

Bright clear skies and a hot sun have given the lie to tales we were told of a severe winter. One can sit out of doors for an hour or so at a time without a British Warm or even a cardigan or waistcoat.

The view from the camp is one of the most perfect you could have anywhere, for situated on the lower slopes of the mountains it overlooks the whole country for miles around.

On the left you have a little bit of a mountain as high as Snowdon, with a picturesque village at the foot. On the right you have the old town, with citadel and ramparts, and beyond the long stretches of the Salonica plain and the Vardar Marches.

Below you, as you stand, you have the modern town, with harbour and shipping.

In the middle of the picture you have the long line of the sea, and at the back a continuous range of mountains, culminating on the left in three huge snow-capped peaks. Olympus, 10,000 feet high and nearly 50 miles away, guards the entrance to the Gulf of Salonica.

It's practically always visible from here, and the effect by moonlight is a sight not to be missed.

I am afraid I have lingered too long on the descriptive side of things, and I must bring my letter to a close.

Yours very truly,
L.B. Clarke.

(This letter from L.B. Clarke from Salonica is a remarkably well-written account of life in the capital city. He has qualities in his descriptions worthy of a professional travel writer. Lionel Beale Clarke had an M.A. from Cambridge and obtained the L.M.S.S.A. qualification in 1914. He was a Divisional Surgeon and President of the Medical Classifying Board, British Salonica Force. He was prior to this a House Officer and Resident Anaesthetist at St Mary's Hospital. He was the author of 'Animal Research: Consideration of its Virtues and Value' in 1914 and 'Active Service and the Unfit' published in the St Mary's Hospital Medical School *Gazette*, in 1917.)

CHAPTER 18

Mesopotamia

Mesopotamia lies between the Euphrates and the Tigris Rivers. It was divided into Lower and Upper Mesopotamia. Lower Mesopotamia stretched from the head of the Persian Gulf to Baghdad and the Upper from Baghdad to East Turkey. In Lower Mesopotamia the world's first urban civilization developed during the fourth millennium BC. The Mesopotamian Empire was established *circa* 2300 BC. With an interest in preserving the Anglo Persian oil fields centred on Abadan but also to encourage an Arab revolt against Turkish domination, a small expedition was sent from India to Shatt-al-Arab at the estuary of the Euphrates and Tigris rivers in the Persian Gulf. The Anglo-Indian troops landed in November 1915 and formed a base at Basra. This was the first stage of a campaign that would take British Forces up to and beyond Baghdad. This campaign would involve over 800,000 men. Initially General Townshend was besieged at Kut-el-Amara and finally surrendered with 10,000 British and Indian troops in April 1916. He was well treated by his captors and his officers adequately, but his men were treated appallingly and over two thirds of them died on the march to captivity, many with heat stroke and want of water, and being abused and beaten by their captors.

Under General Sir Stanley Maude the British Forces re-entered Kut-el-Amara in December 1916 and by March 1917 had captured Baghdad. It was gruelling work and disease was as dangerous as battle wounds. There were few good roads and the Rivers Tigris and Euphrates were used for supply boats with the army advancing up the Tigris supported by gun-boats. Eventually 900,000 British and Indian troops took part in the campaign.

December 5th, 1915–April 29th 1916

Kut-el-Amara

By Captain R.V. Martin I.M.S., M.R.C.S.,L.R.C.P.

On visiting St. Mary's the other day after a long absence, I was immediately tackled by the Editor for an article, so I will endeavour to interest the readers of the Gazette with an account of some of my experiences in Kut.

I was in Mesopotamia from the commencement of hostilities in November 1914, and in nearly all the "shows" up to the advance to Baghdad, Ctesiphon, and the retirement to Kut-el-Amara, which we reached on December 1st, the official date for the commencement of the siege being December 5th, as the cavalry left us by a bridge thrown across the river on December 4th; and that was the last day on which we had communication with the outside world except by wireless. The first week or two were spent making our lines of defence. I was with an Indian regiment and we had three days at a time in the first redoubt on the right of our line, being relieved by the British regiment of our Brigade. The extreme right of our line was the "Fort", a large open space surrounded by a wall about seven to eight foot high, and built as part of the defences of the town against Arab attacks. Before a siege had been thought about, we communicated with the fort by about 100 yards of fire trench, though this was not built till much later on in the siege. The whole three days were spent in making the redoubt. On our first visit there the trench was only about three to four feet deep, and not wide enough for two persons abreast. The digging was done at night, and we could see and hear the Turks digging in opposite us, but no firing of importance was taking place, and so our defences progressed. When not in the redoubt we were busy digging communication trenches and our second line defences. It was continual digging, and everyone had to take a hand at it. The ground being under fire from machine-guns and snipers, not to mention shell fire, made it somewhat exciting getting from one dug-out to another, which themselves were of a very primitive nature, being just large enough to lie down in. On December 20th we took over our relief in Redoubt A, and never left it again until finally forced out by the floods late in March, the reason being that on December 24th the Turks made two desperate attacks on the "Fort", penetrating it, but being pushed out again, and the British regiment which relieved us had to be moved into it as support, and finally remained there permanently till the end of the siege. Our Brigade was the only one which never got any relief in billets, the other two Brigades taking it week about in the front line and in the village, Christmas Day was quiet, the Turks having suffered a severe loss through their repulse. Our Christmas dinner consisted of sausage and mashed potatoes eaten in a dug-out with no head cover, a strong wind blowing, so that we had to have one plate over the other to prevent our food being smothered by the dust, which descended in a continuous stream upon us. I had managed to bring back two or three cases of whisky with us on the retirement, and we found two or three more on arrival, with gin and port, but only one small case of foodstuffs, so though we always had plenty to drink, we had no grub after the first month or six weeks with which to supplement our ration, except a little flour which we sometimes could buy at an enormous price in the bazaar; also, being so far from the bazaar, we were unable to buy any extras which those in the village were often able to buy. It was a good two miles through trenches to get there, and in wet weather it was well nigh impossible – the exercise also made one so hungry! The village was a miserable place, and it seemed like getting out in the country again to be back in our little spot, where we always were cheerful and optimistic. Behind us we had some small sand hills, which, being dug out on the rear face, afforded a safe shelter from which we could watch the "evening hates" from the Turkish guns, and, later on, "Fritz" on his bomb-dropping expeditions. The Fort was about the only part of our front line that was ever bombarded, and none of it was ever bombed. It was a very dirty life, being always in the trenches, and lice were very numerous, none of us being free. We were always in our clothes, though on my birthday I slept in pyjamas, being told off by my C.O. for doing so! Also, we had no beds or any of life's comforts. Fortunately there was no typhus. The Turks in front of us were 100 yards at the nearest point, but at other parts of the line they were much nearer. Unfortunately all my papers were taken from me by the Turks, so I cannot give any exact dates or details of our rations. I think we started horse meat in February, my poor beast being one of the first to go. The meat is not bad, rather tough and tasteless. The trouble was not having anything to eat with it. We would collect various roots and make "spinach" – very nasty. Scurvy soon made its appearance. The Indians refused to eat the horse meat for a long time, making it very difficult to feed them, and one saw far more scurvy amongst them than amongst the British. The treatment was very difficult, as there was nothing much to give them, at least not for so many cases. Towards the end of the siege the aeroplanes dropped dressings and any really necessary medicines. The great difficulty during the whole siege was to keep out the river, which rises extremely high from February onwards. This made it necessary for the men to be always at work making "bunds", etc. I do not think that the men ever got any rest except while in hospital during the whole siege. About the end of February the whole of the front line from about 200 yards on our left were washed out of their trenches by the river coming in suddenly. Fortunately the Turks in front of them were also flooded out at the same time, as our men had to get out of the trenches and get behind the parados, and we should have suffered severely had not the Turks been in the same predicament. After this the line of defence from our left went back in eschelon to the second line. The Turks retired about 2,000 yards, and we had comparative peace. The first day we discovered this retirement we were able to go and inspect the enemy's trenches, but afterwards they placed snipers' posts, which prevented this amusement. On March 8th we were all ready for about the third time to co-operate with our forces downstream for our relief. We had all been marched before dawn from the front line and concentrated in the village, the line being only held by pickets, but we

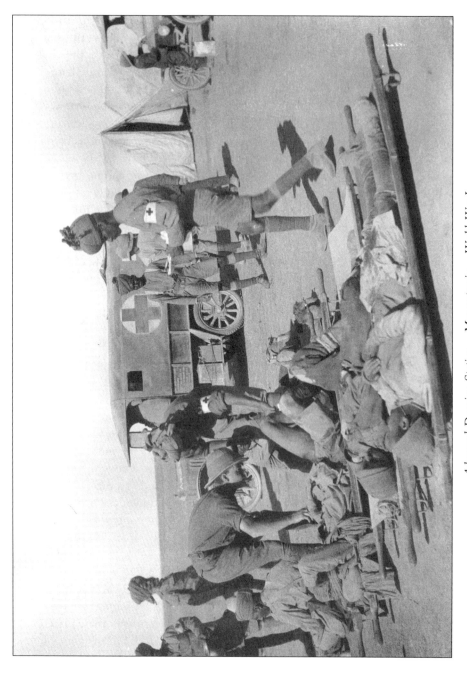

Advanced Dressing Station – Mesopotamia – World War I
Photograph courtesy of the Imperial War Museum, London. Negative no. Q24440

were doomed to a bitter disappointment, as although our force got near enough for us to hear the rifle fire, and we were waiting for the order to be given for us to attempt the crossing of the river, it never came, and the next day we marched back sore at heart to take up our old position in Redoubt A again. Another day previous to this we heard the Turks had been defeated and were retreating upstream, our forces hard on their heels; we even went so far as to open our last bottle of milk punch, which was being kept for the relief, but once again it was a false alarm. So it was one disappointment after another till the end, yet I don't think we ever thought we would surrender, the garrison was always cheerful. The river finally drove us back at the end of March. It rushed in suddenly, unfortunately in the dark, and although about every 50 yards of the trench the length of two traverses were filled in as a "bund", the water came right through so rapidly that we were unable to get everything out of the trenches; however we did not lose anything of much value.

Our place in the second line was much more roomy and comfortable, and we were only troubled by snipers from the other side of the river. In the evenings we could shoot sparrows and starlings and an occasional dove, all of which were most welcome, as at this time we were practically always hungry, being down to 1 lb. of horse meat and 6 ozs. of bread daily, which was at the end reduced to 4 ozs. The days dragged on like this till the end came. Even then our hopes were once more raised to concert pitch, to be dashed to the ground again. The Turks were offered a large sum of money etc., to allow us to go, on parole, and though the local commander accepted these terms, they were refused by the G.H.Q., Constantinople, undoubtedly through German influence. We destroyed everything of military value, and all the enemy got were a crowd of sick and tired men to help consume their food, which was already short; in fact, they were quite unable to feed us at first, and food had to be sent to us from our own force downstream. The day after the surrender we were marched to a camp about 10 miles upstream where we were "sorted out". Here a great many died, mainly British, from severe gastro-enteritis, probably cholera, though it was not diagnosed as such.

The men were all marched away after about five days, having first a medical inspection which was absolutely criminal, men with beri-beri, with a large amount of dropsy, bad scurvy cases, etc., were pronounced to be fit to march. Baghdad, being 100 miles away, and the only food "Turkish biscuits" – a kind of bread with a crust so hard that it was impossible to bite it – the only thing to do was to soak them and make a kind of porridge.

Officers were taken to Baghdad by boat. We disembarked at the British Consulate, and marched in seniority in double file "on show", through most of Baghdad, till we reached the old Turkish cavalry barracks. After two days most of us started off by tram to Shamran, the starting place for our long march of many hundred miles to Ras-el Rin, the next railhead, about 100 miles from Aleppo. But this is another long story, and so I will bring this to a close.

Other Mary's men in Kut were Lieut. Col. Browne Mason, our D.A.D.M.S. exchanged from Baghdad, and Major F. Lambert, who died from typhoid after a very long illness.

(R.V. Martin qualified in 1913. In 1924 he was still serving in the Indian Medical Service.)

The following letter is from V. Zachary Cope.

August 31,1916.
45th General Hospital,
I.E.F. "D",
Mesopotamia
My Dear Kettle,
It is a far cry from Mesopotamia to Paddington, but distance does not dim the vision we have of St. Mary's, and we therefore send you greeting. The plural is used advisedly, for there are six Mary's men in this unit – Pannett, Gosse, Thackray Parsons, Warren, R. de Veil King, and myself. Moreover, one of the first men I ran against was W.L. Hopkins, looking as fit as could be. He arrived a week before we did. Colonel Willcox is also stationed in Basra at present, and has visited our camp several times. He looks very well and is doing most valuable work. I have heard that Alexander and Sharpe are also up this way, but have not come across them yet.

We had a splendid journey from England on the hospital ship "Oxfordshire." True, the monsoon was a little trying, but it only damped our spirits and appetites for a short time. We were permitted to go ashore at Port Said for a few hours and stayed two at Bombay. The heat in the Red Sea and again in the Persian Gulf was trying, but served as an introduction to the heat we experience every day here. We hope and expect that the thermometer will soon lose its habit of running above 100 degrees each afternoon.

At Bombay we met Finlayson, who had returned sick from Me-sopotamia, and whose accounts of the country were not very glowing – or rather they were too glowing. He is not quite recovered from his illness, but is able to get about now. When we reached the head of the Persian Gulf we were transferred to the "Syria", which took us up the river to Basra. On board the "Syria" we were delighted to see and have a chat with Major Whitmore, who was H.S. to Mr. Page about fifteen years ago. He is stationed on the "Syria" for the time and appeared to be in splendid health.

We arrived at our destination on August 20th, and were taken to the Camp at Makina, where we were awaiting further orders. The hospital which we are to look after has not yet been completed, and though every effort is being made to hasten matters an interval must elapse before we get to work.

The whole country around Basra is devoted to the cultivation of the date-palm, and our camp is situated in a palm-grove – in fact several palm trees traverse the roof of the hut which I inhabit – and in every direction are water channels, along which the water courses, or rather stagnates, and feeds the trees of the plantation. These trees are so valuable that as few as possible are cut down. Moreover, they provide a certain amount of shade. The small water channels open into wider creeks, which open into the main river, the Shatu-ul-Arab, or Basra river. Most of the travelling is done by means of "bellums," which are the gondolas of this Venetian region. The roads have been built up during the British occupation, and "bunds" have been built to prevent the river swamping the country, as it generally does at a certain season of the year. These built up roads are abominably dirty, and motor cars, horses, camels, etc., often combine to make a walk more in the nature of a dust-bath. Basra is a mile away from the river. Ashar is its port, but the two towns really form one large town. In spite of the considerable population there is no really good shop in Basra; the best shop would compare unfavourably with a good village emporium in England. The native bazaars are full of interest and odours, and provide one with an object-lesson of the extreme backwardness of Arab civilization. Arts and crafts are poorly developed, and knowledge of sanitary science will (possibly) be a thing of the future. The water supply has to be watched very carefully, and filtration after treatment with alum, combined with boiling or chlorination, making drinking water as pure as possible. In spite of every form of treatment it never approaches the purity of water at home, and often has a mawkish or chlorine flavour. If there is any naturalist who is keen on studying the fauna of Mesopotamia he could do so without exceeding the bounds of our encampment. In a small water-channel close to my hut (not 10 feet off) at low water can be seen hundreds of frogs of every age and size, many crabs, some tortoises, a few water snakes, and fish in large numbers. At eventide an innumerable assortment of winged creatures of every kind press their acquaintance on us, and at 7 o'clock dinner in the open air we spend quite a good portion of our time keeping the grasshoppers from our mugs and trying to pass them on (or make them hop) to our neighbours. Parsons is trying to tame the mongoose which lives on the roof of our hut, and it is credibly related that the sad result of an obstetric achievement of a mother-rat was that the offspring was baptized in the cup of tea which a certain physician of the unit happened to be drinking underneath.

Well, I fear I shall be wearying you with these trivial comments. We are quite cheerful, especially since the war news is so good these days.

Greetings to all at St. Mary's,

From yours sincerely,

V.Z. Cope.

October 31, 1916
40th General Hospital,
I.E.F.D. Hyde Park Corner, Basra,
Mesopotamia.
Dear Mr. Editor,
Perhaps it might be of interest to readers of the Gazette to hear a little news from this corner of the world. You are probably aware that there was some delay in the completion of the hospital to which we have now come, and since idleness, even in a hot country, is not a desirable thing, many of our unit were appointed to temporary duty elsewhere. I have found it difficult to keep in touch with all the Mary's men who are out here. Gosse has been made O.C. or C.O. (I am not quite clear as to the difference between these initials yet) of a large convalescent camp at Mohammerah and is comfortably settled there. Captain Parsons was appointed medical officer on one of the river-convoy boats. Major Pannet was stationed at a hospital at Sheik Saad, but after about a month's work was unfortunately taken sick, and when last I heard was not yet well. Captain King also went to Sheik Saad. I had the good fortune to be attached to a river hospital-ship which was under the command of an old Mary's man, Major E.W.C. Bradfield, and I shall always look back to my month or more on H.S.I. (as the "Sikkim" is officially known) as one of the most pleasant experiences I have had. Major Bradfield is well known to those who were students at St. Mary's about seventeen years ago. He is a distinguished member of the I.M.S., and when war broke out was working as one of the surgeons on the staff of the large Madras Hospital, and one of the Professors of the Medical School at Madras. When it was decided by the people of Madras to equip and maintain a river hospital ship on the Tigris, Major Bradfield was chosen to equip and command the unit, and right well he has done his task.

The "Sikkim" is a shallow draught boat with two decks, and is equipped to carry about 150 patients. The beds are arranged in two tiers on each deck, and every comfort is provided for the sick and wounded. The vessel is indeed a veritable "multum in parvo", and the wonderful way in which things and people are packed constantly excited my admiration. Electric light, electric fans, a very hygienic soda-water factory (and none of you who are at home realize what that means in a land where the water supply is such a great problem), a plentiful tankage to store and sterilize water, a fine bathroom with a beautiful enamelled bath (and here again only those who have had to use the camp-kit bath can appreciate), and a commissariat both varied and plentiful, combined to make life on the boat something of a luxury. What the patients thought of this can be expressed best by what one of the released prisoners from Kut said when he came on the boat: "Why, it's 'Eaven after 'Ell." During the time I was on the boat we made three journeys up the river to Sheik Saad, one trip to Mohammerah, and another short run to Kurna and back. To give anything but a cursory impression of what one saw during the trip would take longer than the patience of your readers would tolerate, but a few facts may be of interest.

Our journeys were all up the Tigris, which is very muddy and tortuous, varying greatly in depth and breadth in different parts and at different times. When the Spring floods have subsided the channel for a time is very uncertain, and vessels frequently bump the bottom – an experience sometimes disconcerting, since it may occur at unexpected moments. Frequently the boats stick, and one boat may block the way for a large number of boats coming behind. I have known eighteen vessels held up at once in this way. When one considers that it may be hours or it may be days before the obstructing vessel clears the sandbank some of the difficulties of transport on the Tigris may be understood. The distance from Basra to Sheik Saad is about 240 miles. As one ascends the river the first 40 miles, as far as Kuona, present a picture of date palms on the banks, then for another 60 miles one sees few palms, but a continuous expanse of plain, of which only the river margin is cultivated for millet etc; the last 100 miles above Amara are very dull and uninteresting – continuous plains covered by low scrub and scorched grass. The country is as flat as a billiard table until one gets above Amara, when far away to the north-east can be seen the beautiful Pasht-i-Kuh hills of Persia. The country is sparsely populated by wandering Arabs, who build their reed-huts or pitch their tents near the river bank. Large flocks of sheep and herds of buffaloes come down to the water to drink, and quite commonly the only signs of a herd of buffaloes are the tops of their heads showing above the water in which they have immersed themselves. In some places the river is very narrow, and here the natives run along the banks holding in their hands, eggs, fish or chickens, which they try to sell to those on the ship.

There are no big towns on the way up to Sheik Saad, but there are several small places which possess some brick houses which entitle us to call them small towns or large villages. Of these Amara with ten thousand and Gumah with five thousand inhabitants merit mention. Both are important stations on the lines of river communication. Gurnah (or Kurna) lies at the place where the Euphrates used to flow into the Tigris; at present the old Euphrates' channel is still filled with water, but no flow takes place there.

Gurnah is the reputed site of the Garden of Eden, and Eve's Tree, Temptation Square, and Angel Alley serve to remind one of the fact. One can still see traces of the damage done by our shelling a year or more ago. I was not impressed with the neighbourhood, which becomes an island during flood-time. A railway now starts from the place. Amara, which will ever be remembered by the medical profession as the place where Sir Victor Horsley gave his life for his country, is the most considerable town on the way from Basra to Baghdad; it is the centre of an area of cultivated land and exports the produce thereof. It is within sight of the Persian Hills, and has trade relations with that country.

The present junction of the Euphrates and Tigris is at Gormat Ali, which is only five miles from the site of our 40th General Hospital; the clearer Euphrates and the turbid Tigris unit to form the broad Shatt-al-Arab.

There were grave and gay elements mingled in our journey up river. In one place there is a solitary camp with a brick building built (so I understand) by a pioneer party whom expressed their hilarity by naming the building "The Leicester Lounge" and writing this up in letters which can be read by all who pass by in the boats. It was not far from here that we lost one of the ship's crew by drowning. He was foolishly getting water from the stream by means of a bucket without following the orders to remain inside the protective railing; consequently he was pulled into the water, and after a few seconds was seen no more, despite thorough search. A few miles from the same spot is situated the tomb of the prophet Ezra – quite a fine structure with a beautiful blue-tiled dome. It lies on the bank of the river midst a small palm-grove, and is an object of pilgrimage for the Jews. I had the opportunity of entering the tomb on one occasion when the boat stopped to take on some sick soldiers from the camp stationed there; the interior was quite impressive.

Some of the features of the river can be guessed from the names attached; thus Pearl-Drop Bend, Mosquito Bend, and the Devil's Elbow signify well the tortuosity, fly-frequency and difficult navigation of respective reaches of the river. It was at the Devil's Elbow that, on my last trip, we fouled a shoal and stuck across the river broadside on, with our stern-paddle touching one bank, and our bow touching the other bank of the river – that serves to show the narrowness of the stream at this spot. It took some skilful manoeuvring to get us clear.

What of the medical work on the boat? We used to bring down a mixed lot of cases, both British and Indian. Surgical cases were in the minority, but there were several very interesting surgical problems. Never before have I seen so many cases of scurvy which, though usually, does not always attack the gums, and when the haemorrhages occur first into the deep parts of the leg or thigh, the differential diagnosis may prove interesting or even difficult. We had many cases of joint-affections, and, of course, fractures of different kinds, but comparatively few gunshot wounds, for little fighting has taken place recently. We carried down to Amara one man who had had a stab wound of the ascending colon successfully sewn up by Lieut-Colonel Legg. The stab was the work of an Arab thieving in the man's tent by night – a common occurrence. There was not much operative work to be done, but the ship was furnished with a very nice little operating theatre, and on those few occasions on which we had to make use of it, we found it served our purposes well.

I am afraid I shall already have taxed your reader's patience too much, so I will close, after wishing you and all those who may happen to read this a happy Christmas, or as happy a Christmas as the war will permit.

Yours sincerely,

V.Z. Cope.

(Zachary Cope had a distinguished career in surgery and was consultant surgeon at St Mary's Hospital, Paddington. He was born in Kingston-upon-Hull on 14 February 1881 and was the son of a Methodist Minister. His early education was at Westminster School from where he obtained a scholarship to study medicine at St Mary's Hospital Medical School. He obtained his medical degree with honours in 1905 aged twenty-four and within two years his M.D. His Fellowship of the Royal College of Surgeons followed in 1909. Cope's progress was rapid: following a period as Demonstrator in Anatomy he was appointed surgeon to St Mary's in 1911 at the early age of thirty. In 1912 he also obtained a surgical consultancy at the Bolingbroke Hospital in Wandsworth.

He held the rank of Temporary Major during World War I, and was mentioned in dispatches, serving in the Middle East from 1916–1919.

He was a Hunterian Professor of the Royal College of Surgeons, a member of the Board of Examiners and in later years a member of Council of the Royal College of Surgeons, and a Vice-President from 1940–1943. His membership of committees was prodigious, covering many aspects of medical practice, including the General Practice Review Committee of 1950.

His publications were many, a number of biographies, including Florence Nightingale, Almroth Wright, notable general practitioners, historical accounts of nursing, medicine, World War II, and an excellent book on the history of St Mary's Hospital Medical School, published in 1954.

In 1921 he published his renowned book on the *Acute Abdomen* which went into many editions and in 1944 followed it with *The Acute Abdomen in Rhyme*.

He was an Honorary Fellow of the Royal Society of Medicine and President of the Medical Society of London. Cope was knighted in 1953.

He married twice and died on 28 December 1964 aged ninety-three.)

CHAPTER 19

Mesopotamia (continued)

Mr. Shaw Crisp writes:

"I have now been in this country a couple of weeks and am stationed at a combined stationary Hospital at Nahramur, a place some 18 miles above Busrah, on the River Start.

We left London on December 4th via Havre, Marsailles and Port Said, and beyond being attacked by a submarine in the Mediterranean, we had a very good voyage out. The medical staff consists of four and the patients are chiefly Persians and Arabs, with a few British troops.

The whole hospital is under canvas, but conditions good at present, later on in the summer the heat will be terrific: at present the days are warm and the nights decidedly cold.

There is a fair amount of work, chiefly medical, with a few surgical cases now and then.

At present I am doing my best to learn some of the language, as signs are unsatisfactory and not easy to follow.

I should like to have gone to France, where the work is more to do with the War; here there have not been any casualties for nearly three months.

I came across V.C. Vickers at the camp at Ashar, on my way up here: He seemed very fit. I trust everyone at Mary's is well."

From Mesopotamia, Captain Cope reports all is well. He sends tidings of Colonel Willcox, very fit and doing most valuable work; Lieut-Colonel Bond, in charge of a field hospital, "it was at this hospital that the Arabs stole three sides of a mortuary tent and left the fourth side with the sentry standing in front of it – an achievement of some merit!" Captain Warren, who is at 40th General Hospital and Lieutenant Hopkins. Captain Gosse has fitted up a fine cavalescent camp, of which he is O.C. with the rank of Temporary Major, at Mohammerah.

Mesopotamian Memories
By A. Hope Gosse, M.D., Camb., M.R.C.P. Lond.
Brevet Major R.A.M.C. (T.F.)

Mesopotamian days are over, and already time is playing its accustomed part and effacing many of the hours of toil or torture spent in the unrelieved elements of air and earth and water, all frequently and intimately mixed as sand storms, muddy Tigris, winter deluges, and summer floods.

In the Mesopotamian prescription doses vary from time to time, but the constituents are always the same. First comes the basis, or active drug proper, which is Sol Concentrata, then the adjuvant, or substance intended to assist, which is the dust, then the corrective, to limit or otherwise modify the same, this is the Aqua Tigris Impura, and finally the vehicle or excipient, to bring the whole into a pleasant form for administration, a British Expeditionary force. The whole constitutes the Mistura Mesopotamia.

One of the most lasting memories will be the hot weather, which can best be likened to the course of enteric fever, except, alas, for its duration. The days of rising remittent temperatures of its onset comprise the whole of the months of May and June. During this period every possible variation in diagnosis as to the nature and severity of the coming hot weather is given. A report is sought from the local Arab, who places his hopes implicitly in Allah, who alone knows. A further report by comparisons of meteorological records gives conflicting evidence. Agglutination tests are useless for, as punkas are limited, all are glued together beneath them. Finally it is expected to adopt an expectant policy.

Then come the days of sustained fever lasting throughout July and August. The daily temperature remains high, 115 to 122 degrees in the shade, and the nightly remission is slight. All the symptoms become aggravated. Tempers shorten as the temperature lengthens. Lips are dry and tongues are dry also. For the rest, bodies are bathed in autogenous baths of sweat. The mental processes are dulled and the aspect is listless and apathetic.

Finally there is a gradual decline of the daily temperature throughout September and October with more definite nightly remissions. The general wasting and pallor is a marked feature, but the tongue is occasionally moist again and a desire for food returns. Failure of application for leave is one of the complications and chief dangers of this period.

One of my earliest duties was the construction of a convalescent depot in Persia some twenty-five miles from Basrah. A political officer warned me that the Sheikh was afraid of our being troubled at first with "petty misunderstandings" or "friction" between our men and the local inhabitants, so an Arab guard was being provided, but whether for our protection or that of the local inhabitants he did not say. They were awaiting us on our arrival; a fearsome looking body of men, thirty in all, with rifles of as many patterns and multi-coloured flowing robes.

They patrolled the periphery of the camp each night in extended formation, and at frequent intervals in the early hours a cry went up from the head guard, which was repeated by each of the others in turn. This ensured that they were awake, and was very impressive. I occasionally awakened in the night and listened for some time to hear, not the shouting of the guard, but the barking of the pariah, the crying of the jackal, and the laughing of the hyena. A gruesome melody which waxed and waned served to mitigate the feeling of splendid isolation. The guard had probably succumbed to the monotony of an uneventful night.

Our protection really lay, not in the power of an Arab guard, nor in our own lack of means of self-defence, but in the prestige of the British race. And this, too, at a time when the tragedy of Kut had not yet been avenged. If they like, let the croakers see in every temporary set back of the British a fatal blow to our prestige in the East, but the success of that prestige has been built up by years of impartial justice and fair play, and it would take years of repeated blows before it could be shattered.

During the early days of March, 1917, an impromptu concert was held in the recreation tent, and about eight hundred men from the hospital and convalescent depot were present. During the evening the Acting Consul for Arabistan joined the audience and at once passed me a telegram he had just received. At the close of the concert I read its contents to the assembled audience and thereby acquired a new insight into the psychology of the British soldier. The first part ran: "Our advanced troops are within sight of Baghdad, which is in flames." A cheer went up which was a joy to hear after many disappointments which the Force had suffered. As the cheering subsided I continued with the second part of the telegram: "All the guns lost at the surrender of Kut have been recaptured." The instant shout of joy is indescribable. I remember the demonstration thrilled me as I had seldom, if ever, been thrilled before. It far surpassed that accorded to the first announcement. Great was the joy of the promise of victory and a sight of the end of continuous trench warfare for the Mesopotamian Force which the taking of Baghdad would mean, but ten times greater the joy at the recapture of the lost guns of Kut. It was more than mere sentiment this inequality of the reception of the two items of news. May it not be that hidden under the cloak of utter indifference to either the British soldier, even in this twentieth century, values honour greater than victory? In the camp there was the Interpreter, a Persian, who had to interpret for the Indian followers, the Arab guard, or the Persian coolies. He spoke all their languages. His Army Form said so, but added "English imperfect." Whatever language that may be, it was not the same as my imperfect English, but we met on common ground by dropping alternate words, omitting the declining of verbs, a liberal employment of gesticulation, and a common determination to understand and be understood.

To wangle a trip to Baghdad I did duty as medical officer on a paddle boat with barges. I was responsible for the care of the sick among several hundred Indians of a labour corps proceeding up river. The first patient foolishly could speak no English, I could not speak (professional) Hindu-stani. An Indian interpreter was commandeered who spoke "perfect English." To my first question I received the reply after the two Indians had had five minutes chatter that it was a pain in the stomach. I then asked when the pain started. For quite ten minutes this vital point was debated before I stopped them and repeated my question. "Do you know?" I said, "Yes, saar," he replied grinning foolishly at me. "Well, when did it start?" I said. His face beamed with pride at his knowledge as he emphatically replied "Tomorrow morning, saar." But my own experiences of the Indian had not been altogether useless for I knew that in Hindustani yesterday and to-morrow are the same. Oh, wonderful Allah! But I asked no more questions.

(Hope Gosse said in this letter that some protection lay in the prestige of the British race. This was undoubtedly so in many parts of the world at the time. Writing this book when in the same part of the world the British are involved in conflict there seems little evidence that such prestige still exists. More's the pity!!)

Mesopotamia (1916–1919)
By W.H. Willcox, C.B., C.M.G., M.D., F.R.C.P.(Lond).
Physician to Out Patients, St Mary's Hospital; Consulting Physician, Mesopotamia Expedionary Force, Colonel A.M.S. (1916–1919)

On returning home on January 25th 1916, after six months spent in the Dardanelles, I received the invitation from the War Office to proceed to Mesopotamia as Consulting Physician to the Expeditionary Force.

The experience gained in the Dardanelles was of inestimable value, for one saw there cases of Dysentery, Enteric Group Disease, Jaundice, Relapsing Fever, and the common medical diseases of campaigns in abundance, and also a certain number of cases of deficiency diseases (Scurvy and Beri Beri). The knowledge gained was invaluable as a preparation for my future medical work in Mesopotamia. In addition the six months in the Dardanelles spent mostly under canvas at Mudros, under conditions which often called for philosophic resignation and could not be described as "picnicking" were an excellent training for the campaigning which formed a necessary part of one's work in the long journeys often necessary in Mesopotamia.

Little attention was paid to the Mesopotamian Expedition until early in 1916, when rumours filtered home that the conditions of the sick and wounded in that region left much to be desired and anxiety was felt as to the medical and general arrangements being such that proper care for the sick and wounded soldiers in that trying climate could be ensured.

The history of the campaign prior to 1916 deserves mention, as it explains to some extent the temporary defects in the arrangements, not only medical, but general, which occurred.

Our troops landed at the mouth of the Shatt-al-Arab, at Fao, on November 6th 1914, under General Delamain, and on November 14th 1914, General Sir Arthur Barrett landed at Saniyah, about 30 miles upstream, on the right bank, and took over command.

About this time the Turks tried to block our progress up the Tigris by sinking three large steamers across the channel of the stream. This device proved of no avail, for the current caused the vessels to swing round while sinking, and ample room was left for large ships to pass between the sunken steamers

Within a month Basrah and Kurna were captured, and a firm footing was obtained in lower Mesopotamia. General Sir John Nixon took command of the force (known as I.E.F.D.) on April 9th 1915, and there followed a series of most brilliant successes. Victory over Turkish forces generally superior in numbers to our own were gained at Shaibah – at Ahwaz, which was the key to invaluable "oil fields" – at Amara on the Tigris, and at Nasiriyah, which gave command of the lower Euphrates region.

Major-General Townshend pushed his force rapidly up the Tigris, and on September 18th 1915, defeated a large Turkish force at Kut-el-Amarah and captured the town. General Townshend advanced up the left bank of the Tigris, and at Ctesiphon, which is only about 20 miles from Baghdad, he again defeated a Turkish force much superior in numbers to his own.

Owing to heavy casualties and to the arrival of strong enemy reinforcements our force could not proceed further, and it was necessary to fall back on Kut, which was put in a state of strong defence, and on December 11th 1915 was invested by the Turks.

The operations from now up to April 29th 1916, were directed toward the relief of Kut, which fell after a brilliant defence of 143 days. General Townshend destroyed all military stores before surrender, and was only reluctantly compelled to take this step on account of the starvation from which his troops were suffering.

When one journeys up the Tigris to Baghdad, which is 500 miles by river, and also travels over the regions as far as Nasiriyah and Ahwaz, over which in the early days our small force was operating so successfully, it appears simply marvellous how so small a force could have accomplished such great things.

At that time the facilities in the way of transport were meagre, and such things as ice and soda water, which are so necessary in a climate like that of Mesopotamia, were unobtainable.

The explanation is that the troops were some of the best of our old army, hardened veterans, well seasoned by service in India, to a tropical climate.

They were finely led and buoyed up by a succession of victories they overcame, not only the Turks and Arabs, but what is even greater, the dangers inseparable from a country of fierce climate and redolent in disease.

Up to January 1917, the Tigris front lay below Kut, a distance of 300 miles by river from the base at Basrah.

The Turks had become heavily reinforced, and they were assisted by a number of trained German troops.

Our force was of necessity considerably increased, and the great difficulties of transport of the necessary supplies in a country like Mesopotamia, with no roads or railways, can readily be imagined. The troops were entirely dependent on the river for supplies, since local resources were at that time few, and river steamers had to be sent out from home and from other countries (India, Burma, Egypt, etc.), the local river transport being quite insufficient.

It is not to be wondered at that great difficulties were encountered during 1915 and 1916, and hardships were inevitable where men and supplies had to be transported such great distances under climatic conditions as trying as anywhere in the world.

The history of the Mesopotamian campaign, together with the difficulties of river transport, and the exceptionally trying climate with its fierce heat and dangers from disease, explain to a great extent the so-called "Mesopotamian Scandals" which were investigated so fully by the Mesopotamia Commission in 1916 and 1917.

I left Southampton March 15th 1916, and arrived via Malta at Alexandria, from where by train Suez was reached on March 29th. Seven days waiting for a boat were well spent here, for one had the opportunity of seeing many patients on their way home from Mesopotamia, and much was learnt from them as to the work which would have to be undertaken there and the diseases to be combated.

While at Suez an epidemic of Relapsing Fever was occurring, especially in the Camel Corps and troops brought into contact with native labour. The two hospitals there were from the Dardanelles, and one met many old friends. I saw a great many of the Relapsing Fever cases, and suggested the administration of Salvarsan intravenously in 3 gramme doses which was most successful in terminating the disease within about 12 hours usually. The interesting fact was discovered that if the Salvarsan were given in the apyrexial period following an attack it usually prevented the occurrence of any relapses.

This line of treatment for Relapsing Fever was subsequently adopted with great success in the outbreaks which occurred in Mesopotamia.

Bombay was arrived at on April 15th and I spent several days visiting the Military Hospitals there which received the sick from Mesopotamia. One thus learnt a great deal about the diseases prevailing in the troops and also as regards the special medical needs of the Mesopotamian Force.

It was obvious that Enteric Group Disease, Dysentery, Malaria, effects of heat and Deficiency Diseases such as Scurvy and Beri Beri, were the chief dangers to which the troops were being exposed. While in India I spent four days in Simla, staying there with Sir Pardey Lukis, who was then acting as D.M.S. of India. I received from him the greatest kindness, help and encouragement, and had the opportunity of discussing fully with him the medical conditions prevailing in Mesopotamia. At this time every effort was being made by Sir Pardey Lukis and the military authorities in India to do all they could to deal with the medical requirements of Mesopotamia. Thus ice machines, topees, spinal pads, and other requirements for heat protection were being collected and sent out. Also Vaccines (T.A.B., Cholera, Plague, etc.,) were being prepared in large quantities in India for the force.

Anti-scorbutic articles of diet, e.g. limes, potatoes, onions, etc., were given special attention to in the food supplies from India. For protection against Malaria and Sand Fly Fever large quantities of mosquito and sand fly nets were being forwarded.

Special attention was paid to the requirements of Mesopotamia in the shape of Hospital transport, such as motor launches, motor ambulances, hospital river steamers, etc.

The Red Cross and St. John's Ambulance Society in India were doing splendid work in sending out medical comforts to the troops through the Mesopotamian Branch.

The hospitals in Bombay for troops arriving overseas were excellently equipped and the D.M.S. of India realised that a great increase in the accommodation for sick and wounded would be required for 1916 and 1917.

Several additional hospitals with all necessary modern equipment were provided, and this forecast was amply justified, for the hospitals in India were, during 1916 and 1917, kept constantly full, but were able to meet satisfactorily the heavy calls made upon them.

Bombay was left on May 4th 1916, and Basrah reached on May 11th. A delightful trip was made on the excellently equipped hospital ship "Madras", and Lieut-Col. Symons I.M.S., S.M.O. and his medical officers, Major Wright, I.M.S., Captain Cruickshank, I.M.S., and Captain Scott, I.M.S. all of whom had served in Mesopotamia, were full of interesting anecdotes and experiences.

Basrah in the summer of 1916 was very different from the city of to-day.

At that time date gardens extended to the river along a great part of the right bank on which the city lies, and these were intersected with irrigation channels which were filled with the rise of the tide.

Several creeks ran from the river two or three miles inland, and formed the main channel of transport for the natives in their boats, called "bellums." As there were few bridges over the creeks the difficulty of getting about at Basrah except by launch or boat can be imagined.

The air was heavy laden with moisture, and insects of all kinds, such as mosquitoes, sand flies, etc., existed in swarms. It is no wonder that one was lucky to escape Malaria and Sand Fly Fever if living in such a place.

Basrah is a picturesque city, typically Eastern in character. Its narrow streets and covered busy bazaars with recesses on each side in which are deposited the goods for sale, its quaintly built houses and the Arab population, form an attractive picture.

The sanitation of the native part of the city was before our occupation practically nil, and but for the purifying power of the sun disease would have made unlimited ravages.

The appointment of military governors for Basrah city, and the part of the river bank known as Ashar, enabled a control of the sanitation of the districts occupied by the natives to be obtained, and any infringement of the sanitary laws met with prompt correction and corporal punishment. In 1916 it is surprising how clean the streets of Basrah and Ashar were kept, and compared with most Eastern cities there was little to offend the olfactory organs.

The Tigris is a magnificent river, and is navigable for large sea going vessels for 30 miles beyond Basrah. Date palms stretch along the banks on each side around Basrah and for many miles below. The beautiful sunsets are one of the most attractive features of Mesopotamia, and are rarely seen to such advantage. On each side of the river beyond the date gardens the flat open desert stretches for miles unrelieved by trees or hills. Camel thorn scrub or wild liquorice are all that will grow on this sun-beaten dried-up soil, but it is marvellous how fertile the desert is if water is supplied by irrigation. The soil is really alluvial mud and deposited from the river floods, and if supplied with water will grow the richest crops in rapid succession.

The possibilities of the country with a proper system of irrigation are very great, and under our administration there must be a most prosperous future for Mesopotamia. Mesopotamia is a country which had an extraordinary fascination for many of us who were fortunate enough to keep fit. The ever changing river scenes, the interesting Arab population, the sense of freedom of the wide expanse of desert, all had an especial charm. It is true that June, July and August were months in which one's resistance to the intense heat was taxed to the uttermost. However, the risks to which we were all exposed, whether from heat stroke or acute disease, called forth a sense of comradeship and mutual helpfulness which usually stood us in good stead in cases of emergency which one was always prepared for.

Major-General Treherne, K.C.M.G., arrived in Mesopotamia on May 13th, and as D.M.S. of the force at once instituted a scheme of re-organisation of the medical units which was at that time much needed. He drew up a scheme for the medical requirements in view of the subsequent increases of the forces so that efficiency could be ensured, and he was ably assisted by Colonel Fell, his D.D.M.S., L.of C. Sir Percy Lake, Army Commander, took the greatest interest in the medical arrangements, and did all in his power to ensure the supply of everything in the way of hospital units, personnel and equipment that was required. This work of organisation laid the foundations of the future success of the Medical Service in Mesopotamia, for in a few months the medical arrangements throughout the force were such that they would compare favourably with those in any other theatre of war.

In May, 1916, the Officers' Hospital at Beit Nama (about four miles below Basrah) was established. It became an excellently equipped hospital of 100 beds, and was afterwards most efficiently commanded by an old St. Mary's man, Major Hope Gosse, and was one of the best hospitals to the force.

During the summer of 1916 the hospitals of Basrah contained a wealth of most interesting clinical material. Numbers of cases of Enteric, Paratyphoid A (which was the type then present), Amoebic and Bacillary Dysentery, Malaria, Sand Fly Fever, etc., could always be studied. Cases of Cholera of a sporadic type were constantly occurring, and not infrequently Plague was to be met with. Constant watch so that diagnosis should be made at the earliest stage, and unremitting supervision by the sanitary departments, prevented these two dreaded diseases assuming epidemic form. Numbers of cases of scurvy in Indian troops were arriving from the front, and these were of the greatest clinical interest. The marked anaemia, the hyperplastic budding with tendency to bleeding of the gums between the teeth, the palate haemorrhages, the haemorrhage into muscles and occasional joint effusions, and brawny oedema of the legs formed a most characteristic clinical picture.

A study of the aetiology of these cases established beyond doubt the Vitamin Deficiency theory of the disease, and thus led to a careful review of the rations of the troops from a Vitamin Deficiency standpoint. New ration scales for the force were introduced in July, 1916, and further improvements were effected in October, 1916, so that a really good ration which was entirely protective against Scurvy or Beri Beri, was established.

Difficulties of transport, of course – were great, and necessitated delay in carrying out the food reforms, but by the end of 1916 Vitamin Deficiency disease, which had accounted for over 10,000 cases of illness, was practically stamped out.

(As was the intention at the outset we have not edited these letters, but this contribution contains long sentences which are often repetitive. To convert the writing to a more modern style, although easier to read, would alter the style popular at the time of writing, and conceal the character of the author.

Colonel Willcox gives a vivid description of the terrain, the climate and the medical disorders of Mesopotamia. He makes no mention of battle casualties, but states that Deficiency disease alone accounted for 10,000 cases of illness. This is a remarkably large number and emphasises that illness causes more casualties than enemy fire. The doctors carry a monumental responsibility!!

Sir William Henry Willcox K.C.I.E., C.B., C.M.G., M.D., F.R.C.P., D.P.H., was born at Melton Mowbray in 1870. His early education was at Wymondham Grammar School. He obtained a B.Sc. London in 1892, and obtained a scholarship to study medicine in 1895. Among his early successes was to qualify with the award of the Gold Medal in 1900. In the same year he obtained the D.P.H. His first appointment was a Lectureship in Chemistry in the Medical School which he held from 1900 until 1904. He was next appointed Medical Registrar and subsequently in 1907 elected to the medical staff of the hospital. In 1910 he was elected F.R.C.P. Soon he began to lecture on forensic medicine and he became Analyst to the Home Office. In 1919 he was appointed Medical Adviser to the Home Office. He gave crucial evidence in the Crippen case, identifying hyoscine in the corpse.

During World War I Willcox served at Mudros and in Mesopotamia and in 1916 was awarded the C.M.G. and in 1917 the C.B.

He served as President of the West London Medical Society, the Harveian Society of London, the Medico-Legal Society and the Medical Society of London.

He was the author of many medical papers, including deficiency disorders, the toxicology of Salvarsan, infective arthritis, parathyroid disease, teeth and gum infections and diabetes, etc.

Among his hobbies were riding and hunting. He was knighted in 1921, retired in 1935 and died in 1941.

Sir William Willcox had a son, 'Dick', who became a consultant in genitor-urinary medicine at St Mary's Hospital. He was a prestigious writer of medical articles, and was a colleague of the authors of this book.)

CHAPTER 20

Egyptian Expeditionary Force

This force consisted of British, Australian, New Zealand, Indian, South African, Italian, West Indian troops and Egyptian labour corps. In the winter of 1916 it advanced against the Turks across the Sinai desert, building a railway and laying a water pipe as it went. By the spring of 1917 it had reached Gaza. Now under the command of General Allenby it continued its advance, taking Jerusalem in November 1917 and thus acquiring a British Palestine (now Israel). Allenby continued his offensive against the Turkish army and on 1 October 1918 Haifa fell to an Indian Division which went on to take Beirut a week later. At the same time the Australian Cavalry entered Damascus (together with 'Lawerence of Arabia' and the Arab army.)

(Edward Henry Hynman Allenby was born in Brackenhurst in Nottinghamshire and was trained at Sandhurst Military Academy. He joined the Inniskilling Dragoons. In World War I he commanded the First Cavalry Division, and next the Third Army in France from 1915 to 1917. He was then appointed Commander-in-Chief of the Egyptian Expeditionary Force. From 1919 to 1925 he was High Commissioner in Egypt. Created Viscount, he died in 1936.)

A note from the editor of the *Gazette* reads:

We are permitted to publish the following extracts from the letter of a St. Mary's man (no name is given), who is serving with the Egyptian Expeditionary Force, though it is with regret that we have had to censor it very freely:

At 7 p.m. we received orders to be ready to move in the lightest possible order at 11 p.m. This meant we had no blankets or coats, just two day's food. At 11 we formed up, and in silence and without smoking we started. We marched until 12.30 a.m., and then had a short halt, and all mounted officers, myself included, sent back their horses. We then started our march again. It was a bitterly cold night, and being in drill shorts we felt it a great deal. At 4.a.m. we reached ——, and formed into artillery formation, and at 4.45 the signal was given to attack the heights. Our battalion led and went forward splendidly. Our guns backed us up and the Turks bolted, leaving breakfast, coats etc., behind. Our advance was so rapid that we had but few casualties and I could not keep up because my mule, with surgical equipment, couldn't get across the waddies, so I found myself behind the — regiment and attended to their wounded. I opened my boxes and dressed the men on the side of a hill, under shrapnel fire, but out of rifle fire except for a few stray shots and a sniper or two. I managed to join my battalion about midday, just in time to help some men who had been injured in a "tank", which was put out of action by five direct hits of high explosive. By this time my mule was about done, and I was glad to get a rest. The regiment had seized the waddi and we dug in on the river bank. All that day and the next the Turks shelled us with H.E. and shrapnel, but except when we took the edge of the "crater" we had almost no casualties. We were now established in a cup-like hollow in the ground, holding the edge, and we had a dry river bed down the centre, which gave us some protection. Next day we were told to advance at 7.30 a.m., and if possible take enemy trenches, labyrinth and two redoubts. We mustered at 7 a.m. and the enemy started shelling. By 7.20 I was at work. The enemy had machine guns and some artillery ready for us as we "came over", and we found we had 3,000 yards of open flat country to cross before we could get at them. Our men were magnificent and got to the trenches, were turned out, took the redoubt, were turned out, and finally fell back at night, having been in the open under fire from 7.30 a.m. to 2 a.m. the next day. They only fell back then under orders from H.Q. I will tell you of my part of the show. I was busy dressing cases as the battalion went over and continued doing so till about 1.30 a.m., when I was about finished, only having some milk and brandy . . . My sergeant and the priest dressed the rest. We were under shell fire the whole time and rifle fire part of it. Water was scanty and the wounded were re-wounded or killed for want of cover. Early on I was struck by a piece of shell on my leg, but it only bruised it a little. At midday we were full up, but had now run out of dressings, and had to pause. An Irish priest brought me some milk, and as I sat drinking I was struck by a bullet on the boot. We started work again and the priest stuck by me splendidly. We were dressing a case together when a shell fell between us, a "dud" luckily. The heat was awful, and the wounded drank my tin of washing water. As I was attending to a fractured femur a piece of shell struck my watch on my wrist and smashed it, and another piece went through the left breast of my tunic, tearing a large hole in it. We went on trying to get the wounded under cover, and my stretcher bearers were splendid. I have got two of them recommended. The rifle fire started again and our men had to fall back to the ridge for a bit, and a shot got me in the elbow, cutting a little place, which is already well. Some of our wounded were between the Turks and ourselves and could not be got out. I went out later to see if I could get nearer them, but as soon as I appeared the enemy opened fire with machine guns and I had to get back to my old position. The wounded with me were splendid; not one of them grumbled even when shrapnel came over them and they could not escape. At 2 a.m. two more doctors arrived. I felt about finished and slept where I was until 4 a.m., when we had to march to our present position. Our men are wonderfully cheerful, and only want the Turks to come on so that they can get a bit of their own back.

Rumania and Russia

The Rumanian Hospital
By D.C.L. Fitzwilliams, F.R.C.S.

The editor of the Gazette pounced upon me immediately on my return from abroad for an account of my doings, very much in the same way that a schoolboy is asked where he has been as soon as he returns from out of bounds, I feel I must give an account of myself, in this case probably a more truthful account than that usually given by a schoolboy.

A hospital was organised for Rumania by the British Red Cross in the month of August, but owing to many causes it was not ready to leave this country till the beginning of November. It was sent as a present from the British nation to the Queen of Rumania, who, as many of you know, is an English woman, being the daughter of the Duke of Edinburgh. It was financed very largely by the miners of England. In the beginning of November the hospital started out. Originally it was to have had a personnel of about 35 people; as it was, we left with only 25 all told. There were four doctors or surgeons, a dentist, seven English nursing sisters under Miss McGregor, the late matron of Paddington Green Children's Hospital, an X-ray specialist from the photographic department of the Daily Mirror, and the rest were nursing orderlies or motor drivers. There were supposed to be six motor ambulances; these however, never got any further than Sweden – even if they got so far – for we never heard what became of them. I may here add that the 200 motor ambulances that were procured by the efforts of the Earl of Lonsdale never reached Rumania either.

We started from King's Cross in the afternoon and reached Newcastle at night, and after the usual delays with papers and passports eventually embarked on the "Jupiter," which was the best boat running between Newcastle and Bergen. Of the crossing we need say nothing – most people were as they usually are when they are at sea. We were three nights and two days crossing, and got into Bergen without mishap, but too late for the morning train to Christiania, and had in consequence to take the night train. This was a great misfortune, as the journey between the two towns is, for scenery, one of the finest in the world, as the railway mounts up a great way along the side of the fiords. We, therefore, were forced to spend the day in Bergen. As the town had been burnt down shortly before this it was not very exciting. The town gave us a forecast of what we were to see in the future, as it was all built of wood. Huge areas had been burnt completely out, and only about a third of the town was left. In the afternoon the medical officers decided to drive up the big hill just behind the town and see the view. The expedition nearly came to an untimely end then and there, for on trying to pass a cutting on the narrow road the front wheels of the carriage went over the side. Luckily for us the two small ponies stood still, and we lost little time in scrambling out. There was a sheer drop of about 300 feet into a conveniently placed graveyard.

Leaving Bergen that evening we reached Christiania the next morning early, and left two men to look out for our stores, which had not been sent with us but had gone by boat to Christiania.

We saw nothing of the capital or of Stockholm, but proceeded directly north to Haparanda, which is situated at the head of the gulf of Bothnia, in Sweden. There was a very marked difference in the attitude of the Norwegians and the Swedes. The first were most friendly and obviously pro-ally; the latter were just as obviously pro-German – they invariably answered you in German if you spoke to any of them. They were firmly convinced at that time that Germany was winning the war, and as they were coining money from Germany they were well content that that should be so.

In those days there was no communication between Haparanda and Torneo, on the Russian frontier – everything had to be carried by sleigh over the river between the two towns. Now the railways are linked up. There were so many stores stacked at Haparanda that the leisurely Swedes would have taken months to cart them across, as their interests were anywhere but with the Russians. I should think that a good deal was still upon the Swedish side of the frontier. However, we got across at once, and owing to the kindly offices of the English Consul we had no trouble with our baggage. From Torneo we got in a train and went south through Finland to Helsingfors, and on to Petrograd. Here we stayed three nights. The morale of the town and the townspeople then struck us all as very bad – they had had enough of the war. The Guards had made a big attack and been terribly cut up in the usual Russian fashion, and as most of them came from the capital, there was great depression on all sides. There was not the spirit in Petrograd that we had left in London. This was not to be wondered at considering, but Russian policy and Russian psychology are not things I can enter into here, or I should never get to the hospital and Rumania. We left Petrograd in a special train for Iassy, and had only one change – at Kiev – all the way. The carriages were very comfortable, with excellent sleeping arrangements – only two in a coupe – a splendid restaurant car, and an excellent cuisine. The Russian carriages are larger than ours, as the gauge is broader. We travelled down with some members of the Anglo-Russian hospital who were going to Galicia, where they had a field hospital. As some of these could talk Russian they were a great help to us. We left them at Kiev.

We got no news of course, but as we approached the Pruth – the boundary river between Russia and Rumania – we began to hear uneasy rumours. After we got into Rumania we heard that the Huns were across the Danube and advancing on Bucharest. When we got to Iassy, which is just 17 kilometres over the border, we had orders to get out and await further instructions. Our hospital was to have been in the new Military Club, at Bucharest, and had been prepared for us on a lavish scale under the direction of Lady Barclay, the wife of the English Minister to Rumania. We began to suspect that we would never see the Military Club; the lack of organisation around us was not reassuring at the moment.

We were put up at different places in the town – the nurses at a hospital – the men at a hotel – while we were separated among the different English residents of the town. My brother and I were together in the house of a Mr. Hould, who was a very well-known shot and sportsman. He gave us all the local news, and also told very much what we might expect to find in the country, as he had lived there practically all his life and knew the people well.

Directly after we arrived there came the victory of the Rumanians to the south of Bucharest, a victory which should have had a decisive effect and thrown the whole Hun and Bulgar Army into the Danube, but a victory, which unfortunately for our hopes, was turned into a defeat by treachery and incompetence. A few days later the General responsible was degraded before all the troops in the town, his sword broken, his epaulets removed, and his spurs hacked off, and marched away by common soldiers to penal servitude. I did not go and see the spectacle.

After this there was a wild panic. The inhabitants fled in thousands from Bucharest they saw the game was up and the only town they could come to was Iassy. Now Iassy is a small backwater of a town, once important and the capital of Moldavia, but since the Russians occupation of Bessarabia and the virtual shutting of the frontier, it has gradually sunk and gone to sleep. It had a rude awakening. It suddenly found itself the capital. And before it could open its eyes properly the whole Government descended upon it, with the military headquarters of, not only its own army, but that of the Russians as well. Then, before it had recovered the shock it was literally snowed under with refugees flying from the Hun. It did not recover for months. How could it? In peacetime the population was about 65,000 people; in less than three weeks it was increased by 100,000 people, and in six weeks time there were close on 200,000 souls in the town. Not only were the houses packed, but think of the buildings needed for the Government offices and the staffs of the armies. In this country we know how the Government has commandeered the houses and large hotels right and left. Poor Iassy only had two decent hotels – very third class they would be in this country. I can hardly go into the complications that arose. There was very little to be bought in the town to begin with. With the stream of people arriving in mid-winter with nothing but what they stood up in, you can well imagine that in three weeks there was nothing more to buy in any shape or form. Food, of course, was not to be thought of. The difficulty of feeding this mass was, of course, immense, and to begin with hardly any pretence was made to do it.

But I must get back to where I was – living in the house of Mr. Hould. I was just going to bed one evening, a few days after I got there, when the bell rang, and Mr. Hould went to the door, and I heard English voices insisting on coming in, and found Mr. Hould humming and hawing in a very constrained manner, but nevertheless giving way.

A lady and gentleman entered and being in pyjamas I disappeared behind the door, thinking it was the usual refugee demanding a room. I was in the only one available. However I soon found out it was Sir George and Lady Barclay, the Minister and his wife, who were seeking where to go, for the lack of organisation was such that the authorities could not even find a place for the diplomatic corps. I emerged and introduced myself – I had letters of introduction to Lady Barclay – and offered them my room. Mr. Hould had another room, though it was not warmed, so we were all right. Sir George and Lady Barclay had nowhere to go, and it was some days before a house could be put at their disposal for a legation. We became very good friends, and Lady Barclay did everything for us later, but I think that at the time, if I had been the sweep and had a room to spare, they would have been very glad to see me. The next day we explained to Lady Barclay our position, for we had arrived, but our baggage had not come with us; we had left men at Christiania to see about it, and we had heard that it had reached Petrograd. But further than that we had not heard, and owing to the evident congestion of the Russian railways, which were pouring troops into Rumania, it was not likely that we would receive it for some time. As a matter of fact a good deal of it did not turn up till six months later. I might explain here that practically all the Russian railways are single lines, just like you have in the highlands and other out-of-the-way places, and therefore the number of trains a day is very limited.

Lady Barclay being an exceedingly energetic woman, set to work at once to buy equipment sufficient to enable us to start a hospital. This was no easy matter, if what I have already said with regard to the shops is taken into account, but by starting at once we were able to buy things before the shops were all sold out. In ten days hard work we had got a minimum, and Lady Barclay was expecting some stores to be sent out to her from the Red Cross, which should arrive very shortly, as they had started long before ours had. I might explain that Lady Barclay was the head of the English Red Cross in Rumania, and chief of the committee which looked after the sending of parcels and stores to the English and Serbian prisoners in Bulgaria. In the meanwhile we had been presented to the Royal Family, and the Queen was impatiently awaiting the time when she might place a hospital at our disposal. In the meantime, also, my brother and the nurses were all working at one of the overcrowded hospitals in Iassy – a hospital with some 500 wounded and one lady doctor to look after the lot.

When we were ready the Queen sent for my brother and myself and asked us to go to Roman and look at and report on the hospital there. We left with the matron the same night and arrived after some sixteen hours journey, where we were met by the Chief of Police and housed very comfortably. This had all been arranged for by the Queen, who had taken the trouble to motor over personally and arrange matters for us. Roman was a small town some 80 kilometres due west of Iassy, and the chief town of the district round about. The main road to the towns along the frontier from Iassy passed through Roman, and the railway divided into two just north of the town of Pascani, one branch going to Iassy and the other to the north of Rumania. It was therefore an ideal situation for a base hospital.

The hospital in the town was a big stone building, much too large for the town and the district. It only had some 60 beds in peace time, but was originally built for 400. It was well planned and fairly modern, and under the direction of the St. Spiridon, which is the large charitable society of Rumania, something like our King Edward's Hospital Fund. We had a good look at the place and came to the conclusion that with a few additions it could be made a first-class hospital for 600 beds, that with a good many additions – for it had a large amount of open ground around it – it could be made to accommodate twice that number. We returned to Iassy, and made our report, and were offered half the hospital, which we accepted with alacrity, for hospitals were badly wanted, and there was something like 700 cases in the Roman hospital and only one surgeon who did, or attempted to do, all the work – an obvious impossibility. Some difficulties were raised by our chief, but eventually we returned to Roman with all the sisters and some of the orderlies. We took over the hospital and started work.

Luckily we had some stores with us, as we could not get many things we were in need of at Iassy. We had chloroform for instance; when we got to

Roman there were only eight small two-ounce phials of chloroform in the whole hospital, and they were only kept for the serious cases. We were able to give them plenty from our stores. We took a house for the nurses, who had no furniture at first and had to sleep in their camp equipment. I am afraid they were very uncomfortable for a time until we were able to collect things for them.

Naturally the work was very hard at first. We had 300 patients with about 180 beds; they were two in a bed, three in two beds placed close together, and many on the floor. We had an operating room, but only one old wooden table; no tables for dressings, and had to be most economical of dressing material; we had reels of cotton for ligatures, and many instruments such as aneurysm needles came out of our pocket cases.

In the middle of this rush misfortune came upon us. One of our surgeons who had come out after us and reached Iassy after we had left, became ill at once, and was sent to Odessa to recover. He later had to go home without ever having been to Roman. Our chief had remained in Iassy all the time. He was an old general practitioner from the Colonies; he knew nothing of a modern hospital, still less of a military one, never having seen any service of any kind. He might have past muster at Bucharest, where everything would have been found for him, but he was too old to rough it, and knew nothing of hospital work where everything had to be improvised or made upon the spot. He decided to go home. Unfortunately for us he took home with him all our orderlies except two.

All this time, too, the Germans were advancing, and the evacuation of all the towns even Iassy was being talked of, chiefly, I thought, by those who were foolish. How we were to get out if they did come was very difficult to see, as we had no motor. But the nurses were very plucky about it, and we held on grimly and prayed for the cold, which was the only thing that could stop the advance. The winter had been so far a very open one, but luckily the snow and frost came in January and when it did come, it came with a vengeance. It was the severest winter known there for many years. The fighting stopped like magic, as everyone went underground to escape the cold. The stream of wounded came to an end, and we had a pause in the work and were able to get even with all the arrears. The pause, however, was not for long. For almost at once the wounded were replaced by the sick. Owing to the huddling which took place on account of the cold, and the prevalence of lice, typhus and relapsing fever blazed out from one end of the land to the other. What this epidemic cost the country in lives will probably never be known. The country rapidly fell into a worse state even of that in Serbia during a similar epidemic earlier in the war. The Rumanian doctors either did not understand or would not recognise the cause of the epidemic, namely lice, and that if you wished to escape you had to kill the lice which carried the infection. This want of recognition on their part cost them dear, for they lost over 150 doctors who died of the disease. One of the first things we did was to build a large disinfector in which we could bake everything in the hospital. Before that was ready we borrowed the mobile disinfector from the Russians, which was kindly placed at our disposal by Colonel Iliine, chief of the Russian Red Cross at Roman. We had very funny experiences using this, as when you disinfect a hospital, you must pass everything through the disinfector that is capable of harbouring lice. Failure to do this thoroughly will only result in re-infection of the sterilised articles from those which are not sterilised. The wardmaids had the greatest objection at first to having their belongings sterilised, and wept like anything when we insisted. However, insist we did. We also got rid of the sentries which were placed over the prisoners who were wounded in the hospital. These were changed daily, and all had lice, and were therefore dispensed with amid grave head-shakings from the wise. But where a prisoner, wounded and with no clothes was likely to run to in mid-winter, was more then they could explain. As the result of our efforts, although we had many cases of typhus admitted to the hospital, we never had a single one of our staff go down with the disease. Another matter which needed strict supervision was the admission of the patients – their bathing, shaving and petroling. This was, or was not, done as convenient when we got there first, and we had to be very strict and see everything ourselves until we had got the men trained to do it. The great fault we rapidly found in Rumania was that excellent orders might be issued, but no one ever saw that they were carried out – hence the failure in very many cases. "Oh, I have given orders," became a stock phrase with us, and we rapidly learned its value and went and saw the man to whom the orders had been given, and told him to report to us when the orders had been carried out. It was the only way to do things, or get them done.

Throughout the whole epidemic there was one person who worked unremittingly, and that was the Queen. She visited the fever hospitals – and all hospitals – day after day, consoling the sick and seeing after their comfort. She always arrived with little presents, such as small icons – beloved of the Greek Church – picture post-cards, sweets which the men loved as sugar was so scarce and the food none too good, and what the men appreciated more than anything – cigarettes, for the Rumanian, even if dying, loves to smoke a cigarette. The Queen always insisted on visiting every ward and speaking to every soldier in it. The men would all shout out in chorus as she came in, "Striets" (it sounded like that), which is the military greeting of a soldier to an officer in Rumania, and each would kiss her hand as she gave him his present. The Rumanian soldier had no luxuries, few comforts, and little attention, as we understand hospital attention in this country, but what he did get was very largely due to the fact that the Queen would from time to time visit his hospital and see that he was properly cared for. She paid three separate visits to our hospital. It is small wonder that the peasants in Rumania absolutely adore their Queen above all their Royal family, though they are devoted to their King and Crown Prince. During the earlier months of the year the morale of the people sank very low. They were beaten, many of them, and had not the heart to stand up to it. "We want peace," "Give us peace," many of them said to me, little dreaming what that peace would mean. "The war must now end," others said, "as we are beaten." You hear the same cry in Russia to-day, and for the same reason. Unfortunately they had entered the war firmly convinced that they had only to march to decide the whole issue and end the war. There is no doubt that many of them held that view, and then when black misfortune and horrible catastrophe overtook them, they could hardly hold up their heads. Russia they hated by tradition – and with reason. The French and the English, both of whom they liked well, were too far off to help them. The French, indeed, sent a very strong military mission which worked wonders training their army, but its effects had not then begun to appear.

It was the firm attitude taken by the Court and Government which kept the country together, and allowed them to tide over their misfortunes. For tide them over they did, and six months later they were a different people again, proud and confident, longing to attack, and the Germans learned to their surprise and cost at Maresesti the metal that the Rumanian soldier was made of. I do not know a soldier in Europe who takes kindlier to training, or fights better on less food, than a Rumanian peasant. After the manner of all peasants he hates shelling, and cannot understand the game. He will tolerate the rifle in his own hands, and that is about all. What he loves is the bayonet, and with that there are few men who are his equal.

With the advent of spring there was another pause in the heavy work. We were now able to push on the buildings that had already been started, to commence new ones, and repaint the wards which needed it sadly. We built a dining room able to sit about 300 wounded men, a long corridor which linked up all the wards, at the same time turning the internal corridor into a large ward. A light railway was run around the hospital, the Belgian manager of the sugar factory kindly lending us the rails. Open-air wards were also started to be ready for the summer. The drains and the water supply both had to be overhauled by us, so that by now, in addition to being a bad surgeon, I am a good architect and a passable engineer. At a later date a large concrete swimming bath was made in the open air, as the summer in Rumania is oppressively hot, and the water supply of the hospital was none too good. At the same time the carpenter we had with us superintended the making of everything necessary for the internal working of the hospital, assisted by the convalescent patients. There is no doubt that the Rumanians are clever carpenters. You had only to show them what you wanted and they would turn out heaps of them for you. The only difficulty was the wood; this was very scarce, as all was taken for building barracks and hospitals all over the country. The rate that some of these were run up was simply astonishing. We made then in the hospital, tables, operating tables, and wooden clogs for all the patients, for we had no slippers. We also made a complete set of machines in wood for easing stiff joints, and these were superintended by our masseuse, Miss Hyde. All these things were for the fitting up of the hospital, but we also turned out good splints of all sorts for the individual patients who were specially measured for them. This was a very great advantage for us, for I never saw a place where the individual treatment of fractures was more neglected. It is hardly too much to say that in the hands of most Rumanian surgeons, especially those in Roman, 90 to 95 per cent of fractured femurs died. This was simply due to the way they had of treating them. I never saw an extension apparatus applied by a Rumanian; even the old fashioned long splints were unknown. They used a wire splint that came up to the site of the fracture, but in a high fracture could not go any higher. The case was dressed every day and for that was taken to the dressing room on a stretcher, taken off the stretcher, and put on the table, dressed, put back on the stretcher, and then put to bed, having been lifted four separate times by orderlies for the most part quite untrained. It was only a question of time when death put a happy end to his sufferings. We took in every fractured femur we could get, and had special wards with Balkan splints and extensions, other wards with double inclined planes etc., all made upon the premises. These cases were of course never moved, and were all dressed in bed.

The nursing of cases was a great difficulty, as our English sisters were all so occupied in the theatres and dressing-rooms that they had little time to supervise this. The Rumanian and the Russian sisters, though very good and willing, were quite untrained as we understand the word training. They would help at the dressings and do this very well, but they never understood nursing or war work and never attempted it, with very few exceptions, and sore backs were a perfect plague. We opened a school for nurses and trained them, but were not very successful.

Any amount of doctors used to come and look round our hospital, and would praise everything they saw, and they used to see a great deal that was new, as we had demonstration brick sterilisers and destructors etc., always going. But I never heard of them copying even the simpler appliances, either because they knew better or were quite contented with their old-fashioned ways, or from lack of initiative. It seems rather bumptious of me speaking of other people as old-fashioned, but you must remember they live still in the cupping age. They cup for everything – a pain in the back, a pain in the tummy, even a vague pain in the limb, all are cured by cupping. How many of you, may I ask, have ever seen a cup applied, or know how to do it? The French sent a strong party of doctors out to Rumania, and I met a great many very able men there and learned a lot of the methods they use in France. They even sent a specialist in the Carrel method, together with his assistants to show the method. This specialist left the country after six months, the only hospitals then using it were his own and ours. No one took it up till they found that the French were using it almost universally as they got their hospitals in order.

But if the upper class were slow to learn, the same could not be said of the peasant. He was anxious to learn – a lazy beggar, naturally, if you let him alone, but if he knew you were always around seeing after things, he worked; if he did not, we got rid of him so that in the end we had a first-class team. I remember one man who knew no carpentering at all when we went there, and used to annoy me by assisting me when I was trying to do some. He was invariable wrong with everything at first. That man built me a barrack to sleep 100 orderlies before I left. Of course he had others under him, but he checked the wood and an engineer showed him the plans and what he wanted, and he did the rest.

The peasant class too were very childlike. They loved to dance to any gypsy fiddler that came by, simple country dances which if you watched for a moment you could join in quite well, and we had a great deal of fun with them. Another point with them was their love of colour – they adored anything bright. We had a lot of flannel coats sent out to us of all colours. The drab colours we gave away to other hospitals, but the coloured ones we kept. Some were bright red brilliant. These were considered very grand, and were only conferred as a mark of merit. They were kept, too, for State occasions, such as visits from the Queen, Royal family, or generals. Any misbehaviour forfeited the jacket, and that was a great disgrace. Those who had them would try and sleep in it, as the others would steal it when they were asleep, for the Rumanian peasant is an inveterate and utterly unrepentant thief. You could catch him red-handed, but it made no difference, he was never in the least ashamed of it. Out of the various other colours we made liveries of different grades. The barbers and some of the chief orderlies had light-blue with dark-blue facings. There were two men, one to each corridor, who did nothing but search the men for lice. They went by the high-sounding title of "Chasseur des poux"; they were resplendent in purple coats. The gardeners and outdoor workers wore pink. The colours never went together, but that did not matter; the more they were, and the more varied they were, the better; and they gave a very cheery aspect to the hospital, and a hospital needs that touch to brighten it.

After a bit we were offered the whole hospital. This we did not really want, but the difficulties of dual control had become intolerable. We had very strict discipline in our half, and the Romanian half had none. There were therefore continual bickerings over nothing. Jealousy, no doubt, was at the bottom of it all, and it ended in some of the authorities of the other half doing all in their power to counteract any efforts on our part. It was all very petty, but we felt that if the hospital was to be a success we would have to take over the whole. This we did after a lot of bother, in which the authorities said they would, and then they said they would not, give it to us. To all this we remained utterly indifferent until it was really given us. We had made all our preparations for taking it over beforehand, as we knew that a big offensive was imminent. As a matter of fact it had begun when we took it over finally, and we had to take it over with the wounded pouring in on top of us. This made it very awkward for us, and I am afraid we had to be very unceremonious with them in the end as they wished to clear out very gradually. But as their hospital was all ready we had to insist on their going at once.

The offensive had been looked forward to by the whole nation. They knew they were ready, the new army was thoroughly trained in the latest French methods, well armed and well equipped with machine guns and artillery. Great and careful preparations had been made, and we had lived on tenterhooks for some weeks knowing that it was coming off. The nightly crop of rumours came in – then at last it had commenced, really this time, and for sure. The Rumanians went forward with a rush. Re-enforcements were hurried down from the interior of Germany and terrific attacks were made by the best Bavarian divisions. They were all crumpled up by the Rumanian peasant, who felt at last he was getting something of his own back. The Rumanian casualties were, of course, severe, but those of the Germans were infinitely more so. There is no doubt that the Rumanians would have taken back their beloved capital if disaster had not occurred elsewhere, and that through no fault of their own. The Russian army in the north in Bukovina had ever since the revolution been in an utter state of indiscipline. What started the panic no one ever knew. Some say they saw the Germans changing the trench guards and thought they were re-inforcing the trenches prior to an attack. Others say that the Russians just got the jumps and bolted. In any case, bolt they did and left everything behind them guns, ammunition, bridges, food, forage, all were left intact. It was the retreat from Tarnpool. There was no fighting – they merely ran, aimlessly and without any knowledge. The Germans could not follow quickly enough to catch them; they put men on motor cycles and cyclists who could speak Russian to follow them, and whenever they stopped these men shouted out that the Germans were on them, and off the Russians would start again. The retreat came to an end when the draft horses of the Germans were quite worn out. I have spoken with men of the armoured cars who were there. They told me they used to go back and search for the Germans 15 and 20 miles behind the Russians and often not find any. The Cossacks tried to stem the rush, but quite in vain. They crucified the motor-cycle Germans when they caught them. The Rumanian offensive stopped at once. It looked as if the Germans would march straight upon Kishinef and Bender, cut the railway and isolate the whole of Rumania. Rumanian troops were drafted to the front at once, and they had no more reserves. The small Rumanian army only held about a third of their frontier, the other two thirds were held by the Russians, both north and south. After this I think we all saw that even for defensive operations the Russian army did not even exist. No orders could be given, but they had to be edited by the committee of illiterate soldiers. No committee could justify its existence unless it altered all the arrangements already made. Staff work became impossible and even regimental work came to an end, for the men no longer obeyed any orders and there were no battalions to be relied upon to put down any mutiny.

Fraternisation was rife all along the front. Schools of propaganda were opened by the Germans, and all men who could speak Russian were sent to them, and when ready were pushed across to the Russian lines. The poor illiterate noujik listened to them and believed them, when they said we are now all brothers, now let us have peace and live together like friends; it is only the capitalist of England and France who are making the war. Capitalist became a stock word among the Russian soldier, who did not know what the word meant. No annexations or indemnities were offered and accepted freely by both sides. Why should the Russians remain? they were asked. They only had to kill a few officers who were in favour of the war, and then they could go home. In many cases they did this. The rot gradually spread until the German got the Russians where they wanted them, and now they are enjoying their peace without annexations or indemnities. Poor deluded fools. But I am running on and am nowhere near the hospital.

During the offensive we had a very severe time for about six weeks. No slightly wounded were sent to us, only the severe cases, and the lighter ones of these were sent on as soon as possible, so we always had a stream of wounded coming in. Luckily we had two motor ambulances now instead of one, and they worked all day and half the night, for they were the only two motor ambulances in the town, and we used them for all the hospitals. Luckily there was a very good French doctor who did duty at the station. He was a very great friend of ours, and used to let us know when to expect the cases in. He also used to send us everything he thought interesting in a surgical way.

Our personnel was curious, for in addition to the English we had many Rumanian nurses. One especially who was over the others – Madame Mazere – was conspicuously helpful, and did everything possible – and that was a good deal – for us all the time we were there. Poor thing, she got into awful hot water with the jealous ones of the Rumanian Red Cross for doing it, and they even took away her Red Cross card for some time. But we got it back for her, but not without a good deal of trouble. Then we had nine Russian sisters and a number of Russian sanitars, who varied in number from twelve to sixteen, according as they got into disgrace for mutinous conduct, and were sent away. I may add that we had many stores of food, cigarettes etc., from home, and used to give these out to the sanitars and patients, so that we were very much better off than any other hospital. The Russians did not like being sent away as there was no food or tobacco to be bought in the town. After the revolution they thought they were going to have their own way, as in other hospitals. They very soon found their mistake, and three were sacked the next day. They all paraded to say that if these three went then they would all go. The Russian sisters were terror stricken. I told them they could go somewhere warm and stay there. In any case the three I said were going should go, and if the others wish they could go too. The three went, but no inclination was evinced by the others to follow them. It is only fair to say that that was the only time I had any trouble with them, and having found their master they were quite contented that it should be so. They always worked very well and very willingly, and later, when we went, they all came and asked to be allowed to come with us to the new hospital. In their own hospital the sanitars did exactly as they liked. If they disliked an officer they would tie him up for the night and demand his dismissal next day, and the doctor would go. All Russian officers were afraid of their men. There were two French doctors who worked with us, one had duties at the station as well, and the other helped with the X-ray work, of which we had a lot, as we were the only hospital in the town where there was an X-ray apparatus. We also had about ten Serbian orderlies, very good well set up men, always smiling. They had been in another English hospital previously to coming to us. The bulk of our orderlies or sanitars as they were called were, of course, Rumanians, usually old men of the militia class. They did very well when they were trained, but knew nothing when they came. Then we had prisoners, both German and Austrian. Only one German was any good, and him we kept for months. He was a carpenter, but was always working, and, what was more, he saw that the other men worked too.

After the offensive was over we had another pause, though wounded were constantly coming in from the more advanced hospitals, which were being evacuated in readiness for the next push. In September we found that we were going to lose all our English nursing sisters, and do what we could we could not induce the British Red Cross to send us out any to replace them. We were told that it was very dangerous for women to be sent out to Russia. This view was largely due to the Petrograd reports portraying disorder and bloodshed. It may have been also due to the accounts given in this country by people who returned and told tall stories with a view to enhancing their supposed dangers.

I have travelled about extensively in Russia since the revolution, and met Englishmen from all parts. They were unanimous in saying that they never heard of an Englishman, much less an English woman, insulted throughout the country. One Englishman was robbed in the dark by hooligans in Petrograd, but when they held him up they had not the slightest idea who he was. Anyway, it was very dangerous to be in Russia; England said so, and, of course, England knew. The Scottish women, on the other hand, renewed their staff without any difficulty, a fact which rather annoyed us. We then had to consider what we should do with the hospital. We invited Dr Clemow's hospital, whom we had heard had very little to do down near the Dobrouja, to come and assist us, but they refused on account of the stress of work. We could not carry on without our English staff and keep the hospital up to the position it held before they departed, so we reluctantly decided to give it up. Just at this time the American mission arrived in the country without any stores at all, without even surgical instruments. They refused to lend us their nurses, so we decided to give them over the hospital as it stood. I am afraid we got very little thanks for our very generous action, for after they took it over they at once assumed that they had made it. They did things on the true Transatlantic style, with a reporter and pars in all the papers for everything, and their beautiful hospital was soon famed throughout Rumania. We had had one poor little par in the papers all the time we had been there. However, they were very nice men, and we got on with them very well.

General Averescu, the Commandant of the Second Army, heard we might all be going home, and very kindly asked my brother and myself to stop on with as many of the staff as were willing to remain, and take over a small hospital nearer the Front under him. To this we gladly assented, for Rumania was in a bad way, and we did not like to seem to be deserting the sinking ship. While we decided on a new hospital we went to Piatra, and stayed at the French convalescent home at that town, where the French were most hospitable to us. There we found a good many French officers who had been in our hospital, and had been sent on to convalescence there. There was some difficulty in fixing on a locality for the new hospital but at last one was found and General Averescu came down with his chief medical officer and gave orders for us to have everything we wanted. The new buildings necessary were just begun, when we were all recalled to England.

We went off to Petrograd from where I was sent to Archangel, and my brother and the matron went down to Odessa, again to join Lady Muriel Paget, who was trying to do something to help the Eukrainist movement. I have not seen my brother since, but heard that he had a hospital in Kiev during the Bolshevik attack on the town, and that he got two shells into his house. He eventually left with Lady Muriel Paget and a large party which included a third brother, who was out there, for Vladivostock, and is not home yet. We very nearly went out by Canada, but none of us thought we should make the round tour of the world in order to get back again. My experiences in Archangel were really most interesting. It was mid-winter, and the sun only came up for about three hours in the day, but the snow reflected the light so that it was not really dark till sometime after the sun had gone down. The cold, however, was too awful for anything. Luckily I had got a pair of aviator boots in Petrograd, long leather boots lined with sheep skin. I also had a good fur-lined overcoat and a fur hat, so was not badly off. I expected to be there a week, and only took kit for that time. Delay after delay took place, and I was there for two months. I went there for the Rumanian stores and tried to take down a trainload of herrings. I had just got the train arranged for when Rumania entered Bessarabia, and the Russians declared war and refused to let the goods pass. So all my efforts were for nothing. I returned to Petrograd to find everyone expecting the arrival of the Germans. Even the dates were given for their entry. I never believed they would come till the late spring, as there was no reason why they should. They had bought the Government and got all they wanted, and if they came they would have had to police and regulate the city. In addition to which they would have had to organise the food supply, a thing which was next to impossible without occupying a large amount of territory in which to collect the food. I did not think they could spare sufficient men, and thought they would concentrate on the Ukraine, where the wheat was grown, and collect what they could there for the benefit of Germany rather than the benefit of Petrograd. This view has proved correct, though no one listened at the time. Still, Petrograd is no place to stay for pleasure. Food was expensive beyond belief. A tin of sardines was 12 roubles, an apple was 6 roubles. Bread, largely made up with straw, was issued at an eighth of a Russian pound – about 1½ ounces a day for each individual. On the other hand, you could get what you liked if you paid the price. But the banks were shut and you could not get money. No one paid any money into the banks, which were in the hands of the Bolsheviks and guarded by sailors. The money in the banks rapidly came to an end.

In my efforts to get out I gave my passport into the Embassy to go for signature and theirs. Knowing the businesslike ways of the Embassy I haunted the door for the next two days, and prayed them not to take mine away if they left suddenly. They went, and my passport was never seen again. This prevented me from leaving with a large party of English who went off next day, and to my great disgust I found myself left behind. That party were all caught on the Aland Isles by the Germans and taken to Danzig and imprisoned. I came to the conclusion that there were worse faults than having an unbusinesslike Embassy. I had to stay in Petrograd three weeks getting a new passport, and left eventually by the Monmansk railway, which runs up past the Artic (sic) circle to the ice free fiord of Kola. It was a two days trip, but we were told to take provisions for a fortnight. We took a week. We were slowed up constantly, and the train had to be broken up to get through, and then we would be left for a day while the engine went back for the other portions of the train. I had a coupe for two, we were seven in it. Two of the men however went and bribed the guard for his compartment, for since the revolution the guard on each carriage has taken one of the compartments for himself. We were therefore only three in the coupe, and very comfortable. Some of the men were in a closed truck for merchandise, and were very badly off, as they had no fire. However we got a stove put in for them at Petrosavodski, and they were more comfortable. Some people who were not so important as we were, for we had a fair sprinkling of officers, and what was more important newspaper correspondents – took more than three weeks over the journey, and as they were all in ordinary trucks, you can imagine their discomfort in the cold of the Artic (sic) regions.

However, I reached home the last of our hospital, after having had a very enjoyable and most interesting seventeen months.

(This is an extraordinary letter from an extraordinary man. He faced untold hardships, starting with his journey from Newcastle to Iassy and Roman, through Norway, Sweden, Finland and then via Petrograd, intermittently without his luggage. This journey was made possible with the help of the Red Cross and various diplomats. He appears to have been a man of immense courage and determination, but also autocratic. Hospitals often had no adequate equipment or sanitation, but he turned his hand to design, carpentry and engineering. He was strong-minded and confident. Surgically he operated with a deficiency of instruments, and though a surgeon, despite lack of drugs, coped with patients medically sick with typhus and relapsing fever. He had an insight into human strengths and weaknesses and carefully handled the aftermath of the Russian revolution with the change in the behaviour of the Russian personnel. A possible weakness may have been an insensitivity to danger. He dismisses the dangers to English nurses in Rumania in the midst of battles, revolution and mutiny.

A strong thread that runs through this letter is that David Fitzwilliams was a born leader.

He qualified in Edinburgh in 1902 and immediately served in the Boer War obtaining the Queen's Medal with four clasps. He returned to Edinburgh and obtained his M.D. and then his F.R.C.S. in 1906. Three years later he was appointed Surgeon to Out-Patients at St Mary's Hospital and also at Paddington Green Children's Hospital and Mount Vernon Hospital. During his time in the war of 1914–18, he served with the Russian Expeditionary Force and was twice mentioned in dispatches and created a C.M.G. in 1919. He also held a number of Russian and Rumanian Crown Honours. He wrote a number of text books, the most famous being *Radium and Cancer*. He was associated with St Mary's for forty-five years and following retirement lived in Jersey until he died in 1956 at the age of seventy-five. John Crawford Adams, now aged ninety-two, the celebrated St Mary's Orthopaedic Surgeon served as his House Surgeon after qualification.)

CHAPTER 21

With the Scottish Women's Hospital

By F.E. Rendel

I joined the Russian Unit of the Scottish Women's Hospital at the end of August 1916. We sailed from Liverpool to Archangel in a boat captured from the Austrians early in the war. From Archangel we went in a special train to Odessa, and from Odessa we were sent on to the Dobruja. This railway journey, exclusive of the time we spent in Odessa, took us just over a fortnight. The train crawled along so slowly that we could jump out and run by the side. Often when the track lay by the side of a road we saw the lucky people in carriages go driving past us.

Soon after we arrived in the Dobruja our unit was divided into two. One became a base hospital about ten miles behind the lines, the other, the one to which I was attached, was sent up nearer the front as a field hospital. This was in Southern Roumania in the first week of October. It was even then becoming obvious that things were not going well.

We were in a little village called Bulbulwick, about three miles behind the enemy lines. Our hospital formed part of the field hospital for the first division of the Serbian Army. Our part of the show consisted of hospital tents and tents for the staff. The Serbian doctors had rooms in the village. The guns were very loud when we first put up our tents, and every day the noise became more ominous. At night the flashes of guns could be seen plainly and a great number of star shells. Enemy aeroplanes paid us frequent visits; they passed overhead on their way to Medjidia, an important railway town at our rear. Most of their bombs were reserved for the station in this town, but they could not resist the temptation of our new white tents, and we always had two or three bombs round about our camp.

Finally the Serbs persuaded us to paint our roofs. We spent a sweltering morning feverishly smearing the tents with pot. permang. and muddy water. That afternoon the guns sounded much closer; that night hundreds of wounded men found their way or were brought in ambulances, to our hospital, and the next morning, after evacuating our last patient, we received orders to strike our camp and retreat.

The Roumanian Army, without adequate guns, ill-fed, ill-clothed, and with ill-trained officers to lead them, had been pushed back by the Bulgars and Germans. The Serbian division had been left unsupported, and after a desperate fight, in which they fought with extreme courage, had been cut to pieces. Out of 20,000 men only 3,000 survived. Only a small percentage of the wounded could be rescued, so hurried was the retreat. The majority of those left behind killed themselves rather than fall into the hands of the Bulgars.

During the following ten days we sat on the hospital carts by day and most of the night and jogged along the country roads in the rear of the retreating armies. The whole countryside was being deserted. We were in a stream of refugees stretching endlessly in every direction. The road was lined four or five deep with tumbledown carts filled with miserable women and children and all their worldly goods. They clung to the most ridiculous rubbish – broken chairs, china ornaments, dirty old clothes, anything they had. The noise was deafening. The peasants shouted and swore and wept. In one cart, beside which we drove for several days, a woman and three small children sat huddled in one corner. In the middle of the cart, lying comfortably on a heap of pillows, lay a fat white sow. Another cart was distinguished for a time by a cock perched on the top of a pile of luggage. One day when food was running short the poor bird disappeared into the family stew-pot. Mixed up with these miserable peasants were the remnants of the army.

Long trains of gun-carriages went past, scattered columns of infantry plodded along. Roumanian officers drove through the crowd at a furious pace regardless of anyone and yelling to their horses to go faster. Our party consisted of three nurses, four "V.A.D.'s," the doctor in charge and myself.

Luckily for everyone the weather was fine on the whole, but at night it was very cold. We had our mess tent with us and in this we slept. Our personal luggage was limited to a haversack each and a "bed-bundle," which contained a rug, a blanket and a few odds and ends. Our tents, camp-beds, and kit-bags, and most of our stores had been sent back to Medjidia at the first sign of trouble.

Food was sometimes a little scarce. We were given army rations of sugar, tea and meat, but we had no time to cook the meat. Sometimes we were on the move all day until 11.30 p.m., and were then too sleepy to wait for a hot meal. During the day we had ship's biscuits, mouldy bread, lumps of sugar and a certain amount of tinned meat. There was no butter and milk, of course, was unobtainable.

Life was made interesting at this time by the alarmist rumours which were always being circulated. We were told that the Bulgars were on our heels, that no one knew the right road, that there were no bridges across the Danube at the place we were making for etc., etc. But all this came to an end only too soon.

In six days we were across the Danube and in Russia and safety, and four days later our wanderings were over. Then came a long and weary time of waiting. We had a hospital for the Serbs who were now in reserve. Later we were moved to Odessa and given a hospital for Russians. Not till the end of March, just after the revolution, were we sent back to the front.

Our unit was at this time rather larger. A second doctor joined us, we had a matron, eight nurses, a secretary and a cook. The Russian Red Cross provided us with 50 horses, 50 Serbian orderlies, 25 carts and an officer to look after the men and buy our hospital supplies for us.

We were under orders to go to Tecuci, a small Roumanian town about three miles behind the lines occupied by Russian troops.

The journey was a nightmare. We were crowded and cold and dirty. Our way lay through Iassy, where we were held up for some days. Iassy was in a miserable state.

The people looked and were actually starving. There was no food to be had in the town. We tried to get a meal in the most prosperous looking of the restaurants open.

On reading the menu my hopes were raised. There were several courses and the dishes sounded most appetising. We ordered soup, cutlets and a salad. Alas, the soup consisted of a few beans floating in water. The cutlets were beans mashed together in a paste, the salad was beans covered with a little salad oil and vinegar.

There was no bread to be had, and we couldn't even get a cup of tea.

The station, in which our train was stuck for three days, was full of hospital trains from the front. Everything in these trains was flung out of the window on to the ground or platform. Old dressings, filthy rags, amputated limbs, every sort of horror lay about the place. We had to lay down planks from our train some yards in length to avoid wading ankle deep in slush and refuse. The inhabitants of Iassy were not only starving, they were riddled with typhus. So was Tecuci, where we at last found ourselves.

Tecuci in peace time must be a dreary enough spot. When we arrived it was incredibly forlorn, dirty and smelly. Dead horses and dogs lay about, the shops were shut or half empty, and the place was full of sick people. There were six typhus hospitals crowded with patients. Men and women lay in the same wards, many of them on the floor. There were not enough doctors, no trained nurses, no soap, milk, or eggs. The patients were fed chiefly on maize porridge and tea. They were nursed by one or two untrained Roumanian girls who had volunteered their services, helped by two or three old crones who had had typhus. In one hospital I saw the worst cases were put in an underground room and more or less left to die there at their leisure. The typhus was chiefly among the Roumanians. The Russian soldiers were better fed and much cleaner on the whole.

While we were at Tecuci we had a hospital in two houses which had been turned into one. It was a tumbledown building with low, dark rooms and narrow inconvenient passages. We did our best with whitewash and soap and water and formalin, but the black beetles remained healthy and lively to the end. We ourselves lived in tents close at hand. It was a very comfortable life in spite of the hot weather. We had our very charming Serbian orderlies to wait on us. They made our beds, brought us hot water, cleaned our boots and waited at table.

Being Serbs they were unaffected by the revolution. The doctors and nurses in the Russian hospitals near us were not nearly so well off. Their orderlies struck work, many of them went away, and those who stayed were extremely insubordinate. One baking day in June some of us met a poor Russian sister toiling along the road carrying two heavy pails of water. Someone said to her "Why on earth don't you make your men carry that for you?" She said very gloomily, "Ah, you see, you have some discipline in your hospital; we daren't ask our Sanitars to do such a thing." On another occasion our Secretary was spending the night in a Red Cross hostel in Berlad, our nearest big town. At two o'clock in the morning a Russian orderly burst into her room and said, "In future you sisters will have exactly the same food as we men."

We had no trouble with our patients. On the whole they were most polite and well behaved and grateful. But when they were better, no matter how slightly they had been wounded, they all wanted to go to Odessa, and no one had the power to stop them. The military doctor in charge of the district merely shrugged his shoulders and said, "They must be humoured."

Our only excitement at Tecuci was aeroplanes. They used to come about 5 a.m. and again in the evening. There were three new English anti-aircraft guns quite close to our camp, and the noise every morning was very irritating. Once two of our Serbs were hit by pieces of bomb, and after that we had a dug out made elaborately roofed over with alternate layers of earth and iron.

In July we left Tecuci and were sent up much nearer the front to a little valley in the Carpathians. For two or three days we had a splendid time, as it was confidently believed that the Russians were really going to make a push. We were told to be prepared for plenty of work, and that we must dig trenches for ourselves and our patients, as the valley would certainly be shelled. This was an impossible order to carry out, as we had no spades or pickaxes, and not nearly enough men to do anything worth while. The order was sent out at four in the afternoon, and the shelling was due that night. Luckily for us and our patients the Russian attack was so unexpectedly successful that the Germans were pushed back over the crest of the hill commanding our valley before they had time to annoy us. The noise that night was deafening. Our camp was surrounded by 30 Russian batteries. They were on all sides of us, and the row was increased by the echoes from the hills. Two days later came the news of the Galician disaster, and the whole Russian line was held up. From that moment until we left Russia a few weeks later there was no more fighting. When the Germans advanced the Russians fell back. The much talked-of offensive was over.

We were moved up much nearer the front for a short time. Very soon after our arrival the Germans began plopping shells over our heads at the Russian battery opposite us. At last the shelling became so continuous that it was obvious we might fall into the hands of the Huns at any minute almost. There was only a low hill, a shallow river bed and a few Russian soldiers between us and them. The whole distance was under two miles.

So one dark night (the road was much too unhealthy by day), we packed up our goods, climbed into our wagons, and made off.

We heard afterwards that three days later, the Germans were in possession of what we always called "the happy valley."

This was the end of our adventures with the Russian Army; we were fated, it seemed, to end as we began, with a retreat.

Africa

The Germans had four colonies in Africa, Togoland, Cameroon, German South West Africa and German East Africa (now Tanzania).

The Union of South Africa with some British troops in support dealt quickly with German East Africa. The troops were led by General Botha who only fifteen years previously had been fighting the British in the Boer War.

May 31st 1915.
Carrier Section,
Base Hospital Duala
Dear Mr. Editor,
I have just received my April copy of the Gazette, and seeing in it that there was a temporary dearth of news from St. Mary's men at the Front, I am sending this short account of the operations in the Cameroons, West Africa. Also as far as I know at present, I am the only St. Mary's man here.

In this world wide war the greatest magnitude and importance of the events in the European struggle naturally mask and obscure the happenings in the more remote parts of the Empire. I may therefore be excused if I mention as a preliminary that the Cameroons is a German colony in West Africa situated immediately to the south of the British colony of Nigeria, and about three quarters the size of it. The Expeditionary Force, under the command of Brigadier-General Dobell consists of (1) Colonial troops from the British West African colonies Gambia, Sierra Leone, Gold Coast and

Nigeria; (2) French Colonial troops from Senegal, Dahomey, and Gaboon; (3) an Allied Naval force.

At the head of the medical side is the Director of the Allied Medical Services, a Lieut.-Colonel in the R.A.M.C.; there is also a Captain of the R.A.M.C. The rest of the medical staff consists of Medical Officers from the various West African colonies, the majority being members of the W.A.M.S., with colonial dressers and dispensers. The largest number of doctors present at one time has been 39; in addition there are 5 or 6 French doctors. At first we served as civilians, but at the beginning of May a step was taken which ought to have been taken seven months earlier – we were given temporary ranks; those who had been in colonial employ three years or more became Captains, the remainder Lieutenants.

The Expedition reached the Cameroons at the end of September, but I did not join until the end of November. The first step was to make a landing, and this was done at the Capital, Duala. Duala is situated on the Cameroon River about seven or eight miles from the mouth. There is here a bar with only a narrow navigable channel. This passage has been blocked by the sinking of vessels and barges, and inside this barrier the river has been mined. The first part was purely naval; the sunken ships were blown up by the "Dwarf", and then the mines were swept. They then proceeded up the river and shelled Duala, which very soon capitulated. The Base of the Expedition was made at Duala, and from here columns have gone out to attack the Germans. Except in a very few instances the Germans have only made a feeble resistance. The usual thing has been that, on the approach of a British column a short action takes place, and the Germans retire to another position further inland. Their policy seems to be not to fight and not to surrender, but to hang on as long as possible. The total British casualties (killed and wounded), officers and N.C.O's up to the end of April has been 23.

The main Base Hospital was also formed at Duala. We were very lucky in finding a very well made and equipped hospital waiting for us. It is only quite lately that extra wards have had to be erected, and I am still using bandages and cotton wool left by the Germans eight months ago. For the first two months one of the Elder Dempster's boats, the "Appam" was used as a hospital ship. The Base Hospital, which has now nearly six hundred in-patients, consists of three sections, the European hospital, the Native Soldiers' hospital, and the Carrier hospital The first two are again subdivided into English and French portions. There are about seven British Nursing Sisters from the various colonies, and five French Sisters of Mercy. The rest of the work is done by locally employed dressers, under the direction of dispensers and dressers from the various Colonial hospitals.

There are several points of difference between things out here and things in Europe. In the first place, Duala is the hottest place I have come across, while I read of frozen trenches. Here we are continually chasing the enemy, there they are all the time at close quarters. Again owing to the fact that the Germans have no artillery here, the wounds are those caused by rifle bullets, and the severer cases we read of in the base hospitals at home are rare. In addition to these, we have to treat the usual tropical diseases, as malaria, anaemia, blackwater fever, guinea worm, jiggers, and tropical ulcers. But perhaps the greatest difference lies in the transport arrangements. It is true that there are two German railways, which are used whenever possible, but still the main work of transport is done on the heads of carriers. With the Expedition came 6,000 carriers from the various West African Colonies. Each man gets about 1s.6d to 2s. per diem, and is expected to carry about 60 to 80 lbs., though this is often exceeded. The whole success of a column going out from Duala depends on the efficiency of the carriers.

Since my arrival here I have been in charge of the Carrier Section of the Base Hospital. I have over a hundred beds (but this number is shortly going to be increased) in my care, in addition to a large number of out patients. As a matter of fact, I see all the non-military natives here, such as clerks, marine employees and engineers.

I have had only four or five cases of bullet wounds among the carriers, the majority being minor surgical and medical cases. The commonest thing I have to deal with are cases of the so-called Tropical Ulcers. The carriers in the bush get small scratches and abrasions on the exposed parts of the feet and ankles; these are neglected and in a few days a large ulcer develops due to infection by a Spirillum. These rapidly increase in size, and when they reach me are large, dirty, sloughing ulcers, exceedingly painful and bleeding easily. They respond readily to antiseptic treatment, but owing to the large raw surface left, it is a long time before healing is complete, and in some cases skin grafting is necessary.

I have had very little surgery to do here. One or two cases of simple hernia, two of strangulated hernia; one I didn't get until the seventh day, this was fatal; the other is doing well. One amputation of the toe for ainhum, one amputation of the foot (Lisfranc), and one through the leg. One case of liver abscess pointing to the front, and radical cure for double hydrocoele. For the rest I have to do the usual minor surgery, and to treat medical cases, the commonest being dysentery, bronchitis, pneumonia, rheumatism, fibrositis, and malaria.

Hoping this account will be of some interest to your readers,

I remain, yours faithfully,

M.C.F.Easmon (Lieut.)

Medical Officer in Charge.

To the Editor, St Mary's Hospital *Gazette*

Sir, – So long a time has elapsed since I last troubled you or your readers, that perhaps I may be permitted, and excused, a brief incursion into your columns. The primary cause of my once more seeking your indulgence was the receipt yesterday of your number for last November, the secondary cause was a curious condition of cerebral confusion revealed in one of your Notes, and in the column headed "St. Mary's and the War." You here state under "South African Rebellion," that Dr W.A.Trumper, of the West African Medical Staff, was captured by the rebels and made prisoner while attending to the wounded.

I am afraid, Sir, that your Intelligence Department, suffering, let us hope but temporarily, from geographic psychopathia of intense virulence, has strangely misled you. By what subtle means, by what prevaricating wile, could this great, but withal somewhat interfering, department, transport a Medical Officer from Nigeria to the Cape? A child-like innocence of all concern with any country or thing not directly contiguous with Praed Street or the Great Western local time-table? or a scornful refusal to permit a specific sub-division of the generic "abroad"? And yet, methinks, were one to state that the Russians were attacking Paris, a German village in Galacia, one would be guilty of a lesser geographical mis-statement. I am reminded of a very unhappy transgression of a well known contemporary of yours. A friend of mine, an officer in a certain regiment, was unfortunately killed in this Cameroon campaign early in the war, and your contemporary, in publishing his photograph, stated that "Lieutenant — of the — Regiment, was killed in East Africa." Except that the officer in question was not a lieutenant, was not killed in East Africa, and that the photograph was not my friend's, the particulars given were commendably accurate.

It will interest many old St. Mary's men to hear how Trumper was captured – not by South African rebels, but by West African Germans. After some rather sharp fighting some way over the Cameroon border, Trumper and another of our men were attending some wounded men, when our troops had to fall back. The two men, refusing to leave our wounded to the tender care of German Negro troops – whose playful habit is to take no wounded prisoners – were unluckily captured. The treatment meted out to Trumper is not a credit to German Kultur. He was sent back from Garua, their great fort which we are still investing, in charge of a few black troops. At first allowed his horse, he was no sooner safely out of sight of Garua than the corporal in charge pulled him off his horse and compelled him to march ahead of him in chains, and with a rope round his neck. Such a thing in Europe would be a gross outrage, but out here, in a black man's country, where many millions are ruled by a few white men, it becomes almost incredible. The Germans in the Cameroons exhibit a bland ignorance of Geneva or other Conventions, which, if less personal, would be positively refreshing.

I will not trouble you with an account of the Cameroon campaign, or the terribly trying conditions under which our men laboured in the early stages of the war, during the rainy season, but I may convey some slight idea of distances and difficulties if I briefly describe my own journey from Lagos to this place (in the northern area of fighting). Leaving Lagos by train on a Monday night I did not reach rail-head until the following Saturday, and I had then to "trek" over 300 miles through the "bush," all my kit – bed, bath, food, clothes – being carried on the heads of natives. That the white population was not dense may be gathered from the fact that I was nineteen consecutive days without hearing English spoken.

My further experiences have been so dull in comparison with those of St. Mary's men fortunate enough to be in Europe, that I refrain from further tempting the censor, and merely remain,

J.E.L. Johnson
West African Medical Staff.
Via Yola, Northern Nigeria.
18.1.15.

Our correspondent should not too readily presume ignorance in others. We over here have even seen officers who have been transported from far further than from Nigeria to the Cape. Perhaps he has been misled by our friends the enemy, and imagines that Germania rules the waves! We gave the facts as we were given them and assume no responsibility for more than their accurate reproduction. – Ed.

14/6/1915.
Nigerian Field Force, Garua, Cameroons

To the Editor, St Mary's Hospital *Gazette*.

Sir, – I wrote to you some months ago describing to you the treatment meted out by the Germans to Dr W.A. Trumper and another medical officer, captured by them at Garua. The facts as then stated rested entirely on native evidence, but this evidence was apparently so genuine that it was generally accepted by us as absolutely correct. On June 10th, Garua defended by several marvellously constructed forts, surrendered to a heavy bombardment, after a prolonged investment by the Allied Forces. On the following day I was able to question several German officers on the subject of Trumper's treatment, and they all, quite independently, vehemently denied the supposed ill-treatment.

The story, according to these officers, was as follows: The two doctors, having been brought into Garua, the Germans would not release them, for fear they would give information as to the defences, but they were not treated as prisoners. On the contrary, they were allowed half the hospital for themselves, and all their propery was restored to them. When they were presently sent south they were not under an escort, but accompanied by five native horsemen as guides. Each officer further told me that they were actually presented with a case of champagne, to help them on their journey. At first sent to Ngaundre, they were later on sent still further south, where, I was informed, they are at comparative liberty, and, far from being treated as prisoners, are honorary members of the Officers' Mess.

The poles are not further apart than the German and native accounts. Which is true, one cannot say, but as the German prisoners here are exceedingly pleasant men, and not followers of the Kaiser's "Frightfulness", I personally believe their statements completely.

As we captured three German doctors in Garua, a possible exchange may lead to the release of our men, and the decision of this painfully interesting question.

Yours,

J.E.L. Johnston.

(These are strange letters from J.E.L. Johnston – in the early ones it is difficult to follow the logic in some of the sentences. In the case of the treatment in captivity of Dr Trumper, the account given by the German officers in captivity does not in any way dispute the treatment Trumper had when he was sent from Garua in the presence of only native guards. It is highly likely that the original account is accurate, and it is not surprising that the German officers had a different story to tell of what took place while in their custody.)

Another letter from Johnston follows:

Sir, Having more than once seen your editorial requests for "copy, and still more copy," it has slowly been borne in upon me that a brief account of the campaign in the Cameroons, as far as I had personal experience of it, might be of some slight use, if not for public delectation, at least as a means of filling some possibly vacant column. Not that I in any way anticipate that your readers will be interested. Far from it. Few will have even heard the word Cameroons, and will possibly hesitate between thinking it to be some new Australian wine, or, perhaps, the latest toothpaste. Most people in England naturally enough consider the war to be comprised in the immense operations in France, and possibly, the Dardanelles; the many other campaigns that are still being fought in Africa and Asia, and even in Europe, being thought of little importance and of utterly no interest. To these a study of a competent map would show the Cameroons to be an immense country of Africa, in which fighting has been going on almost since the outbreak of war.

Much of this has been of a guerrilla type, carried on along the Nigerian border – many hundreds of miles in length – by rapidly moving bodies of German troops, whose ostensible object was usually the destruction of some important post, such as a telegraph station, though it more often degenerated into a pillaging raid. A personal experience may here be instructive. I was for a short time at a small border station, through which ran the telegraph, consisting of a few mud huts, and garrisoned by two political officers, myself, and six native policemen (three of them ill). We had also a few other policemen, who were sent out at various points along the line to defend it against any straggling Huns. Twice some of these men returned hastily without orders, once because they were driven away by lions, and once to report that the line had been damaged – not by Germans, but by elephants! I believe that similar causes of interrupted communications are rare, even in France.

I will only briefly refer to the operations in the southern area. They were brilliantly commenced by H.M.S. Dwarf – on which poor Quick was at one time Surgeon – and H.M.S. Cumberland and Challenger, and later carried on land by large Anglo-French forces, and they have resulted in the occupation of a very large part of the country. Active operations which were impeded and almost stopped by the rains, roughly coinciding in time with the English summer, have lately recommenced, as one can see in the newspapers if one troubles to look.

Up in the north, apart from protecting our immense frontier, the main task has been to capture Garna, a very strong position on the R. Benue. Our first attack, in September, 1914, was not a success, but in January of this year a combined Anglo-French force again invested it.

During the next few months we had a peaceful enough time, although, as we had but little food, not enough clothes between us to cover a cockney guttersnipe, and a temperature – against which our thin grass shelters were of little avail – that would have given heat-stroke to a native of the Persian Gulf, life used occasionally to appear a little dull. However, any excess of boredom was always foreseen, and prevented by a prophylactic dose of marching. To cover twenty odd miles a day, for, perhaps ten or eleven days in succession, under a hyper-tropical sun, or else in a deluge of rain, and without the slightest possibility of getting under cover, with a minimum of food and sleep, may be war, but it is not pleasure. Marching with troops always entailed a large number of "carriers," as ammunition, Maxims and all stores had to be carried on their heads. This might mean a column three miles or more in length, drawn out single file through the "bush," along a narrow native track. It does not need an expert from the Staff College to explain that a column under these conditions presents a delightful object of attack to the enemy. Still, even the best things must have an end, and reinforcements in men and guns led to a ten days' heavy bombardment of Garna and its final surrender on June 10th. Garna was an immensely strong natural position made practically impregnable by German thoroughness. There were four main forts, three of them on small rocky hills, surrounded by a bare plain, with the R. Benue running close by, parallel with the forts. The ground for a considerable radius had been absolutely cleared; at various points beyond were left partially cut down trees, each of which marked a known range, and the appearance of any of our men near these points was instantly greeted by perfectly-timed shrapnel.

Our cultured friends had prepared no less than 7,400 deep pits, each with three or four spears at the bottom, and all covered over with finely-laid grass. The paths through these pits being sinuous and only some six or eight inches wide, and most of them being "dummies," any attempt at direct assault would have been incredibly difficult; even after the surrender, in broad daylight, it was a matter of very considerable difficulty, to avoid a spiky and unpleasant end.

In addition to these pits there were wonderful wire defences, and behind all these one of the forts had a delightful moat, cut vertically in the sand stone, some twenty feet in depth and width, and on the farther side was a really excellent selection of cleverly-concealed machine guns. The forts themselves reminded one of a Tube railway station. It was well for us that our high-explosive shells upset the nerves of the Garnese.

Shortly after the surrender I left Garna and the Cameroons with some troops, and have no definite knowledge of the later operations. It has not, however, escaped me that I have trespassed too grossly on your space and kindness, and that the very least amends I can make is to stop abruptly.

Yours,

J.E.L. Johnston.
London, October, 1915.

(In the earlier letters there is mention of Garua – in the later letter this has been printed as Garna – I think that both may indeed be Garoua in the Cameroons.)

(Unfortunately J.E.L. Johnston died in action.

M.C.F. Easmon qualified in 1912 with Honours in Anatomy. He subsequently became Medical Officer to the Colony of Sierre Leone and lived in Freetown.)

CHAPTER 22

East Africa

Here the situation was entirely different. With only 3,500 whites and 12,000 African troops the Germans took on ultimately 350,000 British (white and African) before they were beaten. Admittedly, sickness was the main problem – with actual casualties amounting to 10,000 and the sick to 36,000.

Two Years a Prisoner of War in German East Africa
"The Capture"
By Surg. B.C. Holtom, R.N.

At daybreak on Saturday morning, 28th November, 1914, two of H.M. Ships were lying off Daressalaam, German East Africa; on shore two large white flags were flying from the signal staff. In response to signal a German official came off and boarded the senior ship, where he had a conference with the Captain and gave leave to send boats into the harbour to examine the shipping, but added he would not be answerable for the attitude of the military, whereupon we threatened to bombard the town if any hostility was shown to the boats. A steamboat carrying the Commander, Two Engineer Officers and an Armed Party then entered the harbour and went up the creek to where two steamers of the D.O.A. Line were lying. Later, about midday, I was ordered to go in and examine a third steamer, the "Tabora," which claimed to be a Hospital Ship, but had not been registered as such at the outbreak of war. Our second steamboat took the Torpedo Lieutenant and myself; we entered the inner harbour by the narrow channel, in which a floating dock had been sunk, thereby blocking the entrance to all big ships. The "Tabora" was lying in the middle of the inner harbour, but we passed her and went on up the creek to the other two steamers. There the German engineers and stewards on board had been made prisoners and were sitting in two lifeboats alongside the gangway. The Torpedo Lieutenant now went on board the German steamer "Konig" and took charge of operations, it having been decided to damage the engines so that this ship could not put to sea: the Commander went higher up the creek in the first steamboat to investigate further, and my boat took the two boatloads of prisoners on tow and proceeded down stream. She put me aboard the "Tabora" and then went on towards the entrance.

The Captain of the "Tabora" met me at the top of the gangway, and I explained to him that I had come to look round his ship to satisfy myself that she was being used as a Hospital ship only. He introduced me to the doctor and sister, neither of whom spoke English, and we all went below. I looked into several cabins, from which the upper berths had been removed and those remaining made ready for the reception of patients, but there were no sick to be seen, and indeed this was hardly surprising for there is a large modern hospital ashore quite capable of dealing with the ordinary sick list, and at this time there had been no fighting in the neighbourhood; but in answer to my query a patient was produced – he was a healthy looking seaman lying in a bunk between nice clean sheets and trying to look at ease. What was he suffering from? He had been operated upon – in the groin. I turned down the bedclothes – the man had his trousers on! I looked my surprise – oh yes, he did not lie in bed all day, he was convalescent now. Ah good, might I see the wound? Yes, it was all right, the bubo had been incised. But then my examination went no further, for suddenly the drowsy tropical afternoon was rent by the quick rattle of a machine gun. We all made a dash for the port hole, and the patient leaped out of bed. We could see nothing, so a hurried rush took place up the companion way on deck. There was the steamboat apparently steaming on her own as hard as she could go through the narrows and the bullets splashing all round her like rain. Not a soul was visible on board her or in the boats she was towing, they were all crouching in the bottom or behind cover. We watched breathlessly, it seemed ages, but in a few moments she was safely out. What would happen now? We listened and in a few minutes heard – Boom – Crash! and the first shells came smashing into the coconut palms, throwing the sand up like a fountain. Our ships had opened fire as retaliation, and with the fourth shot the gunners got their mark. A 12-in. lyddite landed squarely in the Governor's house, and the yellow fumes of the explosion were quickly followed by dense rolling clouds of smoke and the whole house was burning furiously.

The ships then turned their attention to the signal station and we watched shells being planted all round the signal mast, from which the white flags were still flying; little damage, however, was done beyond chipping a corner out of the house. After about 15 minutes the bombardment ceased and at first the stillness and quiet seemed unnatural I was now wondering what was to happen to me, but I kept a look out up the creek, wondering if our second steamboat would appear. About an hour later I saw the pinnace coming down and promptly asked the Captain of the "Tabora" for the loan of a boat in order to board her; this he granted and I started off in a skiff rowed by four natives. We had not gone very far when a maxim was turned on us from the beach and we all dived for cover in the bottom of the boat; one of the natives got a bullet through his heart and died in a few moments almost without a struggle. I heard the pinnace getting nearer and thought she was coming alongside, but the fire was too hot to look up, thus I heard the noise of her engines getting fainter and popping up my head saw her making for the open sea. There we lay helpless in the middle of the creek, and the Germans firing a few rounds at us every now and again. At length the boat drifted alongside the "Tabora" again; when I got on board the Captain was very apologetic, told me the pinnace had got out safely and asked me what I meant to do. I had no idea what to do.

Then the ships reopened fire and this time things became too lively to be pleasant. Shells went whistling overhead and plumping into the water all around the "Tabora," that it is a marvel she was not hit. Naturally I felt a great disinclination to being blown sky-high by a British shell. After about 10 minutes the firing ceased and quiet settled down once again, and by this time it was just getting dark. I realised there was nothing now to be done that night, so accepted the Captain's offer of dinner and a bed in the "Tabora" and hoped for developments in the morning. But with the morning came the Steward, who said, "Your ship sailed in the direction of Zanzibar at daybreak, sir." I had just washed, dressed and had a cup of coffee when an armed guard came off and took me ashore. I was then marched round Daressalaam and interviewed by various officials, who assured me I would be released when the necessary formalities could be settled. That night I was lodged in the local goal, where I found the Torpedo Lieutenant and the two Engineer Officers already installed. They were as surprised to see me as I was to see them. I heard they had been captured on board the "Konig" while engaged on their work of destruction.

The next morning after a breakfast of black sausage, black bread and black coffee, we were all marched to the station under escort. The escort consisted of eight askaris, native soldiers, with a white officer in command. There we were put in a compartment in a corridor carriage with an askari stationed in the corridor to watch us. About 3 p.m. the train arrived at Morogoro, a fairly large town, and we were taken to the Station Hotel, where we had our first meal since our early breakfast. Then we were marched back to the train and journeyed on all night; we managed to sleep at intervals though it was bitterly cold and we had no blankets The askari guard was strengthened at night, and when I opened my eyes I could see two sleepless black figures with fixed bayonets watching us.

We arrived at our destination, Saranda Station, about 6.30 a.m., and there we had breakfast, and quite a good breakfast too – sausage, sardines, marmalade and coffee, with milk and sugar. But after breakfast we were told we had a three hours march before us. Still, we started off gaily and stepped out at a good pace; but soon the lack of exercise after months on board began to tell, added to which the road was absolutely monotonous and uninteresting, bordered on both sides by dense scrub, and finally the sun came out in all its tropical strength. When we at last arrived at Kilimatinde Boma or fortress we were hot, perspiring, dusty, thirsty and disreputable. A few minutes after we had been halted in front of the Boma, the Kommandant came out to meet us, and at the same time many heads appeared at the windows. They were interned British civilians who cheered when they saw us. This irritated the Germans. The corporal ran back, told them all to get inside, and ordered the black guard to shoot anyone who popped his head out. The Kommandant then addressed us, told us we were prisoners of war, and must obey our guards under pain of death, hoped we would give no trouble, and asked us to give our parole. As we had visions of being confined in separate cells if we refused, we gave our parole not to attempt to escape. The Kommandant then walked down the line and solemnly shook hands with each of us in turn. After this we were marched through a small door into the courtyard and there dismissed. The other British prisoners then crowded round, took us up to their rooms and offered us what refreshments they could – a drink of water and some fruit. They were anxious for news, and we were kept very busy answering such questions as: "Was it true the Germans were in Calais?" "Had England been invaded?" and so on.

In a short time the mid-day meal was ready, and we were taken by our new fellow prisoners across to the dining room. The meal was good and sufficient in quantity. It consisted of curried chicken with rice, followed by sago pudding; the bread, however was decidedly coarse. After dinner we retired to our room and slept till tea. We four officers were given a room to ourselves, with a camp bed in each corner, a chest of drawers, a chair and enamelled basin each.

The Boma of Kilimatinde consisted of two long blocks of buildings, with two smaller blocks; in one of the smaller blocks were the Kommandant's quarters. The whole was enclosed by a high wall having battlemented gun positions at opposite corners. Each building was two storied, built of stone, with corrugated iron roof. The lower storey contained store houses, kitchens etc., all the living rooms were on the second storey.

At 3.30 p.m. we went over to the dining hall for tea, the "tea" being always coffee; in these early days milk and sugar were provided, but the brew was always sent up ready mixed. No eatables were provided at this meal. The other prisoners used to save a portion of bread from dinner to eat with their coffee, and we adopted the same procedure. This used at times to lead to some regrettable scenes. One or two with large appetites and small consciences used to get in first to dinner and pocked two or three huge slices of bread, with the result that late comers often found no bread to eat with their dinner, much less any to save for tea, and this naturally led to many wordy disputes upon manners and the conduct becoming in a gentleman. After tea it had been usual for prisoners to be allowed outside the Boma for exercise, but this day a notice was posted saying that in consequence of the cheering upon our arrival all prisoners would be confined to the Boma for three days. Later, when we were allowed out we found we had a small area within sight of the Boma where we could walk, play rounders, or simply lie and smoke. At this time one of the white guards would accompany us, but there was no regular guard over us; moreover, there was no roll call, either on going out or coming in.

One of the prisoners took advantage of this laxity to attempt to escape. He used to carry a cushion out with him every day ostensibly to sit on, but in reality the cushion contained each day small stores of bread, rice, dried meat, etc. These stores were carefully hidden among some rocks until he reckoned the amount was sufficient, and then one evening he simply remained hidden in the bushes when the other prisoners returned, and later, when it was getting dark, collected his stores and made off into the bush. His absence was not discovered until mid-day the following day. Unfortunately he found it harder to make his way in the bush than he had anticipated, though he was a Colonial, and he found it necessary to enter a native village before he was out of the danger area, and as it happened he ran into two askaris (native soldiers) from the Boma, who, with the rest of the village, fell upon him and a few days later marched him into the Boma. As a result of his scrimmage he had two broken ribs and many bruises. And as a punishment he was confined in a small cell about 4 feet by 7 for seven weeks, and for the first 10 days not allowed out at all. Later he was allowed an hour's exercise daily under escort.

Following this attempted escape the rules were much more stringent for us. For a month no one was allowed outside the Boma. In vain I protested that such treatment was bad for our health, the space within the Boma not being large enough for exercise. The Kommandant simply replied: "It is an order from Morogoro." (Morogoro was the seat of the military administration.) Then I and the other officers went in a body and pointed out that we had given our parole, which the other prisoners had not done (the Germans would accept no parole from civilians), and that we had not been concerned in the escape. But the reply was that the order had said "all prisoners." However, we received permission to write to the Governor, and as a result obtained our liberty again after a fortnight. When the others were finally allowed out, they were restricted to one straight path, which was guarded by armed askaris stationed at intervals. A morning and evening roll was also instituted. Some time previously I had been to the Kommandant and greatly surprised him by saying: "Have you had any instructions yet about my release?" "Your release," he said, "no, why should you be released?" "I was told in Daressalaam that arrangements would be made to send me back to Zanzibar, as I am a doctor."

"I have heard nothing of it," he answered, "but you can write to the Governor if you like."

I accordingly wrote, and received an answer about a fortnight later, in which I was informed that my services were indispensable for the prison camps, and I was to consider myself in charge of the health of the prisoners. I answered that I was quite prepared to treat Service prisoners with such means as were at my command, but I considered the German Government should remunerate me for my attendance on the civilians and those who were not British. The reply was that the Government did not consider it necessary to pay me for my services.

In April, 1915, the native "boys" were discharged with the exception of two boys for the officers. Previously boys had been provided for all prisoners, but now the men, civilians, and even the missionaries had themselves to do all the work of keeping their rooms tidy, fetching the meals and washing up. From May also the rations were cut down. The Government had contracted with Frau Mahuke, a local planter's wife, that she should provide food for the prisoners at 2½ rupees a head. It had been pointed out that the value of the food provided did not much exceed 1 rupee per head, so the contract was reduced to 2 rupees, whereupon Frau Mahuke retaliated by cutting down the food.

In June, 1915, we were given an opportunity of writing home, and in August received some letters from Europe; this was the only opportunity afforded us for exchanging a mail during the whole two years that I was a prisoner. Later in the same year we were told we could write again, but about six months afterwards these letters were returned to us: they had never left the Colony.

When we were captured not one of us had a coin of any description. Luckily, we were able to borrow from the interned civilians, and some of us made a little by gambling. There were in camp a number of miners and planters, who were well supplied with cash, and who were inveterate gamblers; at times also a little reckless, when a careful player was able to make a small haul. However, we were not content to exist in this fashion, and after repeated applications the Germans arranged with our Government to make us an advance from our pay of 3 rupees a day, which proved ample to buy tobacco, cigarettes and other small luxuries. At first it was possible to buy imported tobacco and cigarettes, naturally at very exorbitant prices, but at length these stocks ran out and we had to subsist on the native tobacco. This tobacco, when prepared by the Greek traders, was quite smokeable, and some of the cigarettes were really good, especially to a pipe smoker, as they were of decidedly full flavour. But after we could only get the real native "pat" tobacco, which resembled in appearance, and, I should imagine, in flavour, the pats with which the desert Arab builds his fire. At Christmas, 1915, bags of clothing and small luxuries were sent in for the naval prisoners from Zanzibar, and these were passed, but we received no letters, papers or books. Soon after our capture the German Government gave us two suits of khaki each, a pair of boots and some underclothing, for which they wanted us to pay, but at that time we had no money, so were able to get them on the cheap. These clothes were fairly well worn out, however, and the new stock was most acceptable.

During my imprisonment the chief disease which I had to treat was naturally malaria. All the prisoners had malaria at least once, many of them had several attacks, and some became subjects of chronic malaria. Quinine was always available, but in small quantities only, so it was often impossible to give as long a course of treatment as I would have desired. Prophylactic administration of quinine was out of the question. Several cases of Blackwater fever occurred, and the two deaths at Kilimatinde camp were due to this disease. One died of heart failure on the third day, the other of suppression of urine; in the latter case suppression occurred on the second day, and I attribute it to the lack of fluid in the body caused by the persistent and intractable vomiting, which prevented the patient for 20 hours from taking any fluid by the mouth and retaining it. Thus the kidney tubules could not be kept well flushed and became blocked by debris. Rectal and intravenous salines, hot air baths, and diuretics had no effect in removing the complete block. The patient died on the fifth day, but was conscious almost to the last, and had no uraemic convulsions. There were four midwifery cases which I had to attend. Two were simple, straightforward cases in Italians. One was a bad case of placenta praevia in the wife of a planter (British). This woman refused to go to hospital as her husband would not be allowed to accompany her. Labour came on somewhat prematurely, and there were bouts of brisk haemorrhage at short intervals. On digital examination I found the edge of the placenta just overlapping the dilating os. I was absolutely single handed and had a very difficult time, until I managed to deliver the child with forceps. It was still born, but the mother made a good recovery after she had got over the severe loss of blood. In connection with this case I had a bad fright, and learnt that one must consider other factors in diagnosis than one does in temperate climes. On the following evening after the delivery the patient felt extremely ill, vomited violently, complained of severe abdominal discomfort, the temperature was 102 F., pulse 120, and respiration also rapid. The patient was bathed in sweat. I at once imagined that I had to deal with a case of sepsis, and was debating in my mind whether I was justified in doing an abdominal section, should it become necessary, situated as I was with no skilled assistance of any kind, and the next train from civilisation not being due for two days I resolved to leave the case overnight. The next morning the patient was comfortable, cheerful, feeling quite herself, and had made a good breakfast. I at once recognised I had to deal with malaria as a complication and nothing more serious, and was correspondingly relieved.

During our imprisonment the only reliable news of the outside world we got came from recent prisoners. Whenever a fresh prisoner entered camp he was at once surrounded and questioned, and one felt very annoyed with him when he could not give the exact line on the Western Front and all details. The Germans used to impart a certain amount of European news to us, but we never believed them, though I have since found there was always a nucleus of truth in all they told us. They would allow us no news of happenings in the Colony, but we managed to learn a good deal through the natives.

In April, 1916, it was decided to move all prisoners from Kilimatinde, the reason being that our troops were at Kondoa. Here I became separated from the other officers, as the men were sent to a separate camp and I was sent with them to look after their health. From this period, date our walking tours, as we were moved far to the south beyond the railway.

The first "safari" I made was one of twelve days. "Safari" is a word used in East Africa in the same way as "trek" in the South. At first we were absolutely knocked out by the time we reached camp. The average safari was four to five hours. However when we had recovered the use of our legs we were able to enjoy the change and exercise. One awakes at daybreak, often before; sunrise in these regions is about 6 a.m. all the year round. Then after a wash one has breakfast, and during this time the native carriers have mustered with their loads and are ready to start. We were usually on the road by the time the sun was above the horizon. Walking in the early dawn was most delightful and exhilarating, especially as I was allowed a certain amount of liberty and not obliged to walk under escort. We used to march until we reached our next camping place, and the distances travelled each day were naturally very varied; the camps could not be placed at regular intervals along the route, we had to go on till we came to water. In one instance we had to make a safari of nine hours from one stream to the next. When travelling through hilly country water was plentiful, and one came across many little steams of clear, cold, and uncontaminated water, but at other times the only water to be had came from green, stagnant pools.

However, when one made coffee from it, it went down all right.

Our first permanent camp for military prisoners only was at Mahenge. Here we were housed in mud sheds thatched with grass. The doors and windows were merely open spaces in the mud walls and the floor was of stamped mud. The men had to put their bedding directly on the ground with a layer of grass beneath, and it was necessary to air the bedding in the sun everyday, as the mud walls and floor were very damp. The prisoners had not been allowed to bring their bedsteads with them on account of the difficulty of transport. I was in rather a better position as I had been allowed to bring a camp bed with me. However, I succeeded, by repeated badgering in getting native beds locally made, yet it was quite a month before all the prisoners had a bed to raise them off the damp ground.

We had been nearly two months in Mahenge when we suddenly received an order to be ready for "safari." We were moved in batches of 30, with an interval of two days between each departure. I went with the last party, which included all the sick, who had to be carried on improvised stretchers by natives. Our destination was kept secret, but subsequently I heard we were to go to Kissaki, further down the Rufigi river; to get there we had to retrace our steps to within four days march of Kilossa. The rapid movement of the South Africans, however, upset the German calculations.

We had gone six days safari from Mahenge when one night my native "boy" told me that we were to retrace our steps in the morning. I did not believe him, but casually asked our guard if we were going on to the next camp to-morrow. He replied in the affirmative; however, after breakfast the next morning the porters seized their loads and started off back along the road by which we had come. I went to the guard and asked, "Where are we going?"

"You are going back," he answered with a grin.

"To Mahenge?" I enquired.

"Perhaps." "Why?" I persisted.

"It is an order," was the only answer.

Later I learnt that our troops were threatening the road by which we would have had to travel, and even Kissaki itself. Just before the other parties started on the return journey eight prisoners managed to make their escape, and after three or four days in the hills arrived safely in our lines, as I learned later.

We were all most annoyed at being brought back to Mahenge, as we all hated the place. However, after another fortnight or so we were all ordered to be ready to move to another camp. This time we were all to travel in one party, and there were to be no porters for carrying sick. I pointed out to the Camp Kommandant that several sick would have to be left behind: he agreed, and I put in a list of about ten persons.

The District Kommandant, however, wished to have the report of a German doctor. The only German doctor in the place at the time happened to be a drunken old man, who had been doctor on a ship running between

Daressalaam and Bombay. The man, who was known throughout the Colony as "Dr Calomel" – that being the only drug he was ever known to prescribe in addition to quinine – came down to the camp one afternoon after lunch, when he was happy in liquor. He went round all the huts, interviewed all the men, and caused them some amusement, as he spoke English well, and conducted his tour somewhat in this style:- Going up to a man in bed and poking him with his ebony walking stick, he said, "Well my man, and what's wrong with you?"

"Malaria, sir."

"Malaria, I've got malaria. Look at me I'm sixty, and had malaria for the last twenty years. Don't you worry, lie still, you'll be all right."

"Thank you, sir."

"Ah! and what have you got?"

"I've got a headache, sir."

"Headache! Why so have I. It hasn't killed me yet." Then turning to the next man,

"And what ails you?"

"I think I've got rheumatism, sir."

"So have I, had it for years, more years than you've lived. And how are you?" he asked, suddenly poking one of the grinning bystanders in the abdomen with his stick.

The man, a big seaman answered with a broad smile, "I'm all right, sir."

"Glad to hear it. So am I!" answered Dr "Calomel," who had just been avowing himself a victim of every complaint mentioned.

The result of this farcical inspection was that Dr "Calomel" put down thirty-one prisoners to remain behind. I knew this would not be approved, and two days later he came up with instructions to send everyone who was able to be moved. This time he came after breakfast, before he had time to get mellowed, and was in a very bad temper, would speak nothing but German, and refused to recommend any cases to remain. I refused to agree with him; luckily I had the Camp Kommandant on my side, as he did not want to be responsible for moving moribund patients through the bush, and we declined to accompany him on his inspection, and I wrote a strong letter of protest to the District Governor and gained my point; six patients were transferred to the local mission when we left, and of these one died the day after.

We had no idea whither we were being taken when we left Mahenge, but I noted we travelled continually eastwards. By the second day we were in the plains, it was very hot, no cooling breezes, and we were travelling practically the whole time through long elephant grass. This part of the country was very well stocked with game, and we enjoyed the excellent antelope meat and wild pig, which was a most welcome change from tough beef. Luckily the German corporal with us was keen on shooting.

Our camp proved to be at Madaba, six days' safari from Mahenge. Madaba lies in the plain south of the Rufigi river, and is a very desolate place in appearance. It consists of a few native huts, with one or two whitewashed mud-built Arab houses ranged irregularly down both sides of the roadway; scattered about among the huts are mango trees and bananas; these, together with small patches of arrowroot, sweet potato and maize, are the only evidence of any cultivation for as far as the eye can reach. All around is long elephant grass, scrub and small stunted trees covering the plain in all directions. A small river runs through the village, but in the dry season disappears below ground, as was the case when we were there. Water was obtained by digging down in the bed of the river to a depth of about 10 feet.

Our first camp here was formed of long open sheds around a large central square; the sheds were made of a light framework of bamboo and sticks, thatched with grass and palm leaf. There was no privacy, as all the sheds were quite open to the central square, and if one had been so unfortunate to "bag" a place where the afternoon sun streamed in, the only defence was to hang a blanket as a curtain from the roof. The bedding was placed on the bare ground and all one's small belongings arranged round, the fire was built in the open space just in front, and thus one squatted down on one's bed and watched the pot boil or criticised one's neighbour's cooking.

Soon after we had taken possession of this camp it was burnt down. It was about 3 p.m. and a hot afternoon; everyone was lying down sleeping, reading or talking, when suddenly there was a cry of fire. The grass roof at one corner was blazing furiously; those living in that area were frantically pulling their belongings out into the centre of the yard. The guard came running in and ordered us all out; the fire was simply running along the roof, lapping up the dry grass and bamboo. There was only one exit, so the tumult of a hundred men carrying bedding, clothing, boxes etc., stampeding through one narrow opening may be imagined. Another emergency exit was rapidly made by pulling down the wall on the side opposite to the fire. All the Germans turned out with their rifles. At first they thought it was a planned job to effect an escape, but the whole affair was so sudden no one had time to think of escaping, though it would have been easy in the first moment of the excitement. The whole affair was caused by one fellow building his fire too near the inflammable grass shed. Actually we were not sorry that a new camp had to be built, as the original one was too low, an average man could not stand upright when under the roof. The new camp was ready for us in about four days. The whole population was put on to build it, and it was a decided improvement on the old, the shed roofs higher, the enclosed quadrangle larger, and a separate enclosure for the kitchen fires.

The food here was very poor. For breakfast we had mealy pap and black coffee; midday meat if there was any, and when there was meat it was of very poor quality, the beast had been killed probably just before it died of tsetse disease/trypanosomiasis, and there would be very little flesh on the bones. One ox supplied us with meat for one day only, and then frequently the ration would make only one meat meal. Rice or "chirocco", a vegetable somewhat resembling dried peas, was given out to eat with the meat. We made our own bread, which consisted chiefly of maize and rice. The evening meal was similar, except there might be no meat, only broth from the bones, and frequently it was pure vegetarian. The food was so monotonous and poor in quality that one loathed the sight and smell of it, and only when the pangs of hunger became too acute did one eat at all.

After we were here a little time we were given an offer. Any man who would sign an oath not to take up arms again against Germany or her allies in this war would be handed over to the British. We discussed this offer many times and vigorously, but in the end the unanimous opinion of all the able-bodied men was that they would stick it out to the bitter end rather than buy their liberty with such an oath. Those of them, however who were incapable of bearing arms again, or were in danger of succumbing to disease and bad food were advised to take advantage of this opportunity to get back to civilisation. At the same time I was asked if I would care to go. I replied that I was longing to, but I could not give any undertaking not to participate further in the war, as my profession was not combatant, and doctors worked to relieve friend and foe alike. After referring the matter to the Commander-in-Chief, Von Lettow Vorbeck, I was told I would be released merely by giving my parole that I would disclose nothing of military importance. This I gave. I was assured medical attendance would be provided for the men after I had left, so I departed with a cheerful heart. Five men, unfits, were handed over at the same time. We had to travel all the way back to Mahenge, and from Mahenge towards Kilossa, till we met our outposts, a safari of 16 days in all. There was no strict guard kept upon us this safari, so we had a much pleasanter time, and also better food than we had been having in camp.

The last day but one with the Germans we were made to travel at night and not allowed to straggle. During the night we crossed the River Ruaha in canoes. This was evidently one of their defensive positions. I noticed that several large trees had been felled across the path on both sides of the river, but it was too dark to see more than a yard or two in any direction. The next morning we started off early, 7 a.m., after breakfast. Another German officer took charge of us. He had removed all his insignia of rank, but I discovered he was a lieutenant. A sergeant and private also accompanied us, and two Askaris with white flags. After marching an hour or two we came across traces of the British. They had advanced almost up to the river about a fortnight before, but had now retired a few miles. We passed an old camp site, marked by the litter of empty tins and newspapers and burnt-out fires. It was quite a treat to see a printed English newspaper again, though it was months old and trampled under foot. Carcases of dead horses and cattle were strewn all along the road. It looked like a battlefield, but these were victims of the tsetse fly, which in this district were very fierce; indeed, we had to keep slapping our necks, arms and legs to keep them off, and a tsetse gives a very sharp prick like a hot needle.

Just after midday we ran into one of our pickets. The Askari walking just before us gave a shout, and looking up we saw a big South African squinting down a rifle barrel at us. Our hands shot up in a twinkling. The first man was speedily joined by his comrades, then we were called up one by one. When the N.C.O. found out who we were he sent a messenger to the camp, and in about twenty minutes an officer arrived, who formally received us and took us over from the German. This eventful day was October 26th, 1916.

Naturally at first and for many days I felt very strange and could not realise my new freedom. It was strange to be smoking decent tobacco and to light a pipe with matches. The latter we had not seen for months; matches were a shilling a box, and then they could rarely be bought.

Now the time of my imprisonment seems very long ago, and I can look back upon it with less hatred than I had imagined possible; still the two years have gone for ever, and I feel that they are to a large extent lost to me, and I now return to work knowing nothing of modern wound treatment, and feel like a student again, learning with wonder and awe of the modern miracles of medicine and surgery, and of the rival claims of salines and antiseptics in the treatment of wounds.

(Surgeon Holtom, R.N. was in many ways very lucky, especially over the case of placenta praevia in the pregnant lady. He was fortunate that a torrential haemorrhage did not occur following his digital examination, during or after delivery. Also post-delivery the signs and symptoms of pyrexia, rapid pulse, sweating etc., could have been due to puerperal sepsis, and his contemplating an abdominal exploration would have been a strange choice of action. However he wisely decided against this and all went well. This all illustrates the enormous difficulties encountered by relatively young physicians as long ago as 1915, with no antibiotics, and at times no colleagues to consult, and often working outside their particular expertise and beyond their experience, and often under battle or conditions of imprisonment and stress. There are indeed many unsung heroes!!! It is remarkable that the Germans offered the prisoners their liberty if they would sign an oath not to take up arms again against them. Such an oath given under extreme circumstances would surely be invalid, but despite the temptation the prisoners declined. In the days of conscription such an oath would be considered at best ridiculous and at worst an act of treason. Even the promise not to escape was against the conditions of war, when it was held that an officer's duty was to escape from captivity if at all possible.

E.C. Holtom qualified in 1908. He served as a Lieutenant Commander in the Royal Navy, and was awarded the O.B.E.)

CHAPTER 23

Emdem

This fast light German cruiser *Emdem* sailed to the Far East creating havoc off the Indian coast by capturing thirteen merchant ships. It then sank both a French and Russian destroyer before being finally caught and destroyed off the Cocos Isles in 1915 by Australian warships.

To the Editor, St Mary's Hospital *Gazette*.

Dear Sir, – It is more than time for me to try to fulfil a promise I made you more than eight months ago. Material I have in plenty to write more than a letter; it is the serving of it up that does deter, and always has deterred me from embarking on these efforts.

On June 12 of last year I left home for the East, expecting to spend dull periods of time alternately in Singapore and on the Cocos Islands. I had only been in Singapore three weeks when the war broke out, and my Company – the Eastern Extension Cable Company – was ordered to send one of their ships to join the China Squadron. As I was acting as surgeon on the ship at the time I had the luck to go too. We went first to Hong Kong, where we took in stores and coal, and departed within eight hours of getting there under sealed orders. From there we went on up the China coast, and in a snug little anchorage somewhere off the mouth of the Yangtse river, I met Fergusson, serving as surgeon on H.M.S. "Cadmus," and heard of Tozer, who was, I think, on an armed liner, "The Empress of Russia." Fergusson at the time I met him was a spectacle worthy of record: with an eight day's growth on his face and a thick layer of coal dust all over him, his appearance would have been remarkable, even in Out-Patients. Later when I saw him in Hong Kong, the beard had materialised; still later, when we met again down at Cocos, it had been sacrificed. With regard to Tozer it may interest your readers to know that "Tozer Peak," "Tozer River," and some other geological tuberosity or sulcus named after him now figure on the map of China.

Well, from our first rendezvous we went to Shanghai and narrowly escaped being interned there, and later we were even further north than this on business, the nature of which I do not think I am at liberty to tell. Then to Nagasaki, where we saw the Japanese transports leaving for Tsingtao, and after that across to Hong Kong, where we lay for three weeks. Crossing from Nagasaki we had three or four hours about 30 miles from the centre of a typhoon: quite worth while once! From Hong Kong we went south on a cable repairing job along the Cochin China coast, where, in the intervals of bad weather we explored the little bays into which we ran for shelter, and incidentally shot, or shot at, many strange birds. Thence to Saigon for coal, and back to Singapore at the end of October.

It was not till then that I got my medical papers and saw what St. Mary's men were doing; and I felt out of it. With the choice lying between work with the Army and looking after a handful of Chinese and Malays who never got ill, there was not much room for hesitation, but I had considerable difficulty persuading the Company that my duty called me elsewhere. However, they at last consented to let me go at the end of the year, and I was waiting impatiently in Singapore for that time to come when we got news of the Emdem's defeat, and at the same time orders to proceed at once to Cocos to repair the damage she had done and make good her depredations. We were down there a week and were joined two days after we arrived by H.M.S. "Cadmus," with Fergusson on board. The Company's doctor on Cocos at the time was Ollerhead, known to many as Sandy, so there were three Mary's men meeting at this out-of-the-way spot. We celebrated the occasion in a fitting manner, till the officers of the "Cadmus," and my ship, the "Patrol," were sick to death of Mary's. While down there I went aboard the "Emden" with Fergusson and a party from the "Cadmus." She lies on the reef of Keeling Island, about fifteen miles from Cocos. The curl of the swell breaking on the reef comes just about midships of her, so the only place to get aboard is on her quarter, and, with the swell at all heavy this is impossible. However, we had one good day, and it was well worth some trouble to get aboard of her. The most appalling feature of it all was the smell: there had been no attempt to clear off the dead and the fragments, and they had lain for nine days in a tropical clime. It was not a pleasant sight – a debris of clothes and limbs and bodies all decomposing – and the smell seemed to get into one's brain after a time.

The "Emden" is quite a wreck: if she slid off the reef she would sink like a stone. Her hull is riddled along the waterline amidships, in fact, some shells seemed to have gone right through her from side to side; her after part is all burnt out, and an explosion of the after magazine has blown the iron deck up into great rents and craters, till walking on it becomes a precarious proceeding. The bridge and all the upper works are destroyed, the three funnels lying in a heap, the foremost over the side and the bridge a tangle of twisted ironwork: in fact, standing in some parts of her, it is difficult to realise that she is a ship at all. Curiously, in all this wreckage, parts have escaped altogether. The cook's galley, in the very centre of the chaos, is quite whole; pots were on the stove and a tin of macaroni just opened. The conning-tower had some paint knocked off it on the starboard side; inside it was no sign of what had gone on around these few inches of steel plate. Then the sick-bay forward, under the forecastle was undamaged: not a bottle was broken in the little dispensary attached to it, nor was there any evidence of work having been done there. It was, in fact, the most pleasant spot on the ship; even the smell did not seem to penetrate, and the senses had a rest. It was curious how the sight and the smell and the horrible wonder of it all seemed to make one physically tired. The sentimental side did not strike one then; it was afterwards, in the evening and away from it, that the imagination brought home the pity and the tragedy.

On the beach and in the water were men dead. We buried them the next day – all that was left by the crabs on shore and the sharks in the sea. Late in the afternoon we were glad to get back and have a bath. It was a great experience, and I'm glad I did not miss it.

We left Fergusson's ship at Cocos and crossed to Batavia to coal; thence to the other end of Java to Banjoewanji, and south from there some three hundred miles, where we picked up cable out of two thousand five hundred fathoms depth. Then back to Singapore on Christmas day, and on New Year's day I sailed for home. I must ask your readers to excuse this somewhat discursive effort. The past six months have been so full of movement, and of incident, that it is impossible to give anything like an account of them in so brief a space. It seems my luck to see many things and many places.

Yours etc.,

E.C.H.

We are glad to be able to publish the following account of life at sea as experienced by G.V. Davies. It is not the sort of experience we should like, but, then, he always had a capacity for enjoyment.

On Sunday, at 8.30 p.m., there was a nasty explosion forward, and some horrid salt water was thrown up and over my peaceful and contented self as I was reading on deck. This only meant we had been torpedoed. The next result is that everybody put on lifebelts, pale faces and sickly grins; I expect I was the same, but I had no glass to see.

As I was unattached and had no boat allotted to me, I had no work to do, so went and fetched my camera, and started photographing events. When I had finished my film I saw Simpson and went down to our cabin again with him.

He got his camera and then we both took our emergency haversacks, which, at my suggestion, we had packed on leaving Marseilles. I rummaged in my suit-case and found some more films, which we took up on deck with us.

He took photographs while I changed my film and followed suit.

Most of the workable boats had been launched by this time and the vessel was evidently going down.

The two escorting destroyers had each come alongside once and I had a topping photo of each, one with 1,300 men on board and the other pulling men on deck when about twenty feet away. Luckily this latter came alongside again and Simpson and I waded forwards to the forecastle and stepped off on to midships of the destroyer, so you can tell how low our ship was for the transport was a highly built vessel.

We got wet up to our knees wading forward because the well deck between the superstructure midships and the high bow was awash.

At this time all the men left the ship; about 50 got off on this destroyer and it was just as well they did, for as soon as we got way on and moved off, she tilted and sank.

Simpson got a picture of her going down; incidentally he spoilt mine by getting right in front of me.

We have pooled our pictures and made a set of 12, which we have sent off to the Graphic. The Censor at Alexandria, to whom we showed them, will pass all but three.

We cruised about the spot picking up survivors until we were full and then kept the rest company until a sloop and two more destroyers came on the scene.

The new arrivals stayed round the spot all the next day, while we pushed off at 5 a.m and made for Malta. We had thick weather on the way and at 12 noon I succumbed to mal-de-mer, but luckily with an empty stomach; in fact twenty hours empty, so it was not so bad.

We made Malta at 2 p.m. and were sent to various places. My luck was in, for Simpson and I were in a batch sent to Hamrun Convalescent Hospital.

On arrival our first thought was grub, and a bath, which we got at once and then we went to bed, having had our temperatures and pulses taken like good little patients; we slept the sleep of the weary. The emergency haversac which we saved was a great shock to all the other survivors.

Among the men on board were C.C. Harrison and Woodhouse, who were both saved.

Some old Epsonians were on board also viz., Kendal, Day, Shepherd and Wilson; all saved.

We saw and photographed Malta for ten days and then came to Alexandria, which we saw for nine days. During this time Simpson, Wilson and myself got leave for a two days' trip to Cairo.

The most obvious question to my mind about it all was: "Could anyone tell me whether there was a war on?" When one leaves England one's aspect towards the war is similar to that of Nelson when he clapped his glass to his "obliterated optic" and uttered his now famous saying.

I have had a pleasant journey across France; seen Marseilles; wintered in Malta and Egypt, and am now on the Red Sea.

One thing struck me and that is, that the horrors of a shipwreck, especially if it takes some time going down (ours was 45 minutes) are much overrated.

(For the majority, the horrors are not overrated and G.V. Davies was fortunate.)

January 1916

To the Editor, St Mary's Hospital *Gazette*.

Dear Sir,

As I am now at sea, I have the time to write to you on a subject which I have wished to write about for a long time, i.e., German rifle bullets, and some of the peculiarities of their behaviour, and the probable causes of some of these peculiarities. To begin with the so called "explosive" effect of any rifle bullet or even the old slow-travelling round musket ball of our grandfathers' time, has been known and recognised ever since firearms came into use, and innumerable theories, have from time to time been advanced to account for it. More than twenty years ago I made a number of observations of this effect upon animals which I had shot, and found that according to what I had read, two different effects were then comprised:

1. The smashing and comminution due to carrying forward of fragments of bone, etc.
2. A true bursting effect when the bullet struck a cavity filled with fluid or semi-fluid contents, the best instances being a full stomach or a cranium. I then came to the conclusion that the effect was a true bursting of the stomach or cranium due to the hydraulic distribution in every direction of the pressure caused by the impact and entry of the bullet. This explanation is, I believe, now the one generally held. So far as I know, the present rifle bullet, with its small diameter and very high velocity, does not often cause this disruptive effect, or, if it does so, the cases do not reach the Field Ambulance dressing stations. But most of the cases shot through the head have widespread damage to the brain, and considerable protrusion of brain substance on the exit side, both of which are very probably hydrostatic pressure effects.

With regard to the use of rifle bullets containing explosive by the Germans, a belief in this practice is very firmly rooted among the rank and file of the Army, but it is difficult to prove or disprove. I have seen men who positively aver that they were wounded by a bullet which exploded on striking them, and yet whose wounds showed not one scorching, discolouration or other chemical effect of an explosive, and not more laceration or comminution than could have been produced by an ordinary solid bullet. On the other hand, I have found bullets at times broken up into every imaginable form of fragments, bits of lead and distorted fragments of nickel casing being distributed in different directions in the interior, but, curiously enough, these cases have not, as a rule, been those exhibiting a maximum of damage, and I am inclined to look upon them as caused by a damaged or defective bullet, which broke up on impact, and not by one containing an explosive charge.

I have been informed also that the Germans do use a bullet containing an explosive charge, not in fighting, but for the purpose of range finding, as the explosion of the bullet on striking the ground can be seen from the firing point. If this be so, it is, of course, possible that a range-finding cartridge might occasionally be fired in action. A little while ago, I saw in a shop window in France a cartridge labelled German cartridge containing explosive bullet. I had no opportunity of examining it, but the shape of the bullet was cylindrical and blunt ended like the present Belgian or former English bullet, and not in the least like the present German one.

Reversed Bullets: The German bullet is fixed much less firmly in the cartridge case than the French, Belgian or English one, and is therefore much easier to take out and to reverse. That the Germans do use reversed bullets in short range fighting is proved by the fact that clips of cartridges containing such reversed bullets have been found on German prisoners and wounded. One such clip is now in the possession of one of my officers.

The object of this manoeuvre is doubtless to cause the bullet to "set up" or expand mushroom-wise at the end, as the lead is there exposed. It happens, however, that the nickel casing at the base of the bullet is too strong to allow this to take place. I have seen a large number of wounds in which the bullet was found reversed, and probably entered into that position, but I have never found a bullet "set up" from the base. I have also found the bullet reversed inside a wound, when every indication went to show that it had entered point foremost and reversed afterwards. I have, of course, seen every description of wound made by bullets which have been damaged or distorted by striking something prior to entering the body of the soldier. There is another peculiarity about the German bullet, which is well known to all who have been much among them, and that is the sharp explosive sound which they very commonly make while in the air.

I have heard a dozen different explanations of this sound from various officers, not one of which satisfies my sense of physics, and I have a theory of my own which seems to me the only probable explanation.

The sound is a sharp explosive sound; so much so, that when I first heard it, within 200 or 300 yards of the German trenches, I thought it was due to some of our own men concealed around me firing. The sound, however, has not exactly the timbre of a rifle shot, though it is nearly as loud: it sounds more like a hunting whip cracked very loudly. It is not as a rule heard at long ranges, where only the whistle or swish of the passing bullet is heard. The explosive sound is commonest at 200 to 400 yard ranges. I have heard it in the open, but it is commoner where there are trees. The two commonest explanations are: (1) That the sound is really continuous and due to the closing in of the air behind the bullet in its flight, but that it is only audible if the bullet passes vertically over the head of the person hearing it. (2) That it is due to the bullet striking a tree. Neither of these are in my opinion sound. The first is incredible, and as for the second, I have heard bullets strike trees too often to believe it, as the sound produced is quite different.

To understand it, and also to understand the reversal and other vagaries of a German bullet in the body, one must realize that the shape of the German bullet (a very long narrow point, with a very short cylindrical portion), causes its equilibrium in flight to be a very unstable one. As a consequence, the bullet tends to reverse itself while in flight owing to the preponderance in impetus of the heavier base, and the greater air resistance and long leverage of the relatively light front portion. Also the slightest resistance applied to the point, as by striking a leaf or twig, would cause instant reversal. It is this sudden reversal, and the blow to the air caused by it, which in my opinion causes the explosive sound. The sound is absolutely identical with that caused by a sufficiently sudden and sharp reversal of the end of a whipthong. It is certain that an ordinary and not an explosive bullet produces it, since no fragments of explosive bullets are found in positions where bullets making this sound pass by in thousands each day.

Yours sincerely, Wm. Salisbury Sharpe, Lt. Col.
Commanding 84th Field Ambulance, M.E.F.

(This is a plausible account of the noise and explosive effect of the normal German bullet. However, the Concise Oxford Dictionary does mention a dumdum bullet which it describes as 'a kind of soft-nosed bullet that expands on impact and inflicts laceration.' The name is taken from Dum-Dum in India, where it was first produced. In accounts of varying conflicts it is mentioned that such bullets were used.)

Mr. A.J. Hawkridge (Student of Medicine)

It is with deep regret that we record the death of A.J. Hawkridge. He was the younger son of Mr. and Mrs. J. Hawkridge, Sydenham. Born in

Sydenham, he was educated at Sydenham Hill High School, and subsequently at St. Dunstan's College, Catford, where he joined the O.T.C. He
entered St. Mary's in January, 1915, and passed his 1st. Conjoint Board
Examination in September of that year. In October he relinquished his
studies to take up a commission in the Royal Fusiliers. Whilst training in
Fermoy he was called up for active service in the late Irish uprising. He was
then sent out to France in June, 1916. In September he was attached to the
Royal Sussex Regiment. On the 6th of that month, while assisting his
Captain in putting out wires in the front line, a stray shot struck him on
the right side of the forehead. He never regained consciousness, and having
been taken to the Field Dressing Station died the same day. He possessed a
real good public school spirit, and at all times was a thorough sportsman.
He was an arduous worker and a very sociable companion. His Captain
writes: "I am sure that the company and the regiment have both lost a very
good officer, as he was always very keen on his work."

Dear Sir,
I have so frequently seen in the Gazette plaintive requests for copy and
literary efforts generally that I feel constrained to give you some small
account of my doings during the past three months. I left England on
January 24th, 1916, in charge of a Sanitary Section for a then unknown
destination. We were a unit of the British Adriatic Mission, and left
Southampton for a French port in company with other details towards
evening, and arrived safely at our first destination about 11 o'clock at night.
It was then too late to disembark, so we slept on board. I was very struck
with the quite brilliant lighting of the town, which seemed very cheerful
in comparison with London. Next morning I had to interview several
officials, none of whom seemed to have less than five letters after his name.
As a result of their deliberations I learned that we were to march to a rest
camp about three miles out of the town, and this, moreover, before we had
done any work. In this camp we got our first taste of French mud, and
managed to collect a good deal on our persons – it's nice affectionate stuff.
We "rested" for two days in this camp and left about 4.30 one morning.
Apart from leaving nearly half the party in the station at Paris looking for
water no event of much importance occurred till we got to Rome. Here
we expected to be inspected by a General, but this was a "washout" and
instead we found that the authorities had mapped out a good afternoon for
us. The men had dinner cooked by Italians in the station yard, and after this
we marched through the city to see the sights. We visited the Coliseum,
the Palatine Hill and the Forum, and had, moreover, a Staff Major as our
guide. Unless one has seen the Coliseum one can have no idea of its
immense size and grandeur. The view over Rome from the Palatine Hill

was also very fine, with St. Peter's and the Vatican and the statue of Garibaldi in the distance. We saw some very recent excavated portions of Nero's dining rooms with fine mosaic work. After this we marched back to the station, where there was an enormous crowd assembled to see us off. The people of note present included the Countess Cadorna, wife of the Italian Commander-in-Chief, the Staff of the B.A.M. in Rome, and the British Consul. We found out that the men could send postcards, and I heard afterwards that nearly 700 were collected, and that from about 120 men. Lots of local Red Cross ladies brought cigarettes and pencils and flowers for the men. We gave various songs from their repertoire – the more proper ones! We left Rome about 5 o'clock amidst much cheering, and after short stops arrived at our destination about 11.45 p.m. on February 1st. We went up to a camp and pitched tents by the light of one candle and got to bed about 2 o'clock in the morning. I was very surprised next morning to find that the camp was in an olive orchard. The orchard belonged to a chateau, the property of a Greek, but occupied by an Italian Naval Officer. The situation was ideal except for one thing. The water was scanty and impure, and most of it had to be brought by train, and then in barrels on a sort of cart.

We waited here for about one week till a ship was ready to go over to Corfu, and during that time my section was occupied with sanitary work in the camp and heavy fatigue work in the docks. There was not much to do in the town, which was reached by ferry across the harbour, and apart from the two theatres, a so called cathedral, and visits to certain units of the Allied Navies in the harbour, there were no other attractions. The theatre presented a variety show which was peculiar, in that the turns were practically the same, and usually of the song and dance variety. The audiences were as amusing as the performers, and when specially pleased by any turn they hissed and clapped. This was very noticeable when the local George Robey came on. Five of us went one evening and had a box, the total cost being 5 lira – about 3s-4p. On the evening of 7th February we embarked on a ship for Corfu. It had a cargo of hay and petrol, and, as we found out afterwards was towing a sailing vessel with a cargo of explosives! Not very stable, considering the state of the Adriatic then. We all slept on deck on bales of hay, and fortunately arrived without incident about 8 a.m. on February 8th.

The harbour here is very fine, although natural in that it has two islands at the mouth and steep hills on three sides and is of very considerable extent. We lay off a small jetty apparently neglected for about 2 hours, and during that time there was an Austrian air raid. Later we all went ashore to get some food, as we had had nothing on the boat other than what we carried in our haversacks. During the day we saw large numbers of Serbians marching along the seashore. They were just at the end of their retreat, and, as we found out in the evening, were going with us to Corfu. We took about 2,500 of them on a large liner to Corfu, and after transhipping all our stores we lay in harbour till early in the morning of the 9th February. We got to Corfu about 9 a.m. and lay off until about 5 o'clock at night. During this time all the Serbians were taken off in lighters and square box-shaped barges to a camp in the north of the island. This was at a very small village, and was the camp at which my section did most of its work during our short stay.

Later in the day it began to blow like anything, and this made the work of unloading our stores into lighters rather difficult. One of these latter was moored to the ship, and some men left in it for about four hours without any chance of getting off, as there was only a short rope ladder, and the attendant tug had gone off on another job. It set in to rain hard at about five o'clock, and we found we had timed our arrival to coincide nicely with the rainy season. This rain went on pretty nearly daily till about a week before we left, and we were able to realise that Flanders is not the only place where one can find mud.

We landed with all our stores about 9 o'clock at night, and as there was no camp for the men to go to they slept in a barn. This presented the appearance of a miniature Augean stable, as the floor was covered with rat excrement, and there was a small sewer on either side of it. These latter were both damaged by heavy motor lorries before we had been there very long, so it can be understood that the place was not very choice.

In the next week the men did fatigue work on the quay in nearly continuous rain, and with very little hope of getting dry, till one day we moved out to a camp about seven miles off. This camp was in the grounds of a villa in which the officers lived, and as it was situated right up against the sea and on a slope the conditions were much more passable. From here we used to send men to another camp, chiefly for disinfection of Serbian clothing. This was most necessary, but in view of the fact that every one of them was infected with lice, the small amount of work which we were able to do was probably not of much good.

It was a very common sight to see the Serbians sitting by the roadside going systematically down the seams of their clothes picking off lice. Sometimes they would go even better and put all their clothes on one side and work through each garment separately. If these were too bad to be dealt with by digital methods they would crush the garment between two flat stones and then drown the survivors. On one occasion I found a piece of cast-off shirt on a bush. This measured 6ins. by 7 ins., and on it I found 107 live lice and many hundreds of nits. No wonder it was thrown away in disgust! At this place there was also a hospital run by a French naval surgeon, and his morning and evening sick would soon fill up the O.P.D. of St. Mary's.

Some of the scenery in Corfu was very fine, and one could see the snowcapped mountains over in Albania under favourable conditions. I was not able to get into the Kaiser's Palace and the Achilleion, as the French were using it as a hospital. We stayed in Corfu for about seven weeks and then came home again by practically the same route. We had a nine hour stop at Naples, and during that time managed to see Pompeii. This has been very accurately described as "a city of the dead." One's impression after leaving it was that it was very little to be wondered at that Vesuvius swallowed it up.

There were numerous proofs that the inhabitants were a wonderful people. One could still see the remains of lead water pipes in the baths and fountains. The hot baths, moreover, were very ingenious, having a sort of double wall with a space for hot air to circulate round to warm the room and also the bath water. In the Museum at Naples there are to be seen surgical instruments dug up from the ruins, and these include bougie catheters, and a sort of vaginal dilator not unlike Bossi's dilator figured in modern textbooks. There were also small medicine boxes still containing pills made up. Our next stop was Rome, where we had a 12 hour halt, and all the men saw St. Peter's and the Vatican, while the Roman Catholics had an audience of the Pope. Meantime I went off with another officer to the Baths of Caracalla and the Catacombs of Callistus. It is quite impossible for me to take up your valuable space with a detailed description of these and other wonders, so I will conclude by hoping that these few remarks may be of interest to those of your readers who have been less fortunate than myself.

G.B. Argles.

(G.V. Davies qualified in 1917. Following the war he became Medical Superintendent of Park Howard Hospital, Ministry of Pensions and Medical Referee of the Prudential and Pearl Insurance.

William Salisbury-Sharpe, his name is hyphenated in the Medical Directory, qualified L.R.C.P. in 1888 and obtained his D.P.H. in 1901. He proceeded M.D. in Durham in 1908, F.R.C.S.I. in 1909 and the M.R.C.P. London in 1917. He was a house surgeon in St Mary's Hospital, and was Lieutenant Colonel in the R.A.M.C. His appointments included Assistant Surgeon to the Central London Throat, Nose and Ear Hospital, Chief Consultant Surgeon to the G.W.R. He wrote numerous papers on varying subjects including herpes zoster, food contamination, improvement in X-ray tubes, otitis media and the treatment of the ear in the tropics.)

CHAPTER 24

May 1917 – A visit to the Carrel Hospital, France

By A. W. Bourne, Capt. R.A.M.C.

Soon after having landed in France, facilities were granted to me to visit the clinics of Carrel and also of Chutro. The available time at my disposal was unfortunately not very long, but it was quite sufficient to obtain a grasp of the methods employed by these surgeons, and to see the results obtained by them.

The system of treatment elaborated and practised by Carrel is especially applicable to septic wounds of the limbs, and perhaps the best results are seen in cases of compound fracture of the long bones. But it is adaptable to almost any form of septic wound, and is employed with success in cases of head injury, and might be modified for the treatment of certain abdominal conditions. The most striking results, however, are seen in cases of severe laceration with compound fractures, in which sepsis has obtained a firm hold. Inasmuch as this class of injury is perhaps the most difficult and tedious, if not the most dangerous to limb and life, any great improvement on our ordinary methods of dealing with them, will be an undoubted advance.

The hospital in which Carrel works is a small hotel. It consists of small wards, a simply equipped bacteriological laboratory, an X-Ray room, a dispensary and chemical laboratory, and an operating theatre: apart from the ordinary annexes and offices of a hospital. There are 85 beds wholly devoted to the treatment of the septic wounds of war, and there is no accommodation for cases of "local sick." The wards are small and almost overcrowded with patients, but in spite of universal shutting of windows, there is no stuffiness, nor the stale odour due to the presence of large numbers of septic wounds.

In fact, a point that immediately strikes one on entering the wards is the freshness of the atmosphere.

The method of treatment is simple. It is, in fact, merely the modification of the ordinary irrigation of wounds, which aims at a complete, or almost complete disinfection of the wound surface.

The irrigation fluid employed is Dakin's solution, which is a neutral solution of sodium hypochlorite, of which the concentration must not be above 0.5% and should not be below 0.45%. A more concentrated solution is irritating to the tissues, whereas a weaker strength is not sufficiently antiseptic.

The preparation of sodium hypochlorite solution of this concentration requires considerable care, but it is easy once the details have been grasped, to produce in bulk. It is made by the addition of solutions of known strength of sodium carbonate and bicarbonate to a titrated sample of chloride of lime, the precipitate of calcium carbonate being removed by filtration. To the solution of hypochlorite thus obtained, a faint trace of potassium permanganate may or may not be added. It is said to stabilize the solution. Carrel employs permanganate, but it is not used in the Chutro clinic.

The fluid is then contained in a litre glass reservoir suspended at the head or foot of the bed, and connected with the vicinity of the wound by a length of rubber tubing, which at the dressing is attached to a small glass connection carrying several radiating branches. To a certain number of these (determined by the size and depth of the wound) are fixed the so called Carrel's tubes. These are merely small rubber tubes about as large as a No. 8 or No. 6 Jaques Catheter, with the distal end closed, and having a number of small half-millimetre perforations extending from this end for a distance varying from 5 to 15 centimetres. A certain number of these tubes varying according to the extent of the wound are then placed therein, and lightly covered with gauze, the whole being enclosed by a pad of gauze covered wool secured round the limb by tapes or pins. Bandages are not often used.

The actual irrigation is carried out every two hours by day, and four by night, by releasing a clip on the main rubber tube for a period of three seconds at each occasion. Dressings are done daily in Carrel's clinic, but in that of Chutro in many cases every two or three days. The dressing is done with great care and aseptic precautions and always by the surgeon himself.

Apart from the ordinary clinical inspection each day, the progress of the wound disinfection is estimated by frequent bacteriological examination of the discharges. An ordinary smear of the pus is taken, and the mean number of microbes in the field is counted. The figures thus obtained day by day are then plotted on a chart, giving a "graph" representation of the bacteriological content of the wound. It is surprising to see how rapidly the mean count per field falls from 50 or above (infinity) down to one or two, and further to one in every 5 to 10 fields examined. The fall, however, is seldom uniform, and a sharp rise in the curve lasting for one or two days is often seen during the first week. In a period varying from a few days to three weeks the wound becomes "sterilised" and is then ready for closing at operation. Some organisms are more difficult to kill off than others, and the two which give the most trouble are some varieties of streptococcus and b. pyocyaneus, particularly the latter.

In the vast majority of cases the sutured wound closes by first intention, in fact I did not see any case where there had followed suppuration and breaking down. At the operation of closing the wound, any marked loss of tissue causing gaping holes was made up by the use of grafts of fat in bulk; taken from the buttock or thigh.

Of the results it is difficult to write without appearing to betray too much enthusiasm. Large sloughing wounds, with everted edges, and compound fractures were reduced to a condition fit for closing by suture in a period varying from 12 to 28 days. Small wounds are often closed in 8 days from the commencement of irrigation, and fresh wounds are often closed on the fourth day of injury, while it is the rarest thing for a limb to be amputated, and secondary haemorrhage is almost, if not quite, unknown. Since April, 1916, only three amputations have been done on freshly wounded cases. M. Chutro told me that he had only performed one amputation since August, 1916. These are remarkable figures for War Hospitals to shew, hospitals which deal almost entirely with large infected wounds and compound fractures.

The progress and results of the cases are well shewn to visitors by a large series of coloured photographs of the individual wounds, taken at intervals during the treatment from the date of admission to the discharge of the patient with a healed scar. The photographs are grouped with the appropriate "microbobe graphs" and X-Ray pictures. The splints employed are of the wire cradle type, slung by a varying number of pulleys from a Balkan frame-work, giving the maximum range of movements of the patients. Of the ordinary forms of wooden splints I saw none. Extension is obtained chiefly by the ordinary method of adhesive plaster, but in some cases especially at the Lycee Buffon, extension was obtained by attaching the weight to a steel pin driven through the soft tissues immediately above the os calcis and behind the insertion of the tendo achilles. This pin is usually applied for fractures of the tibia, and Chutro also uses it for fractures of the femur. Transfixion of the condyles by the Steinman pin is not performed. Throughout the most noteworthy notes observed were the extremely small quantities of pus in even the largest wounds – not because ordinary amounts had been washed away, for the irrigation is not sufficient in volume of intensity to effect this, but because of very small pus formation. Further the astonishingly rapid progress and cleaning of septic and sloughing wounds, the general well being of the patient, absence of much pain, and low degrees of fever.

While, however, the system is simple and inexpensive, yet it is necessary closely to adhere to Carrel's technique, which has been worked out to the last detail, in order to obtain Carrel's results.

(Carrel's work in treating war wounds is an extension of the pivotal work done by Almroth Wright and his team on the treatment of wound sepsis in their laboratory in Boulogne, described in Chapter 3.)

(Aleck Bourne had immense moral principles. He was the son of a Wesleyan minister and obtained a scholarship to Cambridge and St Mary's Hospital Medical School. Following registrar appointments he was made an Honorary Consultant to the Department of Obstetrics and Gynaecology at St Mary's in 1910. His experiences in the slums of Paddington fed a strong social conscience and this led to his membership of the Socialist Medical Association. He constantly taught the students that the patient should be seen in the light of his or her social state and indeed he was thinking of a Nationalised Health Service before Beveridge. He was also producing successful text books, one being a *Manual of Obstetrics and Gynaecology*. He became one of the most respected obstetricians of his day. He fought hard for an Academic Unit of Obstetrics and Gynaecology for St Mary's. His name became well known to the public in 1935, when a young girl was raped and made pregnant by Guardsmen. Aleck Bourne decided to perform an abortion, thereby challenging the abortion law of the time. He notified the authorities that on a certain named day and at a certain named time he would perform this abortion. This meant certain prosecution and thus the Rex v Bourne trial followed. Aleck Bourne risked imprisonment, the loss of his professional life and future. He was tried but not convicted. This was a most courageous stand for what he considered the best interests of his patient. It was instrumental in eventually changing the attitude to abortion in this country and many years later to actual changes in the law of this country.

When the 1914–18 war broke out Bourne volunteered and he served as a surgical specialist in Egypt and France.

In 1918 he was appointed to the Consultant Staff of Queen Charlotte's Hospital, London and the Samaritan Hospital for Women, as well as resuming his appointment at St Mary's Hospital. Aleck Bourne died in 1978 at the age of ninety-two. Two wards at St Mary's Hospital were named after him − Aleck Bourne 1 and 2.)

With the Armies in France
By S. Maynard Smith, C.B., F.R.C.S. (formerly Colonel A.M.S.)

By way of preface it is necessary to say a few words on the terms I must employ in speaking of the Armies in France. From the middle of 1916 onwards there were five armies. According to the length of line it held, or whether engaged in attack or defence, the number of men in an army varied greatly. At one time I believe over half a million men were in the

army to which I was consulting surgeon. Each army had so many corps –
usually 3 or 4. Each corps had so many divisions from 2 to 5. A division had
3 brigades, latterly with 3 battalions of infantry in each. Then each division
had many batteries of field guns, each corps had masses of heavy guns, whilst
the army had also much artillery under its own direct control. Air craft –
flying scouts, observing planes for spotting for artillery, bombing planes and
so forth were everywhere. Now as to the medical units. Each battalion had
its medical officer, whose duty it was to direct the collection of the
wounded by the regimental stretcher bearers and their transport to the
regimental aid post, where he rendered first aid. According to the stage of a
battle, a regimental aid post might be a shell hole or a comparatively
commodious dug-out in a support trench. Wherever or whatever it was, its
occupants were always in a fair way of being wiped out of existence by one
of the shells which never ceased to fall by day or night. Clean water was
often almost unobtainable, although there was always enough slush to
render life permanently amphibious. From the regimental aid post the
bearer squads of the field ambulances got the wounded back to the advanced
dressing station, which was run by a field ambulance, The advanced dressing
station, usually one to each division in the front line, was situated some
thousands of yards back. The actual distance varied greatly. If possible, it was
sheltered by the lie of the land and placed where there was enough road
remaining to admit of evacuation by motor ambulance convoy – just the
very sort of site, in fact, that the heavy guns wanted and took. So it came
about that advanced dressing stations were always mixed up with "the
heavies." A dug-out, the cellar of a ruined house or chateau, a captured
pill-box, sandbagged elephants under the lea of a ruined barn – from all of
these the engineering and architectural skill of the R.A.M.C. could produce
something in the way of an advanced dressing station. From the advanced
dressing station a stream of motor ambulances carried the wounded away:
the serious cases went direct to the casualty clearing station, the less serious
to the main dressing station. The main dressing stations as a rule – each corps
had one – were in marquees, huts, farm buildings, or a mixture of the three,
with such protection from shells and bombs as could be contrived. Hence
the wounded were taken back to the casualty clearing station. The casualty
clearing station was always at or near a railway siding for convenience of
loading the wounded on to ambulance trains, which took them away to the
base hospitals. After a shorter or longer stay there the cases were sent off to
an embarkation port, and the hospital ship landed them in "Blighty."

I want now to speak of the general principles which governed the
treatment of the wounded.

In the conditions of warfare existing on the western front the great
majority of the wounds met with were severely lacerated, the soft tissues

were extensively crushed and devitalized. Such wounds were heavily infected, not only with the ordinary pathogenic organisms but also with the anaerobes of gas gangrene and gas cellulitis. Fragments of shell or bomb and pieces of clothing, or masses of mud, carried in by the missile, were frequently present in the wound. Varying in proportion with the character of the fighting, clean through-and-through bullet wounds were met with. Even bullets, especially when striking bones at short range or when splitting into myriads of fragments through hitting accoutrements or ricocheting from hard objects, produced wounds which possessed all the grave characteristics of those caused by large fragments of shell.

The results in the early days of the war of treating wounds of this nature by simple aseptic or antiseptic dressings, on the lines adopted in South Africa, caused a rude awakening. In the first place tetanus was rife; the routine administration of anti-tetanic serum had an immediate effect in controlling the incidence of this disease. In the second place, anaerobic infections of the nature of gas cellulitis and gas gangrene – conditions almost unknown to us in civil practice – were nearly universal complications of bad wounds. The measures first adopted, of free opening and drainage, and the avoidance of constriction and undue pressure, had but little effect in the prevention of gaseous infections. Attempts at disinfection in the forward area by pastes and strong chemical antiseptics were notoriously unsuccessful. Almost all severe wounds became infected and foul. Deaths were frequent, and prolonged and painful convalescence the rule.

Excision of Damaged Tissue

Not much progress was made until it became recognised that all but trivial superficial wounds or clean through-and-through bullet wounds needed an early and complete cleansing operation – an operation which involved the free exposure of all the recesses of the wound; the removal of all missiles, clothing, dirt and debris; the methodical excision of damaged muscle and fascia and the paring of damaged skin edges. This operation had to be performed with surroundings permitting of care and thoroughness, with proper aseptic ritual, by surgeons experienced in the technique, and in places where patients, if necessary could be retained for a short period. It was found that when this operation had been efficiently performed wounds ran a course free from complications; that secondary suture was possible in many at an early date; and finally that, under certain circumstances, many wounds could be sewn up right away, and would heal much as the clean operation wound of civil practice. It was everywhere recognised that this operation was the factor in deciding between severe infection, prolonged illness, and eventual crippling on the one hand, and an aseptic course, rapid convalescence, and a minimum of disablement on the other. The operation was termed the excision of the wound. When was it to be performed? Certainly as soon after the infliction of the wound as possible. The longer the delay the greater the chance of established infection. Where? There were not the necessary appliances, theatres, personnel, and accommodation in the forward units. Special hospitals had to be provided for the purpose, as near the line as possible. The casualty cleaning stations, not originally intended for this purpose, were converted step by step into comparatively elaborate operating hospitals. The work of the units in front of them consisted in getting the wounded back as soon as possible, and as fit as possible for the further treatment necessary.

Summary of General Principles
Having these facts in mind, the general principles which governed forward unit work were summarised as follows:
1. Get the wounded back to the clearing station as soon as you can.
2. Dress the wound once carefully; afterwards do not disturb the dressings unless they have slipped or unless there is bleeding.
3. Take measures to avoid shock; if it has already supervened, take measures to treat it.
4. Efficiently splint all fractures.
5. Arrest haemorrhage.
6. Take any special measures needed in special cases. In addition the dressing stations had to fill up the field medical card and give antitetanic serum.

Having given you an outline of the organisation of the Medical Services, I want you to take a tour in Flanders. The pictures are accurate, but I omit all map names. Starting at dusk on the eve of a battle, you get a lift in an extremely muddy Daimler car up the long straight road from P. to W. At first progress is good, but after passing a ruined village about halfway, the ride resolves itself into a monotonous crawl, caught in a continuous single file of ammunition and supply lorries. It is pitch dark, raining of course, and no lights are allowed. It is just possible to see the back of the lorry in front. From time to time a group of returning lorries pass you, and the driver of one remarks to your chauffeur that 'W. is getting it proper'. Unpleasant noises ahead inform you that there is a good deal of hate going on. At last ruined walls dimly seen on each side of the road tell you that you are entering the most famous town in Flanders. The shells have ceased to fall for the moment. A little way on a traffic control man flashes a torch into the car and requests you to have gas masks at the ready. Hereabouts you turn off sharply to the left and get away from most of the lorry traffic. Some ten minutes at a crawl and you see a red and green light hanging on a tree stump – a Divisional H.Q. – your destination. Directed by a sentry you flounder through mud to a dug-out which you learn is excavated in the canal bank. A thick gas curtain of blankets hangs over the door. You join your hosts at dinner. The meal is punctuated at intervals by a 12-inch gun tucked in somewhere behind you, each report of which blows the gas curtain up to the roof. The American M.O. succinctly describes it as "Gee whiz, some gun!" You are relieved to hear the gunner officer goes to bed at 9.30, and the prospects of sleep look brighter. You sleep in another dug-out, and morning tea is brought to you at 3.30. It is still pitch dark. An ambulance car is waiting. You cross the canal and go forward along a road of bumps and holes. It is not long, however, before you have to get out and walk. A big shell has carried the road away, and working parties are hard at it filling in the crater. The continual glimmer of gun flashes throws a fitful light, and from time to time the red glare of an exploding dump, with a resulting fire, shews you a long line of mules, horses and timbers taking shells up to the field gun batteries still some way ahead; whilst on the ridge beyond the gaunt bare stumps of trees are silhouetted from time to time as the sky reddens with the glare. After tramping for half-an-hour you come across a group of ambulance cars held up by the broken road behind you. A great mass of concrete on your left, formerly a German strong point, is the advanced dressing station. You are sure to be offered tea, and at first light of dawn you discard your overcoat and start off on the duckboards. The line of duckboards winds in and out amongst the shell craters — of all sizes and all filled with foul mud and water. If you are wise you keep your eyes firmly fixed on the duckboards, for if you step unwarily the wretched thing up-ends and precipitates you headlong. If you do look up you see as far as the eye can reach a waste of pockmarked mud. Here and there a little group of men is linking up the duckboard walk where the night's shelling smashed it, and a few strings of pannier ammunition mules are making their way back, having dumped their load. One or two lines of telephone wires are being repaired by nonchalant sappers who have evidently developed a fatalistic attitude of mind towards shells. You visit one or two pill-boxes that lie at intervals along your track and are used to shelter relays of stretcher bearers, for no man can carry far. Having left behind in turn both the heavies and the field guns, you come into a zone of comparative calm, and find the regimental aid post in a captured pill-box called for some reason a 'farm.' The atmosphere is foetid. Few wounded are coming in to this particular spot You make your way cross country up to your knees in mud to a push trolley line — Decauville rails laid on the mud serpentining among the craters, with improvised trucks to carry stretchers which are pushed by hand back to the advanced dressing station. If you return by this route you will find a fair number of wounded. In two places shells have carried away the line. The difficulty is surmounted by dumping the stretchers, carrying the truck across the gap, and loading up again. Back at the advanced dressing station you find them hard at work. Bending low through a doorway in the concrete wall you find yourself in a passage some 6 feet wide. A badly wounded man is on a stretcher laid across 2 trestles. An orderly standing beside the top of a box which is neatly laid out with steriliser, tray of needles iodine and bottles of A.T.S., is giving the routine prophylactic dose. Passing a blanket hung across the passage you enter the dressing room. Three pairs of trestles are each occupied by a stretcher: orderlies are busy cutting off clothing. Beside each stretcher stands a dump of dressings; picric acid in spirit for the skin; French cooking pots (marmites) in which squares of gauze have been sterilised; biscuit tins full of squares of wood and neat piles of roller and triangular bandages. Forceps and scissors stand in lotion. The man on this stretcher has had his femur shattered by a shell fragment. His wet clothing has been cut away except for the injured limb, which has not been touched. He is on dry blankets which fall over the two sides of the stretcher. A Beatrice stove is burning beneath, forming a hot chamber. Three orderlies are at work with a Thomas' splint, and, if you have never seen the proceeding before, you ought rather to admire. The limb is fixed firmly by extension over the boot, and slings; a foot piece holds the foot. Then the trouser leg is ripped away and the wound is dressed; supporting Gooch splinting is fixed to the thigh with additional slings; the splint is slung up to a suspension bar slipped over the sides of the stretcher. Feel the limb. You will find absolute fixation in good position of the whole extremity. Three hot bottles are packed round and the blankets folded over; a strip or two of bandage holds everything snug, and the stretcher is carried away through the exit at the far end of the passage to the waiting ambulance. If you have had the curiosity to note the time you will find that 11 minutes have elapsed since the stretcher entered the dug-out. If you ask the men they will tell you they had been trained as a team at the -th Army School of Instruction, and if they weren't too busy they would repeat the drill from 'At the word 1, prepare the stretcher – down to 'At the word 12, apply hot bottles . . .' At the next table a man has an ugly shell wound which has laid open his pleural cavity and air is hissing in and out with each gasping attempt to breathe. The wound has been rapidly cleaned up and 3 or 4 silkworm gut stitches have been passed through the skin and muscle and the wound closed. The improvement is dramatic. The breathing becomes quiet and regular, and the dose of morphia taking effect, the man sinks into comparative repose. The medical officers, as they deal with each case, are dictating and signing the diagnosis and a brief note for the field medical cards. Going out you have a look at another part of the dug–out, where cases waiting for the dressing room are being given the ubiquitous hot tea. Under the lee of the cement blockhouse a sandbagged shelter has been contrived and here the less seriously wounded are collected waiting for ambulances. They will go to the main dressing station on their way to the casualty clearing station and have their A.T.S. given and records taken there, and if necessary be dressed. Sometimes it was possible to do away with the main dressing station, and do all the necessary work and dressings at the advanced dressing stations. When the double line could be dispensed with I think the wounded gained. As you leave the advanced dressing station you will notice stretchers being man-handled across the mud from the flank − a battery of 6-inch howitzers near the advanced dressing station has been badly shelled. You take a lift on an ambulance. It is now broad daylight, and you see that the crater that held you up earlier has been filled in and the road is again passable. You have seen something of the work of the medical officers of the divisions. You have observed something of the conditions in the area which it is their normal existence to inhabit, but to which you are, perhaps, only an occasional visitor. You can breakfast at the main dressing station, and by the time you reach the group of casualty clearing stations for which you are bound, the wounded will have begun to crowd in.

On arrival at D. you find three casualty clearing stations, each formed on the same plan. Marquees are laced together to form a long ward, taking some 30 beds or 60 stretchers each. The accommodation of each casualty clearing station is some 800 patients or more. Each has a hut operating theatre containing 8 tables, 2 of which are in some instances separated off by a partition and reserved for chest and abdominal cases. Another hut contains the X-ray apparatus, and another acts as a sterilising room. As you approach you will see a long queue of ambulances unloading one by one at the reception room and driving away by another road to go forward and load up again at the dressing stations you left earlier in the morning. The plan is for a casualty clearing station to take 300 cases at a time (a stretcher case to account as two), and then to switch off to the next, which takes its 300 and then switches in turn. A group of three casualty clearing stations in battle time might take 5,000 cases in 24 hours. Going to the casualty clearing station that is receiving at the moment you visit the reception room, and you find a constant stream of stretchers entering. You see their records being taken by the clerks and, passing to the far end, you see a constant flow of stretchers into the examination room. Here ranged down the ward are rows of trestles, and the reception room surgeon is at work. He is the pivot of the whole scheme. He need not be a skilled operator, but he must have a quick, sound judgement and any amount of war experience in this particular job. The orderlies are getting the cases ready for inspection. The M.O. examines and decides their destination. He is disposing of the cases as follows:

1. For Operation. These he marks up A, B, or C. A are urgent cases that must take preference. Such cases, for instance, as haemorrhage. B are less urgent cases which, however, must be dealt with before going down the line. Fractures of the femur are typical cases in this class. C are cases that should be operated on at the clearing station, but can, if increasing pressure of work necessitates travel to the base for operation there. A sharp look out has to be kept for the wound of the buttock which has penetrated the abdomen, the wound of the arm which has penetrated the chest or the scratch on the thigh which has penetrated the knee-joint.

   Each case has a slip attached with a few words of information for the operating surgeon. Any man may be marked up for X-ray. From the end of the examination ward the operation cases are being carried through into the pre-operation ward (vulgarly called 'The Dump'). Here the cases are cleaned up and got ready for the theatre – going across to the X-ray hut if necessary. The reception room M.O. keeps himself constantly informed of the size of the dump and regulates his distribution accordingly. There should be news from the ambulance convoy as to how things are going up the line and what numbers are accumulating at the dressing stations. The O.C. keeps himself informed on these points, and at any moment may decide to clear the whole of the C cases out of pre-operation on to a waiting ambulance train. So much for the operation cases. Pass on to the next class.

2. For Resuscitation. – Cases in a condition of severe shock go to the Resuscitation ward (popularly known as 'Resurrection'). Here appliances are at hand for rectal and subcutaneous saline, blood transfusion, gum infusion, special heating appliances for rechauffement (vulgar parlance – 'cooking up') and so on. In some cases special teams are running these wards, but unfortunately the number of M.O.'s available does not permit of this universally. This year, had the war continued, we should have had trained teams of V.A.D.'s for the work. From time to time the M.O. makes a round and marks up for operation all cases that have sufficiently revived. You will notice that the abdominal cases all go to 'resuscitation', even when no specially severe shock exists, but they are sent to the theatre as soon as possible.

3. Penetrating Chests. – These are being sent to the special chest ward, where the physician of the C.C.S. examines them, has them X-rayed, and from time to time fetches the surgeon who is doing this work specially. Together they decide which cases are to go to the theatre.

4. For Evacuation. – These cases are being dressed in the examination room and then carried away to those wards which lie nearest the exit from the C.C.S.

Now leaving the examination room, you will pass through the pre-operation ward and glance into the X-ray room. A medical officer is at work with two orderlies helping him. The number of patients passed through in 24 hours may touch three figures: 60 and 70 are common numbers. Throughout the Army there is a standardized position for every type of examination, and methods of skin marking are also standardized. Endless trouble and referring back to the X-ray department are thereby saved. You will see positions of F.B.'s being measured out on cross-section anatomical atlases. A few steps take you into the operating theatre. There are 8 tables ranged down its length. Four teams are at work, each having a pair of tables at its disposal. The team consists of a surgeon, an anaesthetist, a sister who helps the operator, and two orderlies who clean up, bandage, splint, and fetch and carry. Shortage of medical officers has compelled us to train sisters as anaesthetists, and at three of the four tables they are at work. At the fourth table the special anaesthetist of the C.C.S. is working and is generally supervising. All the abdominal cases and many others are being given gas and oxygen by the 'Coxeter' apparatus. At this nearest table a blood transfusion is being given at the termination of the operation. You glance at the field medical card and see 'Penetrating abdomen, 10 holes small intestine, 2 large, 2 stomach, sutured, wound of the buttock excised, paraffin pack.' You recognise him having met him in the advanced dressing station earlier in the day. The donor of the blood is a convalescent patient who has been tested and found to be Group IV (no others are kept, and that saves testing the recipient). A number of donors are always kept on tap in active fighting times. They work in the C.C.S. until wanted. After one or two bleedings they go to the base, and if lucky, get a spell at home, but no promises are made. The teams come on duty at 10.a.m., and go on operating until 10 p.m., when four more will relieve them for a 12 hour shift. The output of a team averages 8–15 operations per shift, according to the nature of the cases. Multiple shell wounds are so much the rule that such a case as the following is quite common. 'Fracture right femur, lacerated wounds right arm, left thigh and left leg (post tibial divided).' The C.C.S. you are in has two teams of its own: one works in the day shift and the other by night. The six other teams arrived on the afternoon before in ambulance cars from all parts of the country, bringing their operating table, anaesthetic apparatus and instruments with them. Sometimes for six months together a team may be away from the unit to which it belongs, shifting from place to place as need arises. In the earlier stages of the war men have worked in the theatre for 36 hours at a stretch. Later, 16 hour shifts were quite usual, but more than 12 hours is inadvisable (a 12 hour shift often means 14 hours work). The Americans, indeed, adopted an 8 hour shift. As each case leaves the theatre it is marked up 'evacuation when round' (from the anaesthetic) or 'serious case ward' or 'chest ward.' Leaving the theatre you see Engineers at work digging up a bomb, fortunately a dud, which was dropped last night between the theatre and the serious case ward.

You have missed the walking wounded. Step back to the entrance again and you will see they enter a different reception room and pass through a different dressing room. Those needing operation are sent to the pre-operation ward. The rest pass out the back way to their dining tent, are fed, and go up to the evacuation wards to wait for a train. They are thus kept out of the main line of stretcher traffic. You look round the wards already mentioned, and the O.C. takes you to lunch in a hastily erected marquee. He apologises for the conditions, explaining that a bomb fell last night on the kitchen and wiped it and the mess tent out of existence. You understand why the tents in the officers' and sisters' quarters are riddled with holes, and you appreciate the reason for the shortage of medical officers and nurses, which he has been deploring. After a hasty meal you see an ambulance train loading. It is the second to leave that day, and another is waiting to come in. Getting a lift in that Daimler car, which is now more muddy than you ever thought possible, you are taken back to the Army Headquarters. Here is the office of the D.M.S. In a large room you will see two harassed looking men glued to telephones. You will hear impassioned appeals made to someone called 'Traffic' to get another train into X to load at 5 pip emma and depart at 7.30 pip emma. Then you gather that a supply train is off the line at P. and no trains can get into Y. till next morning. The casualty clearing stations at Y. are just ringing up to say they are getting full and wounded are coming in fast. You hear that B. Corps asked to switch their cases off from Y. to Z., and they say their telephone to the main dressing station is cut by a shell, but they're sending off a dispatch rider. More telephoning to someone spoken to very respectfully as "Yes, sir," and Very good, sir." And you hear Y told that an ambulance convoy has been borrowed from General Headquarters to clear them to the C.C.S.'s at W. Then B Corps seems in trouble: the run to Z is four miles further than to Y., and they are short of cars already. This leads to hurried examination of returns of cars. The wretched –th Motor Ambulance Convoy always seems to have half its cars off the road This appears to be due to the unutterable perniciousness of a certain make of car. Still, 10 cars are roped in from somewhere and asked to get a hustle on. Calm reigns for the moment and you look round and see enormous maps covering all walls. Little flags mark all the dressing stations, casualty clearing stations, motor ambulance convoys, sanitary sections, mobile laboratories, depots of medical stores, headquarters of divisions and corps and the rest of it. A string fixed by pins marks the front line. Railway traffic circuits, light railway systems, diagrams of all sorts and kinds cover the walls. In the inner office there are more maps still, marked with blue, green and brown lines indicating the objectives of the morning's attack at different hours. A sheaf of reports give the position from time to time as far as known. Other maps shew the position of the German hospitals ascertained by air photographs. Sketched in on these are lines showing the probable direction in which the railways will be carried forward if the attack succeeds, and schemes for pushing up the casualty clearing stations to take over German sites are worked out. The trouble is that 'Shells' or 'Supplies' or someone else is sure to want the transport at the critical moment; the bridges will be blown up and the roads destroyed. But it will have to be done somehow. Just as you leave you hear the casualty clearing station at W. asking for more surgical teams, and you see one of the harassed gentlemen poring over a big board studded with hooks on which are hung multicoloured labels, apparently denoting the distribution of all the teams, physicians, X-ray plants and so forth in the Army area. A discussion is taking place with a new comer, and you hear cryptic remarks about digging a lady anaesthetist out of the sisters' hostel and sending her up to make a team with B., whose finger ought to be well by now. Something is apparently fixed up when the Sergeant-Major brings in a wire from General Headquarters asking for six teams to be sent off forthwith to another army which has been heavily engaged that morning, and is very short handed. So you leave them to it. When you hear that this sort of thing will go on through the better part of the night you may be converted to the view that even a staff officer works. Curiosity may afterwards lead you to discover that in the 48 hours 3,400 operations were performed in the casualty clearing stations of the Army you have visited, or, if you wish for bigger figures, that in the three and a half months of the third battles of Ypres 61,500 operations were done in the casualty clearing stations behind that part of the battle line. You may get a lift to the base in an ambulance train, but when you embark on this you leave the zone of the armies for the lines of communication, and I must bid you goodbye.

(This is a remarkable letter which paints a vivid picture of conditions at the front and gives the details of the medical care of the wounded. The treatment of wounds described by Sidney Maynard Smith is that originally suggested by Almroth Wright and Alexander Fleming. Likewise the organisation of the movements of the wounded follows the principles also set out by Wright who fought resolutely with the military authorities to establish the treatment of wounds as near to the front line as possible. Thus the establishment of Casualty Clearing Stations and the pattern of patient movement then which extended into World War II. The number of casualties dealt with is staggering and the hours worked by the surgical teams in the casualty clearing stations e.g. a sixteen-hour shift was not unusual, is a lesson in stamina and what can be done when the need arises. Maynard Smith is another example of an extraordinary St Mary's man. He was educated at Epsom College and obtained an entrance scholarship to St Mary's Hospital Medical School in 1893. In 1898 he qualified and subsequently served in the Boer War as a Civil Surgeon. He was awarded the Queen's Medal with two clasps. On his return he obtained his F.R.C.S. in 1902 and in 1904 Honours in Surgery in the B.S. London. He held an appointment as Demonstrator in Anatomy at St Mary's and in 1904 was made Surgical Registrar and Tutor. In 1906 he was appointed to the surgical staff of the hospital as Surgeon to Out-patients. He was also appointed Surgeon to the London Fever Hospital and to the Victoria Hospital for Children, and Consulting Surgeon to King Edward VII Hospital. He rapidly developed a large private practice. On the outbreak of the 1914–18 war he served as Surgeon-in-Chief to the St John's Ambulance Brigade Hospital. He became Consulting Surgeon to the Fifth Army, and was mentioned in dispatches three times. He was awarded the Croix de Guerre and made Knight of Grace, Order of St John of Jerusalem. At the close of the war he was honoured by the C.B.

He wrote many papers on diverse subjects such as Head Injuries, Dislocations, Gun Shot Wounds, Gangrene, Inflammations, Perineal Resection of the Rectum, Surgical Anatomy of the Peritoneal Cavity. He also wrote an article on fractures in the *History of the War of 1914–18*.

He died in 1928 at the early age of fifty-three from a chronic infection from which he had suffered for some years.)

CHAPTER 25

Italian Expeditionary Force

In May 1915 Italy declared war on Austria (a German ally). Italy hoped to gain some borderlands, thinking they were rightly theirs in Trentino, South Tyrol and the coast around Trieste. Their war was waged mainly in the Alps and for the next two years the Italians made several unsuccessful attempts to dislodge the Austrians from their entrenched positions in the north. In September 1917 the Germans transferred seven divisions to Italy and a month later they and their Austrian allies attacked the Italian front. So successful was their breakthrough that they rapidly covered seventy miles before being held at the River Piave by the Italians reinforced by British and French troops speedily transferred to that region. The Italians had lost a quarter of a million men, mostly prisoners, innumerable guns, supplies, horses and transport supply vehicles. Their army then began a slow recovery and although the British and French divisions did little fighting their presence must have given encouragement to the Italians. When the last great German attacks began on the Western Front in France in March 1918 most of these divisions returned there to help. The remainder stayed on to play a part in stopping the last Austrian offensive of the war in June 1918 and then joined effectively in the Italian advance which brought Austrian surrender in October of that year.

A letter appeared in the *Gazette* dated July 1918. It read as follows:

Four Months in Italy
By F.M.Harvey (M.C.), M.R.C.S., L.R.C.P.
(Late Temp. Captain R.A.M.C.)

I stand as a warning to others. From tents, and huts, and duckboards, what greater pleasure than to still find Joe serving his shilling ordinaries? But beware, you on leave, the arm of the press is everywhere and it is precisely at the end of a meat coupon-less lunch they nailed me.

My lot lately has been in the luxurious ease of a Casualty Clearing Station, the envy of the Battalion M.O. and Field Ambulances. For is it not here "real" surgery is done and do not the lucky men live in tents and feed on the fat of the land? The days are tranquil and the morrow is assured. Even a push, a dread to everyone else, merely means more work and the line afterwards further away. Now things have changed. Retreats have broken monotony of the days, rude war has sent us out into the night in some haste, with a pack on our backs leaving all to the Hun. Alas my lost kit! But let me tell you of another retreat, which sent us hurrying to Italy posthaste on November 12, 1917. We just missed the exciting part, arriving in Italy when the Austrian, exhausted from his rapid advance, was held up at last. Still, we did not know at the time that he was securely held, and even prepared for a hurried flit at any moment. Well, as you know he was held on the Piave, and instead of the horrors of a retreat the visit to Italy turned out quite a "joy-ride". Four jolly months under the beautiful blue sky with an easily-held line to hold whilst our troops in France waded the mud and stood up to bombardments only the Western Front knew of. I heartily recommend it to everyone for the next winter months.

The C.C.S. entrained from the Somme for a destination unknown, at least officially it was unknown, though we had more than a shrewd suspicion whither we were bound. The Riviera looked beautiful after "bleeding Belgium", where I had been in team work. The sea was blue and the ground was dry; of the charming ladies who threw flowers what shall I say? Here was the France we had all heard of but had not yet found. This war has become such a monotonous dreary business: there is no acclamation of the hero from his tired fellows: even a Brigadier-General would lose his bounce after a few days of the muddy trenches. Therefore it was quite a shock when in 1917 cheering crowds waited on every bridge and fair ladies ministered to us at the station. We became heroes rushing on to save Italy. There on an open wagon stood our disinfector, the Thresh, looking like a horrible engine of war, which left the people guessing what new invention it could be.

At last we arrived at a town known to all by name, and we at once celebrated our release from the few days passed in a second class compartment by a dinner in which we learnt that chiante can be stronger than the "Vin Blank" of Northern France. In moving one is up against the old argument what should a C.C.S. be. The peace time strength rather resembles a Field Ambulance, but this stationary war has turned it into a hospital. It fills a train with over a hundred tons of material, including the beds and equipment of a big operating hospital. With all this it has no transport but is dependent on outside transport to move. There are some who still hanker for the light C.C.S., a few mule packs, I suppose, and every surgeon with his pockets full of instruments, and on the word "walk march", the whole moves off dressing by the right! A banner would be carried in front with the magic word Evacuate. I know this, that if we had only brought 500 blankets there would have been many fewer deaths on our hands from the cold.

Now, you must imagine the Italian Expeditionary Force thrown into Italy as quickly as the R.T.O. could send the trains through. Each unit detrained at a railhead many miles back, for the front line was still insecure and then approached the line by marches. This war has made for immobility. In an advance quick as on the Somme it was never necessary for the whole army to move at a time. But here was an Expeditionary Force altogether in the air; battalions were marching, Field Ambulances were trekking, and the C.C.S. spent their days at railway stations. Now this is what happened. The men were in bad marching form, the mud of Flanders and trench warfare of late autumn had made their feet soft. Suddenly, after being cooped up in a train for umpteen days they were called upon to do long marches every day with full equipment. Of course their feet gave out in thousands; the Field Ambulances, moving themselves, pushed them on to us. A sore heel is a very real casualty, very few men are fit to march again under a week's rest.

We sat in a railway siding, with our unpacked goods waiting for a move further up. It suddenly became urgent for us to cope with all these bad feet. A curious arrangement was temporarily made whereby I was made C.O. of an Italian Hospital with a few orderlies to help the Italians and meanwhile my C.C.S. went up the line and prepared to open. The scheme worked badly under the dual control. A steady stream of cases swamped the place and everything became chaotic. The Italian director maintained that he was still the doctor of the hospital and insisted in treating the cases. His utter lack of any knowledge of English left him nothing undaunted. His morning round was a pantomime which rapidly showed signs of coming tragedy. Within the first few minutes of receiving Britishers a strangulated hernia arrived. I went off to find our surgical specialist and an anaesthetist and on returning found the case in the theatre and the Italian doctor in the middle of the operation. He operated well but the anaesthetic was very bad. The patient coughed and vomited while the surgeon complacently struggled to reduce the gut as if it was the most natural thing in the world. It is a very curious thing how neglected anaesthetics are in Latin countries; anyone is good enough to give chloroform, and yet there is dissatisfaction with general anaesthetics, for they do as many as possible under local, and often with none at all.

My position was fast becoming untenable with the present arrangement. The men were most dissatisfied with the treatment, and an officer, who had been circumcised under local anaesthetic which misfired, was most eloquent, especially as he was taken to the theatre quite unaware that an operation was about to be done. After some skirmishes I won the concession of treating the cases myself provided I chalked up the diagnosis on a blackboard over each bed. This was for their records, and also so that the nurse, seeing the diagnosis could settle his diet. This took some ingenuity and an Italian dictionary; for example, P.U.O. and I.C.T. in

Italian seemed lost of their glory the way I wrote it up. However, in a few days we were moved to some wards in another hospital belonging to the Italian Red Cross. Here the greatest courtesy and kindness was shown us, and I was allowed full liberty with my cases.

Our men did not appreciate the change from our rations to Italian fare. A breakfast of coffee and a piece of dry bread left them still sighing for something more. The dinner at noon was good, soup and meat or macaroni and a glass of wine. They would readily have changed the wine for tea and the macaroni for pudding. In nothing is an untravelled Englishman more insular than in his food.

We had great trouble in burying one of our men. As is the custom we sewed the body up in a blanket. The undertaker refused point blank to take the body unless it was in a coffin. Never had they buried a corpse without a "box", as the interpreter persisted in calling it, the idea was preposterous and unthinkable! One of our padres was magnificent in reply – it was a privilege dearly prized by us all, he said to be buried in a blanket, a soldier's funeral dead for his country. Really a splendid harangue, though it lost most of its power and beauty by reason of the mixture of poor French and downright bad Italian. However, after much interviewing we won the day and broke all precedents.

The same thing happened again in a village where we had opened the C.C.S. The wily padre had actually got the corpse to the cemetery in one of our ambulances and hastily started the ceremony, when an emissary of the Mayor arrived. A heated discussion in no neutral language ensued and the funeral was suspended what time the great man was won over by interpreters. A further complication then arose, for on the death certificate was "meningitis". The Mayor declared this infectious, and the penalty, he declared, for taking the body through the streets in daytime was 500 lira. Apparently all the Italian dead are buried in coffins unless right in the line. I don't know how they manage it, for fuel was very scarce, we could hardly muster enough to cook our food.

On receiving word that the C.C.S. was ready for cases near the line I evacuated all the cases by ambulance train. There was a tender leave-taking from the hospital authorities; they were genuinely sorry for us to go, we gave them infinite amusement one way and another. In my dealings with Italian hospitals I learnt that when entering an orderly room or office always remove the cap, it is a great breach of good breeding to keep covered.

We had opened up in a school building and were soon full of I.C.T. feet. Battalions were still arriving and marching up the line. I have so often heard the blame of sore feet put down to the slackness of the Battalion M.O.! I agree that a great deal can be done by him to prevent it, but with the men whom we now must necessarily have in the infantry, it is very hard to eliminate it altogether. Take a battalion from the trenches and give them 15 miles a day for 4 days, and you will assuredly have many cases of bad feet. Changes of socks and washing the feet, etc., help enormously of course, and more still the compulsory attendance to the battalion chiropodist on the first sign of a rub. Still, there are bound to be cases, no matter what the Regular tells you. It is moon-shine to talk of pre-war manoeuvres and then blame the temporary M.O. for sending so many down now. They then dealt with picked men and not with bunions, flat feet, old wounds and boots wet through for days. By now Field Ambulances were established and could deal with the lighter cases. Other C.C.S. had opened and we settled down to routine work. In a short time we moved again, this time under canvas; in all we moved four times in four months – rather an undertaking with so much equipment.

I was very surprised to find how cold it was in the plains. The snow-covered Alps looked down on us and made us feel grateful we were on the Piave front. Generally there was a blue sky and bright sunshine; it was possible to keep warm during the day, but directly the sun went down we felt the cold intensely. Fuel was almost unobtainable for fires, and so we were perpetually tramping the hard dry roads to keep warm. We all fell victims to the coffee and cognac habit, especially as the cafes had a nice warm fire and were absolutely airtight. The Italians kept the cold out by wrapping their necks and head with colossal mufflers and carrying in their hands a jar of charcoal. The jar could be carried under the cloak. The beds are warmed by charcoal or cinders put in a jar and then attached to a wooden arrangement on the principle of a bed cradle; it is left in for half-an-hour before bedtime and withdrawn before going to bed. It was quite a common practice for the whole family to sit in the cowshed in the evening so as to keep warm.

The roads in Italy are extraordinary good. They are generally banked up with deep ditches on either side and lined with trees. For the war-time traffic they are too narrow, and an added danger is the slippery surface due to the frost. The results soon showed themselves in the lorries lying upside down in the ditches. The Italians are good drivers but very reckless; the pace of the motor traffic breaks all our own laws of speed; they use a light swift Fiat lorry, often with pneumatic tyres. Our Quartermaster-Sergeant fractured his skull, the ambulance having run into a tree. The roads are well cared for, but in rather a desultory fashion. Most of the road washers are girls; they gave one the appearance of toying with a long shovel and seizing any excuse to lean on it and smile at the passers by. They looked very pretty in their bright colours, and the inevitable scarf round the head. In the dry weather the dust is kept down by splashing the road with water very simply taken from the ditch by a small tin on a long stick. It seems very primitive, but the results are good, for the roads compare very favourably with the French roads.

Our last site was altogether charming. Two villas and their farmhouses made an inconvenient but delightful hospital. The war seemed miles away as we sat in the gardens with Spring just whispering in the trees. The Barons (both owners were real Barons) had left the villas just as they had been, with all the furniture about and the pictures up. The front was quiet, and so we gave ourselves up to a lazy, comfortable time in Italy, our days full of macaroni, chiante, and an occasional fingering of Italian Hugo, which would make us talk in three months, it said. The only rude awakening was the bombing at night. This was really rather bad, and the "blinking moon" had few devotees. The civilians liked less even than ourselves; every moonlight night saw an evening procession of old and young going out to the fields to sleep. They blamed the British for the sudden increase in bombing; our airmen certainly called for a reply, they were most active and worried the Boche incessantly. The increased activity was, of course, due to the fact that since the retreat the enemy aerodromes had come forward a great distance, and also a German squadron was leading the Austrians in the gentle arts of the Western front. He was teaching the lesson well, and demonstrated his ideas of warfare by bombing harmless villages and beautiful old towns, no matter if he gained any military advantage or not. There was a town near us which he bombed to such an extent that it was evacuated by the inhabitants. I loved this town, with its old boundary walls and quaint streets; it seemed a monstrous thing to see its gradual destruction. Among the few who stayed in the town was the old Bishop, an infirm old man. Despite his years he was quite a fire-eater; he refused to leave himself and forbade his clergy also. He insisted on the parish priests staying at their posts, even though attacked by the Austrians, and those who had fled in the recent Austrian advance he ordered back, though it meant crossing into the enemy lines.

Our soldiers enjoyed every moment of the stay in Italy; their only fear was the return to France. The front line was quiet and the billets good, wine and coffee easily procurable; what more can man wish for during this war? The billets were certainly better than in France; the barns are good stout buildings of stone, and not the broken down mud building so common in France. I never saw an Italian unit under canvas, certainly never a medical unit. It took some time to get bathing facilities going, consequently we reaped the result at the C.C.S. in I.C.T. cases. The Piave line at that time was very quiet. It was such a contrast to the Western Front that we all made a point of seeing it, so we could see how pleasant a war can be. The two opposite lines had the wide bed of the river separating them; consequently the distance made accurate sniping difficult. As a sightseer I was invited to walk into No Man's Land at mid-day to see the view. My reverence for the front line is second to none, and I have no desire for the heroics, but I was soon disabused of my fears, for I found everyone walking about in a nonchalant way. We crossed the front trenches by a small bridge and walked on to the bed of the river and stood thirty yards in front of our line for eight minutes or so looking at the Austrian lines. Nothing happened, but then, nothing does happen ever. We then adjourned to the Battalion Headquarters and had lunch in the open with table set and chairs. Those silly fellows the Artillerymen were occasionally sending over a shell to the Austrians and inviting an ill-feeling which would be quite out of place on that beautiful day of heavenly blue. The small stones of the river bed are a serious danger when shells drop on them. Quite a number are wounded by a pebble. One man at the C.C.S. had a compound fracture of the arm, and we removed the pebble from it.

Our reception in Italy was, on the whole, good. On better acquaintance the Italians really liked our men, though I fancied they always considered a Britisher a strange and rather fascinating kind of bird. Our transport was particularly admired. The horses with the fine weather looked splendidly fit and well groomed. The clean harness and polished chains, in fact, the whole turn-out made them think we had just been fitted out for the expedition. They were greatly surprised at the gaiety of our troops; they had always imagined that the Italian was the careless jovial fellow, and that the Britisher was a sour, sullen killjoy. It impressed them enormously to see our troops arriving in Italy, at her dramatic hour of her possible defeat, singing on the march and laughing as if they had not a care in the world. An Italian officer speaking to me one day, started off by admiring my tunic. He thought we were beautifully dressed, but then, quoth he, "yours is such a rich country." And then, "what a magnificent army you have! and to think it has all been done in three years, marvellous, wonderful!" That is quite the opinion of the educated classes. They were always amused at the quick pace we walked, "as if in a hurry." Keeping step tickled the small boys, who delighted in imitating our walk. The Italians do not keep step while on the march. Of course, we were all considered fabulously rich, though it took the shopkeeper quite a time to realise how an officer should be bled. Cigarettes were scarce, but we were quite fair prey for everyone to ask for one.

The Italian is physically a fine fellow, and I am told a brave one, but I never had occasion to see his behaviour under fire. He never looks quite our idea of a soldier, he has no pride of uniform and smart appearance, he doesn't put his chest out or keep step; even a man on sentry makes a very sloppy display of being on duty, more in keeping with a night watchman. Still, he has done some stiff fights and stood the hardships of the trying mountain warfare in winter. In the mountains the cold is, of course, intense, a sentry in the trenches with only a finger and eyes uncovered is changed

every ten minutes, so that he can shelter from the icy wind. The Transport
is poor compared to ours; it gives one the appearance of being tied together
with string. The Officer is very polite. I have been accosted by them in this
fashion: he comes up to me and gives his name and rank and expects me
to do the same; then we shake hands and start the struggle of a mutually
bad French conversation. If an officer enters a train and other fellow officers
are present he announces himself by name and rank and the others do the
same; everyone shakes hand with the new-comer. I was enormously
impressed with Northern Italy. My previous experience had been confined
to the South. Everyone speaks of prosperity, in marked contrast to the
South. The houses are well built and comfortable, the peasantry well dressed
and schools springing up in every village.

The complete story of the Italian retreat has yet to be written. There
were many factors at work; the forced retirement of Cadorna gives a clue
to one of the causes. It must be remembered that only a certain sector
broke, the others very reluctantly had to fall back, and did so in good order.
Whatever the cause they certainly broke down completely. In the general
panic it is pleasant to think that the British Red Cross drivers attached to
the Italian Army drew lots as to who should stay with the wounded. The
unfortunate ones were last seen calmly carrying on with the Austrian hordes
right on them.

The summons came to go back to France, and it was with deep regret
we said "adio" to Italy. On 20th March, 1918, we unloaded in the 5th
Army Area, and then we knew we were well in war again.

German Breakthrough 1918

Between November 1917 and March 1918 the German fighting strength
increased by 30% with the transfer of troops from the Russian front whilst
the British strength fell by 25%.

The German attack on 21 March was a last attempt to break the British
and French armies before the Americans arrived in sufficient numbers to
swing the balance against the Germans. Following a five-hour bombardment of the front line of the British Fifth and Third Armies the Germans
attacked, and by the end of the month eighty-three of these divisions were
involved in the fighting. Within a week they had penetrated to a depth of
forty miles and struck against the French line. By 30 May they were within
sixty kilometers of Paris.

With the Vth. Army on March 21st. 1918

In view of the 20th anniversary of the great German offensive in March,
1918, and of the further fact that the defence of the Vth. Army is to be

commemorated in a memorial taking the form of endowed wards at St. Mary's Hospital, the following account of participation in that action by a St. Mary's man may possibly be of interest.

I was at the time in charge of the Bearer Section of a Field Ambulance and was messing with the Headquarters of the Wiltshire battalion, which, on the night of the 20th March, moved into the redoubt next on the right to that so stoutly defended by the Manchester regiment. The Oise Canal and the French were on the right. The Bearer Section remained in the lines vacated by the Wiltshire regiment's headquarters. At about 4.0 a.m. on the 21st we were awakened by an intense bombardment sounding like continuous beating on drums. We were very soon threatened by gas from gas shells, which we countered in the usual way by donning gas masks and rigging wet blankets over the dug-out entrances. Buried telephonic communication was soon cut off by the heavy shell fire, and on looking out the lie of the land seemed to be considerably altered, appearing more like a ploughed field than the downland it had previously been. After a while one of our men volunteered to visit the store, and brought back with him welcome sausages and onions for breakfast.

At about 9 a.m. two runners stationed by me in the redoubt, either mistaking orders or feeling uncomfortable as to the possibility of the Section having already fallen back to the emergency dressing station, returned, reporting that the redoubt was being heavily shelled. After a while I sent two other runners up to the redoubt, which was about 300 or 400 yards up an incline on our front. These two shortly returned, saying that the barrage was such as no man could be expected to face. Not long afterwards two others were dispatched with similar result. Feeling that I did not care to ask men to do what I would not do myself, I set out with my orderly up the communication trench at about 10.30. By that time the barrage must have lifted somewhat, for it did not seem heavy by comparison with what it had been.

On reaching the redoubt we were challenged and passed through to the headquarters dug-out, which I had seen having the finishing touches put to it the previous day and thought quite impregnable. Altogether it seemed a wonderfully constructed defensive position. The Colonel was surprised to see me and said, "What, are you still here? The enemy are through on my right." The Battalion Medical Officer, strange to say, had no stretcher cases for us to clear, which speaks well for the efficacy of the defence works. The Colonel said "Good-bye," as though never expecting to see one again. It seemed hard to leave such a friend behind with his sacrifice troops, where he was provisioned to hold out for 48 hours in the hope of ultimate relief by practically non-existent reserves.

On return to the Section there was nothing to do but to retire to our emergency dressing station about two miles back with one stretcher case brought in from a field-battery in our rear. The barrage grew heavier as we approached the quarry, to which we were to retire, until it resembled a sort of roof of diverse shell sounds overhead. This was evidently being directed at the battle zone. Smoking gas-holes marked our way and our pace was diminished by the hampered breathing caused by the wearing of gas masks.

The great misfortune of the ill-starred day was the dense fog which blotted out all view beyond a few yards and acted as a defensive screen for the advancing German hordes. Through the fog we saw, in less than an hour after our arrival, what looked like giant figures looming through it on the quarry edge, with hand grenades ready to launch in the event of our refusal to surrender.

That night, as a prisoner of war in St. Quentin, I met the Colonel of the Wiltshires, safe and sound, but heavy of heart after the loss of his redoubt and so many of his men in the impossible task of defending his charge against overwhelming odds. Owing to the fog the Wiltshires were only able to hold this key position until some time during the afternoon of the 21st, instead of the forty-eight hours hoped for. In storming this redoubt, doubtless in the case of the others also, the enemy made effective use of low flying aeroplanes firing machine guns. This I saw happening while being marched past the position on the way to captivity, and the effect was that of a hawk pouncing on its prey.

During the afternoon there was work to be done at the German field ambulance, just out of range of the Manchester redoubt, which was still stubbornly holding out.

C.E. Redman, Late temporary Captain, R.A.M.C.

German Breakthrough 1918 (continued)

Further offensives had little effect and by July the Allies had recovered from their massive retreat and began to counter-attack.

The casualties on both sides had been enormous – over 700,000 in forty days. By the end of September the Germans had lost all their gains and an armistice was in sight.

Obituary

ARTHUR ALLEYNE KINGSLEY CONAN DOYLE
(Student of Medicine)
St. Mary's men will hear with regret of the death of young Conan Doyle, who died at St. Thomas's Hospital on October 28th 1918, of pneumonia following influenza. He was the eldest son of Sir A. Conan Doyle. He joined St. Mary's in October 1911, and in March 1914 took the Second

Conjoint Examination. He joined up on the outbreak of war in the combatant forces, and eventually gained his commission. The following appreciation has been sent by his Commanding Officer, who writes:

"I knew him during the terrible winter of 1916–17 down in the indescribable mud of the Somme. I watched with what enthusiasm he trained his men to prepare them for the first Spring offensive. But it wasn't until April, 1917, during the protracted and bloody battle of Arras, that I got to know his real worth.

He and I were amongst those left behind when the battalion went over the top on 9th April. Rain and a very heavy fall of snow had made the roads a quagmire, yet I remember Conan Doyle asking me for permission to bicycle 10 miles back to buy bread for the men in the battle line: the comfort and welfare of his men were invariably his first thoughts.

On May 3rd it was our turn, and I had the proud honour of commanding the battalion. Conan Doyle was one of the Headquarters officers. Our Headquarters was under a railway arch. The enemy artillery had got the range of that arch to a nicety, judging by the number of direct hits registered upon it. A previous unit had used that arch as a Regimental Aid Post. I suppose they had been relieved unexpectedly, for they had left unburied, and only a few yards away, some twenty poor fellows who had made the great sacrifice. The heat just then was almost tropical: something had to be done: it was one of those jobs that was nobody's job: Conan Doyle did it.

On 11th May, at 7.30 p.m. we were billed to go over the top to take the, at that time, famous chemical works near Roeux: no less than four vain and very costly attempts had already been made. History now relates how the 11th brigade went over that summer evening and dug in beyond their objective, at the same time making almost as many prisoners as the number of men who had delivered the assault. Conan Doyle was just like a great big overgrown schoolboy when I asked him if he would like to come round with me that night to see the men and to find out exactly where they had dug in. It was a joy to have him as my companion as we staggered about from shell hole to shell hole.

His enthusiasm was literally infectious: his loyalty to his superiors, his sympathy with his men, his intense patriotism and his keen sense of duty made him a natural soldier. He did not live his life in vain.

F.W.E."

St Mary's Gazette November 1918 Peace

The noise of the old guns going off at eleven o'clock was the first intimation to most people in the Hospital that the Armistice was signed. It was the same old guns that on many a moonlight night during the past year have turned nurse, staff and housemen cursing from their beds, and filled Casualty with a row of portly policemen very busy doing nothing; indeed, some of the patients required quite a lot of reassuring that it was not the signal for a daylight air raid. Everyone's instinct was to foregather, laughter struggling at first with a lump in the throat. In the space of a few minutes flags began to appear from everywhere, both inside the hospital and out, and the Tommies on the balconies were cheered by staid old ladies, who stood upon the tops of buses and waved flags at them as they passed.

There was an immediate "cessation of hostilities" at the Medical School, and the skeleton, thought by admiring spectators in Cambridge ward to represent the Kaiser was suddenly snatched from a life of seclusion in the dissecting room, and taken for an impromptu joyride round town, hoisted on the front of an army lorry. Newspapers and politicians are urging us to study the problems of reconstruction after the war, and before another number of the Gazette appears we shall probably be plunged into the midst of a General Election, with its urgent appeals for this or that policy. On every hand we have been told that when the men come back from the Front they will no longer tolerate ugliness and discomfort as they did before. For five long years their eyes have been compelled to rest on hideous sights – on ruin, destruction, and desolation.

What can we do to beautify the old place? "If seven maids with seven mops swept it for half a year" the result would scarcely justify the expense (at War prices) of the mops. Nothing short of a bonfire would clear the hallowed dust of ages from the Hospital. We cannot turn Paddington Mews and Praed Street into a Garden City, but there are other things nearer home.

We have an eyesore in our midst, an offence to every aesthetic sense, a stumbling block even to those who would see some beauty in everything – the coal heap. We have tried it from every point of view – from the theatre, from the Squash Court, scrambling over its precarious peaks for balls; covered with springing green sycamore seedlings in summer, with dead leaves and torn pigeon nests in autumn – in the rain – even by moonlight it is always impossible. Let this be the object of our first united effort; secondly, let us co-operate in producing a really good entertainment on Christmas Day in the wards. We can put our whole hearts into it this time, in a way we have not been able to for many years now, and judging by the impromptu impersonations which took place the other afternoon, there ought to be plenty of the necessary talent.

The Balance Sheet

	Numbers mobilised 1914–18 millions	Dead millions	Wounded millions	%
France	8.41	1.35	3.5	60
Gt. Britain	8.0	0.95	2.0	37
Italy	5.25	0.5	?	—
U.S.A.	4.0	0.1	?	—
Russia	—	2.3	?	—
Germany	13.0	1.6	4.0	41
Austria–Hungary	9.0	1.45	2.0	38
Turkey	—	0.4	?	—

(*Authors*: Thus ended a war 'to end all wars', fought by young men in trenches – caked with mud and covered with lice. They died penetrated by bullets and shells – and more so devastated by disease and festered by fevers and gangrene. The politicians' peace was to lead in the end to another colossal conflict within twenty-one years, and to further Middle East enmities as old as history.)

(Frank Melville Harvey qualified in 1909. He was awarded the Military Cross for his army service. He went into general practice, Blaber and Harvey, in London N.W.6.

Charles Edward Redman qualified in 1908. Following the war he was a physician in Winsley Sanatorium.)

CHAPTER 26

World War II (1939–1945)

The New Penguin Encyclopaedia states that 'World War I paved the way for the most devastating war in history'.

Following the end of World War I, Germany became increasingly dissatisfied with the frontiers agreed in 1919 in the Treaty of Versailles. Under the Chancellorship of Adolf Hitler the wish for expansion in Europe was fostered in the German people. Slowly but with determination and skill the German fighting forces, on land, sea and air were increased enormously year by year and the threat of hostilities increased in the late 1930s. The United Kingdom led by Prime Minister Chamberlain was not seeking a conflict but taking every opportunity to have peace with Germany. Germany invaded Austria and then Czechoslovakia in March 1939. Britain and France made a treaty with Poland now threatened by Germany's thirst for land. In 1939 Germany negotiated an alliance with Russia and then invaded Poland on 1 September. Despite the desire for peace Chamberlain and the British government gave Germany an ultimatum that if German troops were not withdrawn from Poland a state of war would exist between Germany and the United Kingdom. As Chamberlain said later in an historic broadcast, 'no such undertaking has been received, and consequently the United Kingdom is at war with Germany.' War was declared by Britain and France on Sunday 3 September 1939. Poland fell to the Germans within four weeks. There followed a lull for some months but in April 1940 Germany invaded Norway and Denmark then Belgium and Holland on 10 May. Despite heavy fighting France was overrun in seven weeks and the British Expeditionary Force evacuated via Dunkirk. Thus Britain at that time faced the might and power of Germany alone. Germany attempted to destroy Britain by aerial bombardment before launching an invasion. Thus began the Battle of Britain, fought in the air by the Royal Air Force against overwhelming odds. Germany's efforts to break the United Kingdom failed due to the resolve and skill of the fighter pilots and the indomitable spirit of the British people, who withstood bombardment on an unprecedented scale, day after day and night after night. In this war the loss of civilian life of all ages was as never before. So the threat of invasion was thwarted and no attempts to do so were subsequently made. Germany invaded Greece and Yugoslavia in April 1941, and Russia in June 1941. Rapid advances were made in Russia aided by massive German tank forces, and successful air support. Soon major cities were under siege, the battle for Leningrad lasted for two and a half years. Casualties were enormous and many starved to death. Eventually the fierce Russian winter and the ferocious and determined fighting of the Russian Army forced the Germans to retreat. Unbelievable atrocities were committed on both sides, a feature of this campaign and indeed others in this horrifying war.

The Japanese expanded into China and wishing to gain more of the Far East attacked the American Fleet at Pearl Harbour on 7 December 1941. Roosevelt in a broadcast said, 'this day will live in infamy' and America joined with the Allies and declared war on Japan and then Germany.

As the war progressed Italy, allies of Hitler were overrun by British and American forces and totally defeated, surrendered on 3 September 1943.

On 6 June 1944 British and American troops with their allies invaded German occupied Europe – D-Day: 130,000 troops landed on five beach heads. A harbour was constructed and towed into place to facilitate the landing of more troops, guns, ammunition and supplies that were necessary for this force. The battle toward Berlin was under way. By 28 April 1945 these forces met with Russian allies on the River Elbe.

Germany surrendered unconditionally at Reims on 7 May 1945 – VE Day.

Fighting with the Japanese, who now controlled S.E. Asia and Burma, continued.

The Japanese were forced to retreat late in 1945, but while fighting was still in progress the United States of America dropped two atomic bombs, on Hiroshima and Nagasaki, with horrendous and devastating effect on 6 and 9 August.

Japan surrendered on 14 August 1945 – VJ Day.

(*Authors Note*: It is disappointing that the number of letters to the *Gazette* in World War II are so few. There were about thirteen Editorials, but only a handful of letters. We have tried to account for this, and it is our opinion that there are many causes. During World War II there was a large number of professional war correspondents, serving as such with the military forces, and accounts of the progress of the war appeared daily in the newspapers. Additionally, broadcasts were frequent and some even from the battle-front. Film crews also served in war zones and in the cinemas the news was occupied by scenes of battles on land, sea and in the air. Thus the events taking place in Europe and elsewhere were brought directly to the civilian population. It is a fact however, that the news was carefully selected for civilian consumption. Censorship was extremely severe and even family letters home were critically observed and whole passages thought to be inappropriate for general knowledge were removed. Letters describing events in the battle zone were not encouraged. Another rather sad reason for the sparsity of letters was that the art of letter-writing was also disappearing and there was little to match those literary skills seen in the letters written by earlier medical men. There also developed in the armed forces a reluctance to talk about the war, and the horrors and atrocities that were witnessed in Europe and the Far East.)

September 1939 Editorial

These remarks are penned while the Sword of Damocles hangs poised by a very slender thread over the issue of Peace or War, and no useful purpose is served by making any comment on the tragic situation in which we find ourselves twenty-one years after the war to end all war. The life of Europe may be passing peacefully to its close, as a cynic has put it, and only one thing can prevent its decease – the conscience of Herr Hitler.

Let us make no mistake over this threatened war. Whatever the slogan may be this time, "The Defence of Freedom" or the "Curbing of the Aggressor," the reality of war and its trail of disaster will far outweigh any of the advantages gained by the nominal victors. Medicine has the task of clearing the human debris and doing what it can to repair the human wreckage. Those concerned with this task will assuredly have no delusions about its misery and futility, and we feel that they have an especial part to play in their contact with the people, healthy or wounded, in allaying what are very natural feelings evolved at such a time – blind fury at the German people and impassioned hatred of everything German, and also what is equally dangerous, an unthinking faith in the complete "Rightness" of everything done or said by their own nation. Surely such an obvious lesson must have been learnt from the last war, but (on the other hand) there is no evidence to show that human reason has advanced one step since then.

We make an urgent plea that in every individual, reason may override passion, whether the present situation be "solved" by war or negotiation.

The hospital itself has taken on a mantle of warlike and repellent aspect. The glass dome of the main hall "stains the white radiance of Eternity" with various thicknesses of black paint. Lewis Lloyd Ward has again been transformed into an operating theatre with six tables. Allcroft is to be a receiving and pre-operative room for casualties. The garage has been connected up with the tunnel under Norfolk Place by means of a large hole in the wall, so that ambulances can drive into the garage and discharge their patients under cover. The function of the hospital is to serve as a "front line" casualty station, whither patients are conveyed from first-aid posts, and are later transferred to "base" or outlying hospitals, those in the sector serving St. Mary's being Ealing, Hanwell, Hillingdon and Harefield and

Basingstoke. The staff of St. Mary's is under the charge of Mr. Bourne and Mr. Porritt, and consists of registrars, housemen, trained nurses and thirty-three senior students. All duties and hours have been allocated, and whatever deficiencies may be found in the large scale organisation of the London Medical arrangements, our own local scheme seems to be as complete as it can be. A feature of the arrangements is the organisation of the Blood Transfusion Section which has been busy during the last months "grouping" the Voluntary Blood Donors (or life Donors, as they have been so inaptly described in the Government propaganda).

There is grim irony in the fact that the Norfolk Place entrance at the moment bears all the signs of heavy fortification, scaffolding, blocks of stones and large baulks of timber completely obscuring the doorway. The explanation is, however, that the Fifth Army Memorial is to take the form of an entrance porch, replacing the country station awning which was such a distinctive memorial to our Victorian founders. Comment seems superfluous.

The indulgence of readers is asked on behalf of this month's issue of the Gazette. It is of necessity an emergency effort which needs must be somewhat scanty. We have no leading article, but what we have seems to be predominately of a frivolous nature with, we venture to suggest, even grains of wit scattered here and there. That frivolity should be the distinguishing mark of our contributions received during these dark times is not a little interesting. We only hope that the sources of humour will not dry up in the hum-drum days of peace which we earnestly hope are before us. The general state of unrest precludes us from marking in a worthy way the retirement of Professor Langmead from the post of Medical Director at the end of September. We hope to do justice to his work for St. Mary's and Medicine in our October issue.

September 1940

Thus pleasantly the summer shortened its days. But a change gradually came on; warnings became more frequent, and although we gave them scant respect, it was apparent that things were warming up. Preparations which had been going on for months took on a more lively tempo; fewer patients were admitted; the strategists were active at all times, and illustrative crockery fairly flew around the club. Then on a Saturday afternoon less than a fortnight ago came the first mass raid on London. A number of people watched it from the roof; their feelings were compounded of excitement to see the aeroplanes wheeling, now black, now silver, in fight in the distant sky, and of distress and indignation to see the great clouds that rose from the fires in the East End.

That week-end fifteen clinical students dossed down in the Hospital in the Housemen's sitting-rooms; though two bolder spirits, by simulating fearful immorality, managed to persuade one of the Housemen that his own bedroom was no place for him! Soon the clinical students were organised for duties in the Reception, Pre-operative and Primary Dressing rooms, Theatre and Wards. To one of the Home Guard fell the sad distinction of helping to bear in the first air-raid casualty to Mary's; but the man, alas, was dead. This – stretcher-bearing – is one of the jobs of the Mary's Home Guard; and they do it very well. They also watch the roofs of the Hospital during air raids, to give warning of fire or any other danger wherewith the Hospital may be threatened.

In the next few days the resident colony was augmented by a number of people. Most of the Hospital inmates sleep in the waiting-hall of the Inoculation Department Outpatients Clinic, Dr Hope Gosse among them. Others – for example Mr. Cokkinis – sleep in the basement of the Lindo Wing; a few in the tunnel at one end, some of the nurses being at the other. The Restaurant staff had been dealing with more and more people over longer and longer hours, and doing it with great efficiency and charm; and now left some of their number to sleep in the Medical School. We are fast learning to sleep at odd times and in odd places, for we have found that lack of sleep means loss of morale, and we will not play Hitler's game for anything. The barrage was a heartening innovation whose effect has not been dulled by time. The shrapnel may keep us indoors, but it does keep our chins up. Many patients have been evacuated altogether; one day Extension was emptied, and the next evening Thistle and Manvers followed suit (Extension, Manvers and Thistle are wards). So now Mary's is ready for what may come. We are full of sympathy for those other hospitals which have suffered already, and naturally thankful that we have been more fortunate. It is raining as I write; the guns boom when aircraft are heard, and occasionally shrapnel splatters on the roof and in the court outside; sometimes one hears the hiss and thunder of a bomb. One does not feel entirely safe, yet there is a sense of comfort in knowing that around one are many men and women gathered together for one purpose, in a place in which all are at home. It is a good feeling; it is a good purpose; it is a good place.

(This letter demonstrates that St Mary's Hospital itself was in the thick of battle, this time from bombardment by German bombers. The casualties were predominantly the civilian population on a scale as never before. This battle was to be fought for a long time and each civilian called upon to face the uncertainties of life in wartime, and the horrors and distresses of injuries and death that were the inevitable consequences of war. The civilian doctors and nurses were to play a crucial role at home while the uniformed colleagues played their part elsewhere.)

Monday, December 30, 1940
Daily Express

Bombed-in-a-Bath Doctors should receive the G.M., say Patients. Took 10 minutes to carry it 200 yards.

Daily Express Staff Reporter

Visiting day at one London hospital yesterday afternoon became a game of "Spot the doctor." Patients found that visitors, having asked about their health, wanted to see the doctors who had saved their lives and the hospital by prising an unexploded bomb from a ward floor and carrying it out in a tin bath.

The bomb-in-a-bath heroes are Dr Daniel Crawford Logan, a thirty-two year old Scotsman and Dr Mustapha Kamill, aged twenty-seven, an Egyptian.

When the bomb fell on the corner of the diphtheria ward it knocked down a wall and buried itself in the floor.

Dr Logan, as medical officer and Dr Kamill, as house surgeon, ran to the ward to superintend the evacuation of the children. But they had no place fit for the children to spend the night.

PUT BOMB IN BATH.

They decided to remove the bomb so that the children might return.

Gently they prised the bomb with their fingers from the floor. Dr Kamill ran to the kitchen, brought back a galvanised tin bath big enough to take the bomb. They packed the bath with blankets from a bed, put the bomb in it, and carried it out to a field.

The field was only 200 yards away, but the journey took ten minutes of sweating labour. Three times they had to place the bath down to ease their hands and straighten their backs.

Because medical etiquette forbids self advertisement the two doctors talked to no one outside their hospital about their feat. But the Royal Engineers who disconnected the bomb presented the detonator to the doctors.

The medical superintendent saw the detonator on the sideboard of the Doctor's lounge. He reported the doctor's courage to the local civil defence committee, who have reported it to regional headquarters.

Yesterday patients told their visitors the story for the first time, suggested that the doctors deserved the George Medal.

Dr Kamill was on duty. Patients said "That's him," as the tall lithe doctor did the round of the wards in his neat tweed suit and rubber-soled shoes.

Soft voiced Dr Kamill would not tell. He would only say how brave the children were, how they "never turned a hair."

Only his colleagues knew that the day the bomb fell was probably the most exciting day of his life. He qualified that day.

George Medal
Flying Officer K.L.G. Nobbs, R.A.F.V.R.

An aircraft caught fire in the air one night in November, and crashed in the vicinity of an aerodrome. Flying Officer Nobbs hastened to the scene, and although the aircraft was burning fiercely and machine-gun bullets were flying in all directions, he at once entered the wreckage.

He pulled out the trapped air-gunner, and after carrying him to a safe distance extinguished his burning clothing just before the petrol tanks exploded. Although the air-gunner subsequently died of his injuries, Flying Officer Nobbs displayed the utmost courage and an entire disregard of danger in his efforts to save his life.
Captain G.O. Brooks.

For conspicuous gallantry in carrying out hazardous work in a very brave manner.
Mustapha Kamill, House Surgeon, Clayponds Emergency Hospital.

A time bomb penetrated the roof of the diphtheria block at the Clayponds Hospital, coming to rest on the floor of the bathroom without exploding. Dr Logan and Dr Kamill arranged for the evacuation of the patients. They carried out their duties with coolness and courage, regardless of any danger to themselves, and prevented the possibility of great damage being done to the hospital buildings and to the houses adjoining.

December 1940

E.M.S. at S.M.H.

(Emergency Medical Service at St Mary's Hospital.)

Life at St. Mary's these days is quite simply classified. It may be divided into:
(a) Day Life
(b) Night Life
(a) Day Life. This starts at any time from 8 a.m. to 9 a.m. Some people have a swim and some don't; everyone has a shower or bath when there's any water, and a few people still do when there isn't. Then breakfast: the routine is for a very senior man to arrive in the restaurant, take up his position at the head of the E.M.S. table and quickly become absorbed in the "Daily Telegraph"; then, a few students in a more or less regular order, some with papers and some without; strategic places are taken up with due regard for whether you want to overlook the "Telegraph" or the "Daily

Mail." Enter other senior men at intervals, some officially present, others bombed out, others here just because it is a good place to be. The official commentator (who hasn't a paper of his own) gives his own news bulletin, complete with tactical advice on how to invade Italy, etc. Finally (very late), enter the "Times," but there's no one else left to read it.

From after breakfast until 6 p.m. life is just as it used to be, with full Out-patients and some positively marathon teaching efforts which are beyond all praise. The only grouse is the filling up of beds with some forty chronic cases – beds which, if they can be filled, should surely be used for our own out-patients to come to; but that is rather outside the province of this communique, because most people have seen Mary's in the daytime, while few, except local inhabitants know how the hours of darkness are passed.

(b) Night Life. Starts at 6 p.m. in the Annexe. Plans for the evening are made; it's all so simple really, as there are only two alternatives:

1. To go out
2. To stay in.

To go out entails four possibilities, i.e to stay in the one you're in, or go to the other three down the road. People have fairly regular haunts in this connection, and the Lodge are thus sure of being able to find Dr So-and-So at any given time; all very convenient.

To stay at home means dinner in the Club, which entails several short bridge meetings, "Craters I have seen," "Bombs that just missed me," and such serious discussions as the cure of Spasm.

After dinner one can

(a) Work
(b) Not work.

Not working means sitting, sitting and thinking, sitting and talking, playing bridge, playing billiards, or going in for aeroplane construction. The latter is being done in a big way, though one can't say much about it without giving away vital secrets. Room 3 is the largest factory, with subsidiaries in various rooms, from 1 to 20. Manufacturers are somewhat reluctant to fly their own machines, and at least one producer snoops round and flies other people's models when they're not looking, which is generally considered rather bad form.

At any time during these proceedings, of course, casualties may come in, and the whole place buzzes with activity, and on some nights a beautiful pair of little white gum-boots may be seen trotting busily round the Reception Room; Puss-in-Boots is on duty!

The lights go out occasionally, too. If you possess a torch you've somehow mislaid it or the bulb's broken, but it doesn't really matter, because when you've just finished helping Sister light one of those things that looks like a time bomb, smells like poison gas and makes a noise like "that one at Tussaud's," the lights are sure to go on again; another certain way to get the fuse mended is to put down your H.J. and P. (Handfield Jones and Porritt text book) with a contented sigh, and say, "Thank God, now I can leave my kidneys till to-morrow."

Everyone is immune up here, too. We've been filled up with millions of this and that which is most useful; there is, however, no truth in the rumour that there is an anti-gastric serum available, but we're full of hope and are all believers, though someone was heard to sing:-

"Lay a culture of pneumos
At my feet and my head;
And if I don't sneeze
Then you'll know I'm dead."

And so to bed, to join in the chorus of Amphoric Honorarial snores in the basement of Inoculation, with a silent prayer that the whistlers won't whistle too close.

(There is no signature to this composition. It may have been an editorial. I doubt if it paints the correct picture of what life was like at St Mary's during the war – it is certainly on the frivolous side.)

December 1940

To the Editor, St Mary's Hospital *Gazette*.

Dear Sir, – You ask for matter, and here is matter. Maybe it is not what you want, being too moralising and sentimental, but maybe it will help one or two of your readers in these times.

I qualified some time ago, no matter how long, and the years have rolled by, no matter how many, and what has the bottom of the tankard brought forth? War! Yes, but that is no topic for a Christmas Gazette. It is futile to talk of black-outs in conjunction with turkey, dancing, carol singing and all the brightly-lit, Yule-log, Dickens atmosphere. Who wants to hear of my bomb? You know, the one that fell with the noise of a bleating sheep and landed right on the top of Keningsea Church spire, and it is impaled there to this day. And, my dear, it is still ticking and strikes the hours ever so melodious. Who wants to know my adventures coming back from Dunkirk? How I was surrounded on all sides parrying Tommy gun bullets with my Spencer Wells, but still carrying on dressing the wounded. Who wants to know about my remarkable Grand Slam in the Edgware Street Air Raid Shelter? In fact, who wants to know anything about anything that I could write about? We are so hemmed in by war and its secondary advantages and disadvantages, that we are apt to forget that anything exists outside the framework of war-time England. But it exists. Go into the country and talk to the people there. They still do the same things, though they may do more of them. They still taste peace, see peace and feel peace. The fields and woods are the same to them now as they were in the sunny days before September 1939. But they have a great advantage over the Londoner. They see every day what we are fighting for, while we, who are working in London, tend to see only what we are fighting against. We all know what we are fighting against: brute force, bad faith. But we forget what we are fighting for. Freedom in thought, the Bible, and all great authors from Plato to Galsworthy, from Jane Austen to P.G. Wodehouse; freedom in art, from Praxiteles to Rodin, from Raphael to Van Gogh; freedom in music, from Bach to Stravinski. Think of the mighty who are on our side, the fighters for freedom, the writers and creators for freedom: Shakespeare, Chopin, Goethe, Michael Angelo, Homer, Beethoven, Lister, Lincoln, names of all races and creeds, all times and all places. We are fighting for the freedom of peace, freedom to be ourselves, freedom to create ourselves. But most of all we are fighting for the spirit of Christmas. Let us fling care and rising income tax, futility and danger to the winds, and remember there is something more vital, more human and more everlast-ing: the spirit of Christmas.

Cast away the tyrant Reason
Let one season
Be free from this exaggerated rush.

Remember this Christmas that happiness is given, not like a present with a demand for a thank-you letter on Boxing day, but by an unconscious effort on the part of everyone in the home, in the hospital – yes, and in the Air Raid Shelter. You must enjoy yourself. Stop talking Hitler and bombs, and if you must talk war, remember the Rio Plate, Narvik and Taranto, September 15th, and Churchill's inflection on the word Nazi. Remember that Victory is coming to-morrow, and not like the to-morrow of the White Queen's jam. And when Christmas is over do not forget that though Christmas is only one day in the year, yet what Christmas stands for is every day in the year. Therefore be happy this Christmas and every day in 1941. Then and only then will you have beaten Hitler to the ground, for his most potent weapon is not the bomb, or the tank, or the submarine, but pandemic unhappiness.

                                        Yours Sincerely, D.Y.

(We cannot identify the author from the initials. He thinks his letter may be too moralising and sentimental. We leave that for the readers to decide, but one message is open to doubt i.e. that those in the country were in some way remote from the war and 'still taste peace, see peace and feel peace.' During World War II no matter what part of the country civilians were in they felt the war in many different ways, knew all about it and indeed tasted it, unlike in World War I. Additionally overhead fighters and bombers allowed you to see it, and in many cases the Home Guard, the fire fighting forces and air raid wardens permitted you to be serving in it. In this war civilians played an enormous part and suffered in every country that the war touched.

Daniel Crawford Logan qualified in 1931. He obtained his D.P.H. in 1938. Following the war he was in general practice and was Medical Officer of Health in Whittlesey.

Mustapha Kamill qualified in 1940. He was awarded the George Medal. He served as a Surgeon Lieutenant in the Royal Navy Volunteer Reserve from 1943 to 1947. He was a Divisional Surgeon in the St John Ambulance Brigade.

Kenneth Leopold Nobbs qualified in 1936. For his bravery in the war he was awarded the George Medal. He served as a Wing Commander in the Royal Air Force Medical Branch and was a medical specialist. He obtained his M.R.C.P.Ed. in 1950 and was a general practitioner in Edgware, Middlesex.

Geoffrey Olivant Brooks obtained his M.A. in 1933 and his medical degree in 1936. For his war service he obtained the George Medal and was awarded also the Military Cross.)

CHAPTER 27

Editorial

May 1941

This editorial is penned as the last fires die away, leaving London licking its wounds after the most savage of raids, and St. Mary's breathing a sigh of relief as the last bus of the convoy disappears round the corner from Norfolk Place, bearing away to safety the victims of the night's terror raid. Readers in Bombay, Baluchistan, and anywhere else that circumstances have led them, please accept this, the only intimation, that St. Mary's still stands. It has not been bombed, blasted or burnt, and ugly whisperings are said to be heard in our less fortunate fellow teaching hospitals: "St. Mary's again, they must have friends over there."

During the two recent widespread raids in London we have had between fifty and seventy casualties on each occasion. From the administrative point of view the air raid organisation has worked pretty well. On both these occasions three tables have been in operation at the same time in the theatre. Nearly all cases received were admitted, and by the next afternoon the majority had been evacuated by convoy to base hospitals. Sincere tribute is paid to the work of the almoners in receiving cases throughout the night, and in settling up the manifold distressing problems which arise amongst those who have suffered as a result of the raid; and to the work of the nursing staff in reception wards, theatre and general wards, where many did an almost "round the clock" shift, and were still as efficient at the end of it.

From the clinical point of view certain interesting and instructive points arise. One is struck by the value of adequate resuscitation in rendering what appear to be hopeless cases fit for operation, by the importance of full detailed examination of every case, not in reception room but when undressed in bed, and by the great properties of sulphonamide powder, applied locally to wounds, in combating sepsis. Another interesting aspect of the injuries is the manner in which for each raid there seems to be a predominating type of injury – on one night a large proportion of head wounds were found, the causative agent being glass. With this series were also found quite a large number of eye injuries. In the most recent raid the injuries were more typically "war wounds." A large number were caused by bomb fragments, and these were lodged in the abdominal, pelvic and perineal regions, with a consequent high mortality. Four abdominal cases were operated upon that night, whereas up to that date only four such cases had come to operation during the whole time of the "Blitz." Much more could be written in this vein, for Air Raid Casualties have at least been instrumental in teaching all who have dealt with them much of which they knew nothing before. It is to be hoped that an adequate record is kept as a permanent memorial to the work of the hospital and also as some contribution to the advance of medical knowledge.

We heartily congratulate Hodson, Jackson and Kemp on achieving the Membership of the Royal College of Physicians.

1942

Tropical Tales

The usual answer to requests for news from the Services is that it is so difficult to write anything that is not secret. It was certainly my first reaction, and is probably a natural protective instinct which provides one with an easy and plausible excuse. However, on further analysis I found that a year away from the old pile in Praed Street had not been entirely devoid of items which might be worthy of comment. Admittedly, half the time seems to be spent in doing things which are so secret that we don't know what they are ourselves, like those blitz time convoys used to be to Harefield. Anyway, herewith some harmless trivialities. Within a few weeks of leaving Mary's I found myself sitting in the most tropical tropics of West Africa. It looked horribly real with a few palm trees silhouetted on a sandy shore, and I was assured that if we got sunk and had to swim to the beach, we should be greeted by horrible black men with large iron cauldrons. However we anchored in pseudo-civilization in Freetown, capital city of the White Man's Grave, Sierra Leone, and a lot of other very rude names as well. There we stayed for several months. To say we lived would be an over-statement; mostly we just existed. The first thing to do was to dispose of the 18 stone chief steward, who had tried very hard to have acute appendicitis when we were seven days out in mid-Atlantic. The surgeon consulted suggested waiting for three months. I've never known three months pass so slowly! I hope one day someone will write a book on clinical indications for operating at sea for the use of inexperienced House Physicians. Then we made our acquaintance with the Dark Continent. The rainy season had just ended, and as the days went by the sun rose as a dazzling disc, and travelled over a monotonously leaden sky, which seemed to act as a gigantic reflector focussed maliciously on us. The earth dried up, the lush vegetation wilted, and only mad dogs and the Royal Navy went out in the mid-day sun – the latter to work or bathe if an opportunity arose. In the ship, of course, it was just like living in a radiator. It wasn't long before I was sorely regretting my ignorance of tropical diseases. I had always regarded those portions of the text books solely from the point of view of whether the examiners could be trusted to avoid them. My sentiments were shared, and in many cases now regretted by many of my contemporaries, as I have since found. Prickly Heat was the first Bete Noir; it was only the fact that the first patient – an old salt of much experience – announced the diagnosis as he entered the sick bay, that prevented me from ruining my reputation forthwith by exclaiming "Good Lord, German Measles."

Then there was Dhobie itch; at least, what one called Dhobie itch in the absence of a microscope. Some may have been a form of Sweat rash, though most cases showed definite circinate elements. I think nearly everyone had it eventually. Treatment became an important problem; any form of ointment was far too extravagant on a large scale. Iodine was effective in some cases, and sometimes my sick berth attendant got excellent results with tinct. iodi. fortis. The latter, however, the patients were liable to object to, as it often removed large chunks of epidermis as well as the fungus. Eventually we found a most effective and economical treatment was a lotion of hydrarg. Perchlor gr.3, acid salicyl. Gr.25, and s.v.m. The patient paraded twice or three times a day, and the lotion was sprayed on with a throat spray. The exact mode of spread of this curious condition remains something of a mystery to me.

Then, of course there was Malaria. In this connection I was speedily taught a sharp lesson. My first case was a cerebral type of Subtertian, and I regret to say that I "sat on it" for two days. The patient was an old Petty Officer, and it wasn't until he announced that he had a propeller attached to his bows and showed signs of meningeal irritation that I discharged him to hospital for proper investigation. I was kindly but firmly told that all sick men must be regarded as having malaria until it was proved to be otherwise.

As far as mosquitoes in general were concerned, we were very little troubled with them lying offshore. Number One, whose aircraft identification abilities were greatly respected, announced one evening that he had had an Anophelene reconnaissance type in his cabin, and he brought it down with a rapid burst of fire from his flit gun. He swore he could recognise them by the fact that they made a dive bombing approach, as opposed to a steady run up on the target, and they had a retractable pair of legs astern.

The Tumbu fly was not uncommon; I never saw an adult fly, but its progeny shook me not a little when I first saw it. The larvae bore their way into the skin, and one day when a boil was ripe and I gave it a gentle squeeze, I was amazed to see a head pop out, take a quick look around, and pop in again. Once the maggot was removed resolution quickly followed.

Diarrhoeas were prevalent and at times proved most exhausting. I was told that B.Aertrycke was a common cause. Some M.O.s swore by

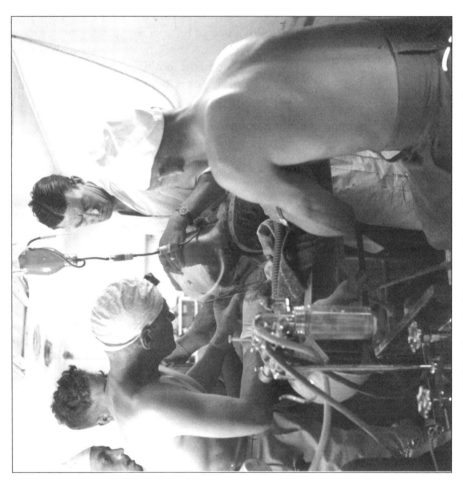

Mobile Operating Theatre – Western Desert – World War II
Photograph courtesy of the Imperial War Museum, London. Negative no. E14996

Sulphapyridine as a routine, investigating bacteriologically and cytoscopically after two days if symptoms persisted. My impression in a small series was that there was little difference in time of disability with that or symptomatic treatment. Of course, one always had to be on the look-out for the amoeba, which did not leave us entirely alone, at least one case occurring three months after we came home.

Some trivial abrasions took a phenomenal time to heal, and the question of choice of dressing was interesting. Once a wound was clean, a 1 per cent. Zinc Sulphate solution seemed more effective than most application. The method of fixing the dressings was always a problem; adhesive plaster was always badly tolerated, causing an irritating follicular rash. This was liable to occur too with firm bandaging, but could be prevented to a large extent by applying some antiseptic like "Dhobie lotion" to the area whenever the wound was dressed.

I had no personal experience of Heat Cellulitis, as described in the Gazette last year, though our environment seemed to supply all the requisite extrinsic factors. I did, however, meet one Mary's man in a destroyer who had had several cases, all occurring within a few days of each other on the outward trip. Otitis Externa was always with us, and was generally most painful and troublesome. A treatment advised by the local E.N.T. Specialist, who dealt with many cases, consisted in packing the external ear very tightly with plugging soaked in 10 per cent argyrol. It was moistened at night and repacked daily. Relief from pain was always marked, and the cases responded rapidly.

So much for some trivialities which may be met by any innocent abroad. I might add that in travelling, one is constantly amazed by how far-flung are the outposts of Mary's these days. Wherever you go you always meet someone with whom you can recall the good old days in the various annexes; in fact, I have heard that well known ballad, the song of the Virgin Sturgeon, sung by a rather senior Naval officer on a particularly steamy night under a tropical sky – and it was prefaced "with apologies to S.M.H."

R.R.H.L.

1943 Obituary

SURG.-LIEUT. IVAN SEYMOUR JACKLIN, R.N.V.R.

It has now to be accepted that Ivan Jacklin lost his life at sea on March 13th, the day he was posted as missing on active service. He was on a large liner which was torpedoed by an Italian submarine with the usual and useless German brutality. Many foreigners on board and not enough boats to go round were circumstances such that a man of Jacklin's character was likely to lose his life, and from survivors' stories it is plain that in his last hours he performed many incredibly brave and noble acts. One saw him going below when the boat was settling down to bring up a sick steward; another saw him swim three times from the sinking ship to rafts carrying service women who had been left behind. Later when the ship had gone down, he was still to be seen rescuing people in distress and it was while doing this work of rescue he disappeared and was seen no more, and all this in a sea alive with sharks and blue fish!

Jacklin came to us in 1934 from Cranleigh School, he was a South African, and had started his education at the Arcadia in Pretoria. He came with one of the Dean's nomination scholarships and he was just the type for whom these awards were designed. He had passed all his examinations at school, had been a Prefect, enjoying a popularity with schoolfellows and masters known to few and at sports he had excelled, playing not only for his school in all games, but also in representative School Rugby.

At St. Mary's we all remember his charming manners and shy smile, they endeared him to all; he was straightforward and true in all his dealings, a demon for work and great sportsman in the Rugger field where he won many a match for St. Mary's. After qualification he was Casualty House Surgeon and the department ran smoothly under his care; no complaints were heard during his tenure of office and he was always quick to consult when he felt a case was getting beyond his powers. He was House Surgeon to a very strenuous firm, and it was obvious that he was full of surgical promise and destined for a great career. His management of patients and anxious relatives was perfect, and he took great trouble with his dressers and gave complete loyalty to his chiefs.

His training over he was quickly in the Navy; at Portsmouth he did some good work in air raids, losing all his belongings on one occasion. In H.M.S. Kent he chafed at inactivity and transferred to a destroyer, H.M.S. Griffin, and in this ship he had some stirring times with the inshore forces along the Libyan coast during the blackest days of that campaign. Later he transferred to H.M.S. Express on the South African Station, and while there he was married. Three weeks later he sailed for England for shore posting, and after two weeks at sea his ship went down and his bright, promising life came to a premature close.

When Jacklin came to us from school, aged 17, his headmaster wrote thus of him: "He is a gentleman by birth, breeding and instinct and his influence on all around him has always been for good." To these words those of us who knew him at St. Mary's can only say Amen.

He was the most outstanding man St. Mary's has seen for many a long day and it will be long before we see his like again. A.D.W.

(A.D.W. are the initials of Arthur Dickson Wright)

From the Middle East

The following is an extract from a letter we have received from Lieut-Col. S.A. McKeith:

"I was pleased to see Croyn's letter in the May number. Also to read news of Furnivall, Lloyd Owen, C.D. Evans, G.S.N. Hughes, Perkins, etc. Isn't Corbin in the Middle East, too? I met him at Aldershot in 1940 at the Cambridge Hospital, but I think he went overseas soon afterwards.

I have met several Mary's men here and I expect there are many others I haven't seen.

I have run across T.C. Hunt and Reggie King, commanding the medical and surgical divisions respectively of the same hospital. Also A. Cokkinis (O.C. Surgical Division), Campbell, Embleton, and Gideon. And my brother's hospital ship calls here at intervals.

Can the somewhat cryptic remark in the July "Gazette" that Graham Jones "has been swimming in a big way recently" be related to the latest news we have heard of him?

He was shot down into the sea off Sicily and was hailed in the darkness by a passing ship. To the enquiry as to his identity he replied "I'm airborne."

We are indebted to Dr R.R. Wilson who handed us this letter from Captain W. Wynne Willson just as we were going to print. It makes part of the editorial seem a little redundant but that is all to the good and anyway we can't write another one now!

21st August, 1943
B.N.A.F. (late M.E.F.)
My dear Robbie,
The rag which I believe you still edit might like to have news of some old members of the hospital which I have run into during the past year in Africa. Most of last summer and autumn I was a "base wallah" at Cairo and at various hospitals in the Canal Zone, plying my trade as a bleeder of blood donors. Here I saw a lot of Pen Corbin and his wife (also "Pen") when he was in No. 9 General Hospital. Recently I have also seen him on occasions during the Tunisian Campaign, when he was with first a C.C.S. and then a Light Field Ambulance. By last Christmas, having personally produced several hundred gallons of blood and plasma, I thought it time to get back to the more general side of Army doctoring, and got myself transferred to a Light Field Ambulance in time to take part in the Tunisian Campaign, which I must say I enjoyed considerably. I was in charge of our M.D.S. which meant getting the casualties anything from one to 12 hours after they had been wounded. Multiple wounds from mines, bombs and shells formed the majority, and I saw very few serious burns. This was because we served

the Motor Brigade of our Armoured Division and the other Field Ambulance belonging to the Armoured Brigade got most of the burns from the tank crews. My transfusion experience came in very handy and I soon had the men trained to do them themselves; it was a common sight in those days to see eight or ten plasma transfusions going in a row. For a time we had a Field Transfusion Unit attached and so could give stored blood (taken in Tripoli and flown up). Resuscitation in fact is the great thing in the M.D.S. of the Light Field Ambulance. Only the most simple surgery can be done, and with good R.M.Os in the brigade there is no point in disturbing dressings and splints in these days of sulphanilamide prophylaxis.

We joined the First Army a fortnight before the fall of Tunis, and who should I run into but David Gideon, in very good form, cough and all! He gave me an excellent lunch (we couldn't believe our eyes when we saw First Army rations), and most of the S.M.H. news.

In the far off days before Alamein I saw a good deal of Car Young, a medical specialist to a C.C.S. Morris Lloyd-Owen was with a C.C.S. which took a lot of our casualties during the battles and we used to exchange rude notes. More recently we shared a bottle of gin while on leave in a Tripoli hotel. I've also met Dick Lawson who was a terrific fellow with the L.R.D.G. and has a very well deserved M.C., and old Beemer, who was in a hospital in Alex. Bill Ross I heard a lot about but never met.

Here is the end of the page, so I must stop. All the best.

Yours,

Bill W.W.

(T.C. Hunt was a consultant physician at St Mary's Hospital with a special interest in gastroenterology. Car Young also was a consultant physician with a special interest in diabetes. Morris Lloyd Owen was a consultant anaesthetist. 'Cocky' Cockburn was awarded the Military Cross for his war service. He became a much respected Medical Superintendent of St Mary's Hospital, a post he held until retirement. All four were colleagues of the authors of this book.)

17th April, 1943
H.M.Ship
To the Editor, St. Mary's Hospital Gazette.
Sir,
I read with interest the letter dated 3rd January from "Per Ardua ad Astra," who deplores the fact that doctors in war are not used outside their province. He is lucky.

In a small ship the doctor's duties in order of importance are:

I. WINES. To maintain a good supply of gin, whisky, beer, etc., for the Ward Room. See the stewards don't steal any and the members don't exceed their limit, which is carefully laid down for each rank in "K.R–A. 1." (King's Regulations). Keep a complicated set of account books, which purport to state exactly what each member drank, when he drank, how much he should pay, how much it cost, and the profits, and when each bottle was opened. The daily, weekly and monthly totals are each checked and cross-checked. This cumulates every four months in an audit which lasts several weeks, while the inquest into a few tots of gin or missing empties is being thrashed out.

II. MESSING. This is similar to wines, although the books are not so complicated. He must strike a balance between those who say the bills are too high and those who say the food isn't good enough.

III. CYPHERS. Although officially a non-combatant, the doctor is expected to be cipher officer. Ciphers are brought to him from the wireless office at all hours of the day and night. They take a considerable time to work out, and may relate to anything from orders to chase an enemy raider to the need for economy in sea boot stockings (99.9 per cent, are of the latter category). One does not mind being roused from one's bed at Mary's to see a case of appendicitis, even if it only turns out to be indigestion, but it is exceedingly trying to be roused from one's bunk at sea and spend the early hours at simple arithmetic, only to find that a buoy off the coast of Scotland has been moved a few yards northward, and again, perhaps the following night, to find that the said buoy has been replaced in its original position

IV. MAILS. He is responsible for mails carried to and from other ships and bases, involving endless small, tiresome details. In harbour he is expected to censor hundreds of badly written letters and arrange for their dispatch, and the major catastrophe of the captain's letter missing the post must be avoided at all costs.

V. MEDICAL DUTIES. Except when there are casualties, his work as a doctor definitely comes last. As such he is considered useful for finding medical grounds for getting rid of some unwanted member of the ship's company, and passing officers as fit for promotion or punishment. Those he sends sick are invariably "key men," and the doctor is sometimes regarded as if he were personally responsible for their illness. The above is not a complete list of the duties undertaken by a naval doctor. Some keep a watch at sea, others take over the responsibility of the confidential books. But the more executive jobs he does the less is he regarded as a doctor and more as an unskilled clerk put there for the benefit of the captain and first lieutenant to be ordered hither and thither, to hunt out old signals and explain new ones, to add up accounts, entertain visitors, or sell stamps, until the medical side of the ship is completely neglected.

Sick men need a clear, sympathetic mind to deal with them. They need someone who can devote his time to them. There should be no struggle on the part of the doctor such as " Shall I do that cipher or try and make that splint more comfortable." Hours of idleness there are admittedly, but rather hours of idleness as a doctor than hours of labour as a stooge.

Yours faithfully,

NELSON EXPECTS.

(This is a sad letter from a disappointed man. I doubt if all naval doctors have this experience, but perhaps at sea there is indeed much time on the doctor's hands except when casualties have to be dealt with. The morning sick parade with a ship of healthy men would not take up much of the doctor's time.)

October 1943
O.H.M.S.
This is not really an article, for it is too loosely knit and rambling, and it is not a letter, for it is too long, but is what I prefer to call a Contribution, which term covers a multitude of sins and is, after all, the thing which the Editors always mention after articles and letters in their regular and often eloquent appeals for "copy" for the Gazette.

It had been my intention to write a concise letter containing my views on two letters that appeared in the May issue of the Gazette, one from Flight-Lieutenant Pugh and the other from "Nelson Expects." But those views have now been merged into the formless blind structure of the Contribution. (Authors Note:- we have not found the letter from Flight-Lieutenant Pugh.) To be a doctor in the Forces is not half so satisfactory as being a doctor at St. Mary's, the main reason for this being that there is no "doctoring" in its narrowest sense to do. No doubt "Nelson Expects" has discovered this and is finding a little difficulty adjusting himself to a mode of life very different from the one he must only recently have left, that of being a houseman, or some other lesser form of medicine man, all day and every day. Every person who has joined up must have envisaged this change, and most of them luckily have compensated themselves to meet it, finding in the entirely new life unimagined opportunities for learning something about the Human Race which is really very much the same, whether it be dressed up in a uniform or not. This is not the kind of pill-gilding which John of Gaunt had to hand out to his banished son:
"Teach Thy Necessity to Reason Thus,
There is no Virtue like Necessity,"
But it comes from my own experience − a very limited one incidentally compared with that gained by those in the Army or R.A.F. The cosmos of the Naval doctor is naturally limited by the size of his ship, and 250 men (the complement of my little vessel) may hardly be an adequate number for

a statistical survey, but is enough in these days of conscription to provide a very true cross-section of the community. To many of us this war time experience is our first launching out from the confines of wards and out-patients into the world where people are normally healthy and where if a man is unwell there are no labels stuck on or near him with the Latin name of a disease on it, and perhaps above this the name of an eminent consultant whom one knows has got to take the responsibility in the end. Here are no convenient X-ray or Physiotherapy departments, no Dispensary with plenty of exciting alternatives should one medicine become monotonous, and no bright nurses to answer and cope with those distressing practical questions of bowels and diets and dressings. In a hospital so much is taken for granted, and for those of us who have not had the advantage of a period of general practice, the Services have been the means of showing us that there are more than two classes of human beings, patients and non-patients, that there is quite a difference between prescribing Mist Dyspeps. and making up your own, and that scabies is more than just sending the case round to the Town Hall. For myself I can say, though much has been forgotten and already the articles in the learned journals are almost unintelligible, I am in many ways a better doctor. I have lived among other people and performed many other tasks hardly included in the medical curriculum − and that without becoming the "unpaid clerk of the Captain and the First Lieutenant," that state of affairs which "Nelson Expects" alleges is the status of the Naval medical officer.

The same plaintive writer's somewhat piously worded dilemma, "Shall I do that cipher or make that splint more comfortable?" is one that, it hardly needs stating, should never be allowed to exist. It would indeed be rare for two such pressing obligations to occur at the same time, for no one in a seagoing appointment is going to pretend that medicine pure and simple takes up more than 20 per cent of his working day. The doctor, besides the routine chores allotted to him which most of us take on willingly, can make himself extremely useful and busy in his capacity of being an officer, yet not bound by the same rigid code of his executive colleagues. He is in contact with the troops and should feel himself responsible for doing all he can for their mental as well as their physical health. The Navy's "ceaseless vigil" in practice means almost ceaseless boredom, the boredom of oft repeated routine, of crowded mess-decks and the same unchanging faces, of bully beef and Bing Crosby on gramophone records. The organisation of entertainments and activities should not be considered too unmedical to be undertaken by the doctor, and the results are well worth the trouble.

Flight-Lieutenant Pugh has said all this in his admirable letter, and as I have said this to be a contribution and not a letter, it behoves me to quit controversy and become anecdotal.

A Naval doctor stands or falls by his Sick Berth Attendant (it is he who is called "The Doctor" on the lower deck: we are just "The Quacks"), for Naval medicine is a pleasant combination of history, tradition and an unbounded faith in the efficacies of the doings of Nelson's time. A Vandal gaudy with still bright gold on his cuffs, walking in to its time honoured ways, knows nothing of "Having the Honour of Submitting," of those amazingly worded documents Hurt Certificates, of the mystery of the Nosological Table, or of the intricacies of Surveys and Supply and Demand. A well trained S.B.A. (Sick Berth Attendant), does know these things, and if he is an expert you will do well not to question his words or actions. Yours not to reason why – just sign on the dotted line. You will be told how to sign, what to sign, when to sign, and all you have to do is – sign, if necessary in quadruplicate. I had a preliminary training for a few months under one of the real old stagers. No case of constipation, "foot-rot," Dhobie Itch, sea-sickness or obvious lead-swinging ever passed through his mesh to darken the door of the Medical Consulting Room. The Navy had its own methods of coping with such, and I never dared enquire further. I signed and asked a few questions just for information and we got on very well. However, on joining a destroyer I found the squarest of pegs in the roundest of holes waiting to be my right-hand man. He had been a miner in peace time, and at the ripe age of 43, by some strange turn of Fate's wheel, had become an S.B.A. He came from a part of England that produces an accent I never could understand without great concentration, and quite early in the commission he lost his false teeth in an encounter with the dust of the coaling jetty at G——, after a quiet run ashore. Accordingly conversation was difficult and, as writing did not come as second nature to him (his writing resembling the track of a tabetic spider) communication was a slow and tedious process. Spelling was to him a waste of time and he took a fiendish delight in medical malapropisms, perhaps the best being a case of Anxiety Neuroptics which necessitated a visit to the Phyzziatrist. The labels on the bottles became a source of great joy to me: there was "Idine" and "Miss PetroF" and, best of all, "Mis. Soddy Sally." There is a lot of whittling yet to do on that square peg. Amongst the trivialities of the daily sick parade one is surprisingly often confronted by a good case, and one realises how easy it is to miss the gold amongst the dross. One rating who had unsuccessfully applied for compassionate leave to marry his fiancee who was in the family way, came complaining of pain and "tiredness" in his left leg and knee. I thought I had here a clear case of Plumbum Pendens, but examination revealed a small swelling which turned out to be a sarcoma, the leg being amputated a few weeks later.

A whole article could be written and should be written on Naval Skin Diseases, for unquestionably they merit separate classification from the ordinary run of "Civvie Street" epidermal eruptions. There are fantastic permutations and combinations of macules, papules and pustules with an infinite variety of colours. The trouble is that they are all the skin diseases which haven't got Latin names, the ones you really meet outside out-patients and textbooks, and one's ignorance of their aetiology and treatment is prodigious. Children, take this solemn warning – learn something about skins before coming out into the great wide world. Spots and rashes are so painfully obvious on board ship – and they are there all the time, you can't tell the patients to get right out of your ken until next Monday or Thursday. Benzyl Benzoate is a gift from heaven for scabies in a small ship. Cases seem to clear up after two applications and in those which don't investigation usually shows that the application was only a dab: a few sharp words to the applicator and a cure is effected. The treatment of casualties is, needless to say, the main reason for having a doctor in a small ship, but so far, luckily, I have had none in my own ship's company. On various occasions, however, casualties and survivors from other ships come under one's care and, in addition to numerous honest-to-God sailors, I have coped with two Russian dock workers (one, I think, was a female), several German and Italian prisoners, six nurses (who got very wet, but were lucky no worse off), one Arab, whose toe I removed, and a dog who, a few hours after being torpedoed, gave birth rather stormily to a litter of four. The dog is still with us after nearly a year, and is about to produce another, Anglo-French, generation.

The Contribution, I have decided, is the easiest and laziest – therefore ideal – form of literary composition there is, for the Author or, I suppose, the Editor, can stop short where he likes with no epilogue or conclusions.

Excellent, the moment has come, and my only effort at Finale shall be to wish the best of everything to all at, or of, St. Mary's.

R.P.M. Miles, Surgeon-Lieutenant, R.N.V.R.

(This Contribution is a very fitting answer to the letter from 'Nelson Expects', and indicates the manner in which the varied activities of a Naval doctor on board a small ship can be accommodated into the doctor's life under the circumstances in which he finds himself.)

(Cecil John Hodson qualified in 1939 and obtained his M.R.C.P. in 1941. He served as a specialist Radiologist in the R.A.M.C. In 1954 he obtained his Fellowship of the Faculty of Radiologists (F.F.R. later Fellowship of the Royal College of Radiologists in 1975). Hodson became the Director of the Department of Radiology in University College Hospital, London. He was the author of many distinguished papers on radiological topics. He emigrated to America and was appointed to Yale.

Thomas Arthur Kemp qualified in 1940. He held the rank of Lt. Colonel in the R.A.M.C. In 1949 he obtained his Fellowship of the Royal College of Physicians. He was appointed a consultant physician at St Mary's Hospital, a post he held until retirement. He wrote many medical papers. Kemp was a superb rugby player and captained England. Uniquely he played for England before the war as a student and subsequently after the war.

Arthur Dickson Wright was a Consultant Surgeon at St Mary's Hospital and one of the last great general surgeons of the twentieth century. He qualified in 1922 and obtained his Fellowship of the Royal College of Surgeons in 1922 and his Diploma of Tropical Medicine and Health D.T.M.&H. in 1924. He was a surgical specialist in Singapore in his early career. Dickson Wright was the Hon. Treasurer of the Imperial Cancer Research Fund. He was Vice-President of the Royal College of Surgeons, President of the Harveian Society of London, President of the British Neurological Society and President of the Medical Society of London. He wrote a large number of distinguished papers and gave lectures internationally. He was said to be the best medical after-dinner speaker of his time. He supported St Mary's Rugby Football Club and was one of the most popular of the consultants with the student body.

Stephen Alexander McKeith O.B.E. McKeith qualified in 1932 and took his D.P.M. i.e. Diploma in Psychiatric Medicine in 1935. He held the rank of Hon. Lt. Colonel in the R.A.M.C. After the war he was Consultant Psychiatrist to the Norfolk and Norwich and King's Lynn Hospitals. He was the author of many clinical papers.

William Wynne Willson qualified in 1937. He held the rank of Temp. Captain in the R.A.M.C. He obtained his Diploma of the Royal College of Obstetricians and Gynaecologists in 1946. He was appointed physician in the Henley and District War Memorial Hospital and Obstetrician in Townlands Hospital.

Roger Paul Meredith Miles qualified in 1940. He obtained his Fellowship of the Royal College of Surgeons in 1947. For a time he worked at the University College of West Indies, Jamaica and later was Consultant Surgeon to the Chichester Group of Hospitals.)

CHAPTER 28

Extracts from Stalag IVG, Germany

Extracts from Jim McGavin's Letters written from Stalag IVG., Oschatz, Saxony, Germany (present address)

24.4.44.

"I am at my new hospital. I left the Stalag on a tractor with 11 tons of Red Cross Parcels for Leipzig where I visited the other area M.O., Captain Webster. We delivered the food there and I was dropped at this small hospital 20 miles outside the town. It is an old health resort, Bad Lansick, where people come to take the water. The hospital holds 110 beds, 20 British, 20 French, Dutch, Poles, Russians and Italians. I have taken the place of the British M.O. who is being repatriated with heart trouble. I work with a Frenchman – a good chap who speaks about as much English as I do French. I have some interesting chests and hearts. There has been a lot of rheumatic fever in Italy amongst the Russians. I have two British Nephritis, a Prolapsed Disc, Graves, Addisons, and lots of deficiency trouble. The country round here is very nice. To-day I saw a chap with a carp weighing 4 lbs. The only game we get here is an American one called volley ball. It is good fun – a court about as big as a Badminton one and 4–7 per side."

22.5.44.

"I have arrived at a new place but address the same. There are only 50 beds and a French doctor. I am hoping to get more work visiting the British in the area. I've had some good walks. The French Surgeon in the main hospital and the French physician are both good chaps. I met two Kommand Work Parties who had just finished playing football. Our people always look very fit and smart, morale very high. Captain Wright came back as he failed to pass the repatriation board. That is why I am at this new place. My French is improving a lot. I wish I could speak Russian as I would like to do a job there after the war."

4.6.44.

"Marvellous weather. Writing this in the sun by the river, where I have had a good bathe. We had a German film to-day with British captions. All the area Kommandos came, the distant ones in carts pulled by horses. They looked great – as if going to a picnic. We all enjoyed it a lot tho' the actual film was typical of the country. I have been playing chess. There are some good exponents here, especially the Russians.

12.6.44.

"We were all thrilled on Tuesday (D–Day) and are confident it will soon be over. Nobody talks of anything else, tho' we all know what a bloody business it will be. Well, I have moved again, still the same address and town. The place is the proper hospital for the P.O.W. of the district. It is run by a French Surgeon, his assistant and a French Physician. All my cases have to be written in French so I am improving rapidly. There are 150 beds and about 20 to 30 English ones. I get out more. The hospital staff run a team with matches once a week. The building, part of a biggish hotel, is pretty scruffy, but it works fairly well. Passing a shop the other day I saw an advertisement for Worcester Sauce. They eat it a lot round here!"

2.8.44.

"We got about 200 books from the Oflag. The older patients are especially pleased as they never get out of the hospital, and the exercise space is only about two tennis courts for 120 patients. I am hoping to get permission for some walks for them. We had a French film last night and a good contralto."

22.8.44.

"Very hot weather indeed and very hard on the patients as their rooms are so crowded. The black–out is always down in spite of many protests. I have quite a bit of work at the moment. I have now got a Dutch interpreter who is very good in French and his English is rapidly improving. He translates my French notes into Dutch and then German. I think he will soon have English taped.

5.9.44.

"I have got some very interesting cases now. We had a film "Sherlock Holmes" in German, with English captions. It is surprising how well known Sherlock is here and in France. They have a rum idea of what Englishmen are like! I enjoyed it very much tho' it was taken from a very German angle."

12.9.44.

"I have had four letters including one from Mr. Dickson Wright – and very welcome too. I am writing to them next mail. We have got some invasion prisoners here, and it is a treat to see them. They look so full of life and so fit after seeing the prisoners from Italy."

3.10.44.

"I am quite busy now with many things to do and getting ready for a repatriation board with eleven patients. Big thrill. The other day we got three Americans – nine days prisoners from near Metz. We have lots of British Paratroops in this area all taken in the last month.

31.10.44.

"The letter supply is good now. Everyone is full of hope for a quick ending tho' the pessimists are talking of next year. This week-end I had a very pleasant trip to a British hospital to see the repatriation commission. I had seven from this hospital who all passed – four from another, one of whom was referred to the next commission. One comes from Clitheroe and will either write or call if they get home before us. I very much doubt it tho'. The hospital is a good one and I much enjoyed meeting British doctors, tho' we were not at the place very long. We were away for two days. I met Bill Law again, a South African whom I knew at Annaburg, and lots of old patients. The weather has been muggy and wet, but I have been so busy I hardly notice it."

(This letter paints an acceptable picture of a P.O.W's life in a German P.O.W. camp. I doubt if it is typical of all such camps, but is a sharp contrast to the treatment prisoners of war had in the hands of the Japanese.)

June 1944 Editorial

To-day history is being made at a rate which leaves us bewildered; we are in any case incapable of doing justice to the great events which are leading this war to its climax. Once again we feel our remoteness from the scenes of action and by contrast our work seems dull and unreal and concentration on study is increasingly difficult. Whatever our feelings this is our work and only in this, and in those special tasks associated with the Hospital service can we play our part.

All his friends and particularly everyone at St. Mary's Hospital will join in congratulating Professor Fleming on the honour of knighthood bestowed upon him in the recent Birthday Honours. This national appreciation of Professor Fleming's work comes at a time when penicillin is being used with such effectiveness in the Western Front and other medical services. May he long continue to make contributions to scientific knowledge in happier days.

Postcript

In a snow storm H.M.S. "Activity" came across a Carley float in the artic. It was tightly packed with seventeen seamen, the survivors from a sunken destroyer. In the high seas it was thrown about like a cork threatening at any moment to throw its occupants into the icy sea. With great difficulty the men were got aboard in a dreadful condition and when they had been attended to and were able to speak told their story.

Their ship was struck in the darkness by a torpedo and came to a standstill so injured that the Captain ordered its abandonment, and as the ship's complement stood along the side waiting to leave a second torpedo struck amidships, and all were thrown into the sea. The sea was terribly rough with a blizzard blowing and the overcrowded float threatened to capsize every minute. It seemed to one of the small group that if one man left, the others might be saved, and that man, the doctor, was heard to say "I seem to be in the way here," and before anyone could expostulate he had disappeared over the side in the icy seas and was seen and heard no more.

That doctor was Peter McRae.

Officers' Mess, R.A.F. Halton, Bucks.

30-7-44.

Dear Sir,

Mrs. Barratt has written to me to say that she has had some messages from her brother, Dr L.J. Clapham, who was taken prisoner in 1941 by the Japanese in Sarawak. He was in the Colonial Medical Service. She has asked me to let you know, and would be glad if you would publish as much of the news as you think fit in the next issue of the St.Mary's Hospital Gazette. The following were cards written in his own writing.

(1) Excellent health. Removed from hospital. Voluntary agricultural labour main camp. Best wishes to all. No letters received yet. October 1943.

(2) Health remains excellent. Enjoying vegetable kitchen gardening – no responsibilities . . . censored . . . optimistic. Give best wishes whereabouts all friends. No letters parcels received yet 25.12.43.

I believe the main camp he refers to is the "North Borneo Concentration camp." I must say the idea of taking an experienced doctor off medical work and letting him do kitchen gardening is curious to say the least of it.

Yours Faithfully,

F.J.G. Jefferiss 2/Lt.

(Dr Clapham was one of the lucky ones in Japanese hands as most of the prisoners of the Japanese were treated very badly and most suffered from severe malnutrition.)

20 Ind. Ambulance Train, South East Asia.

July 3rd

To the Editor, St. Mary's Hospital Gazette

Dear Sir,

From time to time you ask in your columns for news of St. Mary's men abroad, news of which is all too sparingly given. In my own small corner of the globe I have met a few and hear of others; which is my excuse for taking up your space. The Japanese some time ago caused quite a concentration of Mary's men by inconveniently cutting our lines of communication; it was a pity that life was a little too hectic, or was it that drink was a little too scarce, for us all to get together. Bruce Stanley was there, commanding a mobile surgical unit, he claimed to have recently had the highest operating theatre in the world. Johns, who was well before my time at Mary's, was second in command of a Field Ambulance, and was kind enough on one occasion to present my mess with a quarter of beef which had perished in somewhat mysterious circumstances. Cocky Cockburn I had frequent news of, though we never actually met. Phillip Willcox I have since discovered was medical specialist at a nearby hospital. Now it sometimes falls to my lot to read his clinical notes, masterpieces of meticulous observation which leave one in awe when he concludes that the patient should be evacuated for further investigation.

Just when the ubiquitous Jap had got uncomfortably close the powers that be rang me up and said still higher powers had demanded my immediate posting to take over an ambulance train, and so it was that feeling more than a rat I boarded a plane, the only channel of escape, and flew away. Here I do not have my patients on long enough to practice much doctoring; it was de Swiet who asked me, before mutual recognition had taken place, whether I was in fact a doctor at all. He was engaged in loading patients on to my train. He told me that "Colonel" Flowers was at the same hospital as himself awaiting an appointment as D.A.D.M.S. which has since come through. Mary's must indeed be proud to-day to be associated with the name of Sir Alexander Fleming. I thought that the magazine "Time" hardly did justice when in the course of an article on Penicillin and its founder it referred to the Fountains as a potted palm pub. "Time's" correspondent should visit it again on the night of the conjoint results, would that I might do the same.

Yours Faithfully,

T.R. Maurice, Major, R.A.M.C.

Editorial September 1944

The end is in sight. The long-awaited moment is at last here, the moment for which the nation has battled, endured, and patiently waited. The armies of the 3rd Reich are running pell-mell in a disorderly rabble across the face of France and the low countries, while the Allied Armies sweep triumphantly on in pursuit in a gigantic tide of artillery and armour.

Never has there been a finer Allied army, never in the annals of the British Army has the efficiency and bravery of its units been greater. Between the Battle of Britain and the Battle of France lies the greatest symposium of national achievement in the history of the world.

On the home front, less spectacular, but equally important, there have been, as in the armed forces, long periods of boredom interspersed with shorter periods of excitement and danger. But there has been no slackening of effort – no softening of the determination to see the business through to the end. Mary's has reflected this attitude, and, fortunate in being scarcely touched by enemy action, has not once closed her doors. With the end of the war within measurable distance we can see the cheerful prospect of the hospital functioning at full capacity once more, with all wards in use and a full honorary staff.

Throughout all the air raids Mary's has carried on her own work as well as the reception, treatment and evacuation of casualties. After a long lull, the air raid casualty organisation has again functioned smoothly and efficiently during the incendiary blitz earlier in the year and the present flying bomb infestation. Among the many factors which have contributed to this efficiency must be mentioned the E.M.S. (Emergency Medical Service) student stretcher-bearer organisation. The E.M.S. stretcher-bearers have done a first rate job, and a very important one. It is not easy when working for final examinations, to spend most of the night carrying loaded stretchers to and from ambulances and the theatre. Stretcher-bearing is not merely a form of unskilled labour – it demands gentleness, promptness, and skill, and gentleness and dispatch are of the first importance in dealing with badly shocked casualties: the E.M.S. students have never been found wanting in any respect. The Hospital was honoured by a visit from Her Majesty the Queen on August 9th, an account of which will be found elsewhere in this issue.

The kaleidoscope of war is changing its pattern with astonishing swiftness almost daily, as the allied armies rumble on towards Germany. Already the flying bomb menace is receding, and by the time this editorial goes to press untold new victories will probably have been won. And when it is all over the fighting men and the prisoners of war will come back – back to England. One of the many problems of the post-war years is that of the rehabilitation into civilian life of the men from the Services – many will remain, but many will return, and they must be rewarded for their services with the prospect of security and congenial work – especially those who have been prisoners of war and who have had the hardest lot to bear of all. After the last war there was a great deal of cant about "a land fit for heroes to live in." All men are not heroes, but the vast majority have risked their lives and endured mutilation, discomforts, privations, and separation so that Germany may finally be taught her lesson. They have earned the right to look forward to post-war Britain with confidence and excitement. Let us hope with all our hearts that they will not be disappointed or disillusioned. Rupert Brooke died, and was buried in the Aegean, in 1915, but his poetry lives on:

God, I will pack and take a train,
And get me to England once again!
For England's the one land, I know,
Where men with splendid hearts may go.

Extracts from a letter written by Capt. A.C. Porteous R.A.M.C., from a Field Ambulance with the British Liberation Armies,

16th September 1944.

". . . We have covered 230 miles in the last two days, and are now in another country and will very soon be in another. It is very tiring travelling from 7.30 a.m. to 9.30 p.m. with 15 min. halts every other hour only. We have had a colossal welcome – greater than anything we experienced in France. Fruit was literally showered into the trucks, beer also, and the streets were lined with masses of cheering people . . .

I don't know whether I have told you before, but we can tell news up until a fortnight back. Briefly, our division took the leading part in the battles round Eterville, etc., We then switched to another part of the front and fought and captured Mt. Pincon and forced a crossing over the river Noireau. We then made the bridge-head over the Seine at Vernon – the first British troops to cross . . . I have been to Paris and Rouen, and had a very good time in the former place – which is little changed by the war, except for the food and transport situation. There is nothing short in any of the shops but the prices are fabulous. We were more or less mobbed, being the few British Officers in Paris. . . . We are advancing on a front from Antwerp to the Belfort Gap. We are sleeping above ground these days, but I don't think it will be long before we are digging in again . . .

(We are indebted to Dr A.B. Porteous for very kindly sending in these extracts from his son's letter.)

October 1944 Editorial

These days of victory before the final destruction of our enemies are days filled with hope not unmixed with anxiety and sorrow. The campaign of the last few weeks in Western Europe has been the most brilliantly successful of the war; the advance across France from the original beachheads into the Low Countries and into the very bastions of the German fortress was the most extensive of all in this war of swift and mobile strategy. The men of the mild, and as some thought, over civilised democracies have fought boldly, and have well beaten the professionals at total war. That the Germanic traditions, intensified in the forcing-house of the last ten years, should successfully produce efficient fighting machines in place of good citizens is not surprising. But the determination and hard physical courage of the soldiers reared in the peace loving, easy-going spirit of the Western democracies are a source of wonder and respect. The men of Arnhem and Nijmegen were the ordinary citizens of this land with no thoughts of conquest or of violence. Their gallantry should be an incentive

to the ever-watchful guardianship of the personal liberty and the freedom
to order their own lives which they have temporarily relinquished. They
have fought for their freedom from direction and control and when the war
is over, having faced fiercer enemies, they will be determined to have it.

We hear of many St. Mary's men in action at this time, but get very little
definite news that could be published. We know that news is always eagerly
awaited and we should be pleased to think that information of Mary's men
in these columns might relieve the anxiety of their friends or bring to mind
happier days.

October 1944

We wish to thank Dr Harold C. Lees, Arkendale, Darwen, for sending us
the following extract from the "Northern Daily Telegraph."

Among the treasured souvenirs of the Glasgow Highlanders' stay in
Belgium during the war will be a beautifully executed tapestry portrait of
King George VI, which was presented to the battalion by the Mayor of the
village of Bellingham. The tapestry had been kept in hiding during the
German occupation. The officer who received it on behalf of the C.O. was
Captain H.W. ("Bill") Lees, third son of Dr and Mrs. H.C. Lees of
Arkendale, Darwen.

Captain Lees told a reporter that the Mayor could speak quite good
English, but that the rest of the imposing array of officials could speak none
at all. They simply smiled their approval of everything which took place.

"The Mayor came up to me," said Captain Lees, "and solemnly unrolled
a magnificent piece of tapestry, which he handed to me. He made a short
speech, in which he said he wished to give it to the chief man of the
regiment, on behalf of the people of the village. I accepted on behalf of the
C.O., and made a speech of thanks, and everybody was highly delighted. If
we had let them, I think they would have brought out a brass band to
welcome us, but we had to push on."

The Battalion of the Glasgow Highlanders had been diverted off the main
axis of advance and were the first British troops to enter the village. In fact,
German patrols were only a quarter of a mile away when the Jocks entered.
The local inhabitants went almost mad with joy at their liberation and the
whole column was held up.

Captain Lees handed the trophy to the Commanding Officer, who has
written to the Mayor thanking him for the spontaneous gesture of
friendship. The tapestry is now in Scotland.

Captain Lees has been in the Army since 1939, and in 1940 he ran a
hospital on the coast of France just before Dunkirk. The evacuation of the
patients took longer than anticipated, and he was one of the last to get away.

He heard afterwards that the hospital ship in which he had intended sailing had been lost in the Channel. He served in England until returning to the continent just after D-Day.

Before joining up Captain Lees was in practice with his father for a time. After leaving Tattenhall, near Wolverhampton, he went to St. Mary's Hospital, London from where he took his M.R.C.S. and L.R.C.P. degrees.

Dr and Mrs. Lees have five sons serving. Two are in the Army, and the others are in the Indian Army, the R.A.F. and the N.F.S. A son-in-law is in the Navy.

(James Grant McGavin qualified in 1941; there are no details of his subsequent career but his address was in Shropshire.

Lawrence John Clapham qualified in 1935 and took his M.B.B.S. in 1938. He obtained his D.T.M.& H. in 1940 (Diploma in Tropical Medicine and Health) and his D.P.H.(Diploma in Public Health) in 1952 and also his M.D. in 1952. For a time he was in the Medical Services in Sarawak and became the Director of Medical Services in North Borneo.

Frederick James Gordon Jefferiss qualified in 1935. He was Temp. Squadron Leader in the R.A.F. and subsequently became the Director of the Special Clinic at St Mary's Hospital, London. He was the author of many papers on Venereal Disease. He was a colleague of the authors of this book.

Thomas Richardson Maurice qualified in 1941 he was a Major in the R.A.M.C. and following the war was in general practice, Maurice and Wheeler. He was the medical officer of Savernake Hospital, Marlborough.

Alexander Calvert Porteous qualified in 1942. He was a general practitioner in the Isle of Wight, Kennedy and Porteous.

Harold Cruickshank Lees qualified in 1904 and practised as a surgeon in Blackburn and E. Lancs. Royal Infirmary.)

CHAPTER 29

April 1945 – Editorial

Once again the lights are shining in London and over the country. Through the dark years we have often thought of this day, when the destruction and troubles of war would be past. Gradually the immediate dangers have receded, and more and more we are becoming aware of the enormous task awaiting us in the peace. The German plan of wanton destruction of life and the means of life in Europe, which, out of spite and hate for their enemies and the wish to embarrass our victories, is their one remaining activity, faces us with the most pressing problems now and, it can be expected, for future generations.

We will not speak of the horrors deliberately inflicted on thousands of innocent victims, but the plight of millions of survivors is of such urgency as to demand our utmost efforts, lest the loss of life after the peace be greater than before. Relief to Europe now and until the crisis has been overcome must be on a scale equal to and carried on with the energy of the greatest efforts of the war. Only by the provision by the Allies of food, amenities and expert assistance, will the great tragedy of Europe be lessened and an even greater tragedy be avoided in the coming months.

NOTE
We were delighted to see Graham Jones and Douglas Scott, both recently freed by U.S. Forces in Germany. They looked remarkably well, due in great measure to then-hospitable treatment by the Americans.

A dozen students left for Germany on April 28th to help in the rescue work at the concentration camps. We feel it is out of place to wish them bon voyage, but we hope their experiences will not be too grim and that they will have some lighter moments.

August – September 1945

Belsen
By John Hankinson

Just before the Easter week-end a most interesting notice appeared in the Medical School headed "Holland," asking for twelve St Mary's students to join a party of one hundred from the London schools to aid in feeding severe cases of starvation in the liberated Dutch cities. This met with an immediate response, and unfortunately many had to be disappointed, but in the course of the next week twelve were inoculated, instructed and equipped with enough Army impedimenta for an extensive campaign. We now experienced a method of organisation with which we were eventually to become very familiar, characteristic of Army movements as we experienced them. I refer to the preliminary alarm and frantic preparation, the long latent period with its crop of wild rumours and cheerful indifference, followed suddenly, in the twinkling of an eye, by the hasty departure. Throughout April the latent period lengthened until the most sanguine shook their heads and spoke of false alarms — we had a lot to learn!

Friday 27th was the day of the Rugger dance and naturally of all days the one of which we were told to be ready for immediate departure. However, for better or for worse, we were able to take part in the festivities, and next day in varying degrees of fitness we made our way by taxi to the meeting place at Red Cross Headquarters. Here we did nothing for three or four hours, but heard with considerable interest that Belsen and not Holland was to be our destination. For the first time we met the assembled party, which, despite khaki and British Red Cross flashes, in some cases achieved a bizarre lack of uniformity.

Eventually we found ourselves in Paddington (which we hadn't expected to see again quite so soon) and thence off to Cirencester. We were destined to spend the night, and more nights than we imagined, in the Rover staging camp a few miles from Cirencester, and our arrival there was memorable. The snowstorm which had greeted us at Cirencester was blowing with increasing violence as, laden with kitbags and blankets, in pitch darkness we blundered madly through the wood in which the Nissen huts stood. The bellowings of the appointed Hospital representatives, as down in the dark wood they called together their struggling and benighted flocks, were reminiscent of Teddington and the cry "Mary's" vied with "Guy's" and the rest until all were gathered in a hut to each hospital. I think we provided a few minor novelties in Army organisation. Everyone appeared quite accustomed to the cafeteria method of dining and the distance from the cookhouse to healthily ventilated marquees resulted in an unusual addition of snow to food which didn't really require it. In the days which followed the cook proved himself thoroughly convinced of the high nutritive value of baked beans and spam.

For the next four mornings we were awakened at 3.30 or 4 a.m. according to the whim of a sergeant with the cheerful appearance of a man who had been waiting all night for that pleasure and would soon be retiring for a good day's sleep — as a night sister before retiring from the scene might urge into consciousness the newly risen day staff. Going for breakfast by moonlight was not a entirely new experience, but as a routine it soon began to pall.

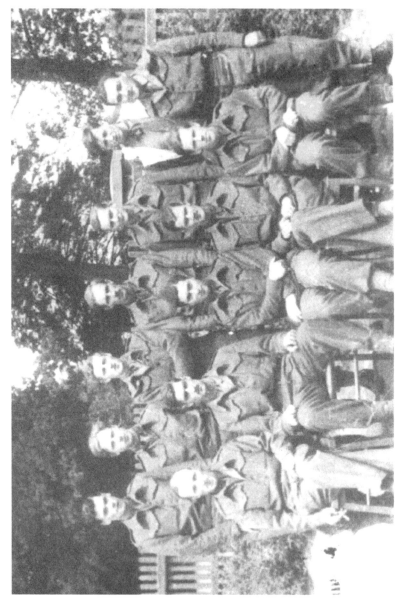

Belsen 1945. Back row: R. Armatage, T.C. Brown, T.D. Hawkins, R.W. Watson, A.B. Matthews, G.C. Thick, A.V. Price
Front row: J. Hankinson, J.L.C. Whitcombe, G.W. Korn, P.D.C. Jackson, J. McLuskie

Photograph courtesy of Dr Desmond Hawkins

Twelve medical students from St Mary's Hospital Medical School who volunteered to work in Belsen caring for inmates

I think the idea of arriving at the aerodrome at 6.30 was to avoid the possibility of the 'planes leaving without us, which on the return journey I was to learn was a very real one. Sunday was very bright with a bitterly cold wind and, after watching the ice being scraped off the wing and a few other unenthusiastic preparations made, we heard about noon that all flying was cancelled for the day, due to icing. We were soothed by W.A.A.F.s who made cups of tea and gave us the Sunday papers. It was little consolation to read there that the party of London medical students had already been flown to Belsen and would be starting work the next day. A reporter's life seemed a very enviable one.

As our stay in the camp appeared likely to be prolonged, such enthusiastic attention was given to the heating of the huts that chimneys glowed red–hot under forced draughts, much to the Camp Commandant's alarm. It was Sunday night, I think, that I was awakened by wild cries to a scene like pictures of the lower hell. Through the smoke, flames showed the terrifying figure of Whitcombe leaping madly backwards and forwards as he fought the fire with an empty biscuit tin. The general feeling was that he might have made rather less noise about it, and the gallantry of his action in getting out of a nice warm bed to perform this service for the community tended to be overlooked at the time. Thanks were rendered at a more suitable hour.

Monday was memorable in that six Dakotas took off, indeed one of them completed the full journey to Celle and another delivered its much envied load for a night in Brussels. It would not be proper for me to give a second-hand account of life in that ancient capital, but I am told it is still full of interest. Two 'planes returned directly to Cirencester and two landed at Croydon. After long journeys by train, truck and 'plane, Paddington to Croydon in two days was a depressing rate of progress; but we had a good lunch before returning to Cirencester, which, however, was fast losing all its charm for us. The following day we tried a different aerodrome, different only in its locality and improved catering; like the other, 6.a.m. was the appointed hour, but flying was not on the programme.

By this time we were quite resigned and had the hotels in Cirencester well organised for baths, and dinner in the evening, and our reappearance was expected and called for a round of drinks. They must have been quite surprised on Wednesday evening when we were not forthcoming. I will visit Cirencester again some time. On Wednesday evening we dined at Belsen. The flight was very calm and straightforward. I slept most of the time, early rising not being a habit of mine. The moment in the flight which always thrilled us most was as the 'plane stood still at the end of the runway with brakes on and both engines roaring at full throttle. For a few seconds everything vibrates and then we are rushing across the aerodrome to clear the fences and hedges by a few feet and soon all sensation of speed is lost. All I recognised was the Channel, the Rhine with its bridges destroyed and a few very battered German towns. We arrived in Celle at 10.30 a.m., after four hours in the air. We waited five hours at the aerodrome for transport to Belsen for, although R.A.F. trucks were going there soon after we arrived, we had to await R.A.S.C. trucks from Belsen. I suppose these letters painted on the side do make a difference, but to our undisciplined eyes they all looked like empty trucks going in the same direction. Belsen was very fortunate in that about two miles away were very large, well built army barracks. Part of this was already a subsidiary Camp II, housing 27,000 male internees; the rest, about half a mile distant, was first used by the army and people like ourselves. Later this became Camp III for fit internees evacuated from Camp I, the original Concentration Camp. So we had quite good quarters in two of the barrack buildings, and a very comfortable mess in a handsome building which we called the "Chalet." This had been an officers mess of this great German military training establishment and was now occupied by the H.Q. Staff of Belsen Camp. The surroundings were delightful; pine woods stretched on either side and a lake, complete with swan, made a very pretty picture. The whole area was enclosed by barbed wire fences, which again was fortunate, as in some measure it prevented our flock from straying over the countryside.

On the evening of our arrival some of us visited what became known as the "Round House." This appears to have been the main army mess. It was a combination of the Halls of Valhalla and Blackpool Tower Ballroom. The main banqueting hall was a lofty room with musicians' gallery and long tables strewn with glasses and bottles and the remains of the last dinner. The place looked like the morning after a colossal debauch; and there, measuring the potential bed-space by pacing out this great hall, with the abstraction of one engaged in mental arithmetic, was an R.A.M.C. colonel. I think he had calculated to fit in about three hundred beds. Eventually this showy Nazi palace was made to accommodate five hundred sick internees from Camp I. The building had been designed on magnificent lines and the kitchens and cellars were very fine, but there was too much plaster about and the woodwork was veneered. It wasn't built to last, but nevertheless outlasted the builders.

The following day we were provided with a contrast to this heroic way of life, when for the first time we saw the victims of German glory. Before I describe our impressions of the Concentration Camp, I will quote from the Medical Appreciation written a fortnight before (18/4/45) by Lt. Col. J.A.D. Johnston R.A.M.C., O.C. 32 (Brit), C.C.S., and Senior Medical Officer at the Camp. This was a review twenty-four hours after the Camp had been liberated by a truce asked for by the Germans, who had completely lost control of the situation.

"General Layout:

"Camp I consists of huts-housing 22,000 females and 18,000 males.

"Camp II of brick buildings housing 27,000 males. All European nationalities are to be found but chiefly Russians, Poles, Czechs, Belgians, French and Italians.

Conditions Prevailing. It is impossible to give an adequate description of the camp when entered on 17/4/45. Camp I was full of emaciated and apathetic scarecrows – without beds or blankets and some completely naked. The females are worse than the males and most have only filthy rags. The dead are lying all over the camp and in piles outside those blocks; miscalled hospitals, housing the worst of the sick. There are approximately 3,000 naked corpses in varying stages of decomposition. There is no sanitation, but there are pits, some with perch rails. From apathy or weakness, most defecate or urinate in the huts or anywhere. No running water, no electricity, and all water brought by water trucks. Death rate not known. Camp II is better, but there are 600 housed in buildings of 150 capacity. Death rate 10 per day. These internees are better clad and less emaciated and attempts are made to bury the dead.

"Diseases Prevalent.

"Camp I Riddled with Typhus and T.B. Gastro-enteritis common. No cholera or dysentery diagnosed. Erysipelas, scurvy and starvation prevalent.

"Camp II Enteric, T.B. Erysipelas. No Typhus.

"Rates of Sickness. Seriously ill requiring hospitalisation but excluding starvation cases and those who will inevitably die:

"Camp I Males 900, females 2,600 Camp II Males 500. Total 4,000

"Medical Personnel – Internees fit to work:

"Camp I Doctors 42, Nurses 33. Camp II Doctors 7, Nurses 50

"Medical Stores, Negligible.

"Urgent Measures to be taken:

(a) Bury dead

(b) Evacuate patients from Camp I to suitable clean buildings in Camp II with plans for reception, de-lousing and cleaning.

(c) Evacuate fit from Camp I to Camp II

(d) D.D.T. all inmates.

(e) Arrange suitable feeding for patients – death-rate has increased since abundant food became available.

(f) Pile and burn masses of rubbish, rags and human excreta which litter the camp.

Work has started on all these projects and in addition a hospital area in Camp II has been earmarked and is being evacuated and cleaned prior to the reception of seriously ill patients from Camp I. This is to be for 7,000 patients, and the following are urgent minimal requirements: blankets, 14,000, stretchers 5,000, paliasses 7,000, bedpans and equivalent 700, cooking utensils for 7,000.

This then was the gigantic task which faced a small medical team consisting of 32nd C.C.S., 11th Field Ambulance and 7th Mobile Bacteriological Laboratory. The camp was garrisoned by Light A. A. Regiment. They were later joined by 30th Field Hygiene Section, 9th British General Hospital, 163rd Field Ambulance, 35th C.C.S., Medical Students at the beginning of May and 29th General Hospital at the end of May.

When we arrived, a fortnight after the liberation, the dead had been buried in common graves containing 3,000 or 5,000 corpses each. The original estimate of 3,000 was too low, as large numbers were found to be lying in the huts with the living. The official figure of 10,000 unburied corpses at the time of liberation was later given. It is hard even for those who saw the camp after such a short time to imagine the difficulties and chaos of those first days and to appreciate the miracles of organisation performed by the R.A.M.C. and the army authorities at the camp. The almost complete lack of communications and the isolation from higher authority, a state of affairs which was little changed even at the time of our departure, permitted a free play of the most inspiring energy and initiative. I was particularly interested to meet Capt. "Frosty" Winterbottom, R.A.M.C., a Mary's man, who was anaesthetist to the 32nd C.C.S. "Frosty" was certainly one of the best known of Belsen personalities. He was officially in charge of hospital stores and his fame is well founded on his achievement in equipping the 7,000-bedded hospital area proposed in Col. Johnston's first report. With knowledge of only negligible stocks of medical ordnance stores available, by scouring the district and "freezing" all he could lay hands upon, Capt. Winterbottom equipped 7,000 beds in a week at the rate of 1,000 each day. Naturally with this reputation everyone came to him with their supply problems. He was always to be found in his "flat", a little room in the caves of the stable which formed the stores building. The divan bed and cushion were brightly covered with the material from a large silk Nazi flag. Everything was very cosy – I suppose the furnishings had been a very easy matter to one of Capt. Winterbottom's genius. Sleeping in a chair was his Czechoslovak interpreter, who was easily awakened to deal with some difficult linguistic problem; like all the internees she had lost all appreciation of time and would fall asleep at the oddest hours. Subsidiary concerns in the Winterbottom combine were "Harrods," where thousands of sets of new clothing and footwear were distributed to internees who had been cleaned; a hairdressing establishment with Hungarian staff; plumbers and carpenters for the buildings under his control in the hospital area; internee seamstresses who mass-produced a standard Belsen nightie for the sick — very utility and too much like a shroud for my taste; wirelesses and bicycles were serviced in this hive of industry, and last but not least, "The Coconut Grove," a night club, well in the Mary's tradition, flourished sporadically — Capt. Winterbottom and his enterprises were the most heartening things in Belsen.

The camp when we arrived was fairly orderly, but the state of the sick in the huts was appaling. In the huts in which I worked about 200 to 300 people were crowded in enough space for 80. They were in three-tiered wooded bunks with barely space to pass between; there were in addition many lying on the floor on piles of dirty rags. The three great troubles were typhus, starvation and almost universal diarrhoea. The two latter conditions were allied, in that the food provided after the long period of starvation was unsuitable for weakened digestive tracts and resulted in severe gastro-intestinal disturbances. The psychological condition of the internees was also of importance and with the language problem added greatly to our difficulties. And even here, in these sorry circumstances, nationalistic prejudice caused trouble, particularly between the Russians and Poles. Amongst the fit, even doctors and nurses, there was at first, an almost complete indifference to the fate of the sick. Those who were well enough to get food over-ate, with a great increase in the rate of diarrhoea, while those who were too weak were left to starve.

Our primary function, therefore, was to ensure the proper distribution of suitable food to all the internees. In this we worked under the direction of Dr Meiklejohn, an old Mary's man working for the Rockefeller Institute with the U.N.R.R.A. His calm, diplomatic handling of students and the higher authorities greatly added to the effectiveness of our efforts. We first of all kept a record of the numbers feeding from each kitchen (about 5,000) and also each day provided figures of the fit, sick, typhus cases and deaths. The death-rate was about 500 a day and dropped to 80 after 10 days. A student attached to each cookhouse correlated this information and saw that the correct amounts of the different kinds of food were prepared and distributed. It was equally important for a student to be present in each hut at meal times to see that the sick were fed.

I have nothing to say about the use of protein hydrolysate or intravenous plasma and serum in starvation. Dr Janet Vaughan has already spoken of these and official reports will be forthcoming. In the huts intravenous work was impossible and only extremely limited use of hydrolysate was practicable. Those who could take nothing else, because of weakness or diarrhoea, were given a glucose vitamin mixture. Many required great urging to take anything at all. There were various gruel-like concoctions made with dried skimmed milk, the most famous being the Bengal famine mixture. This consisted of dried milk, flour, salt and sugar, according to the Bengal recipe. Strangely enough, although the proportions of sugar was decreased and salt increased, and although the patients' energy reserves were so sadly depleted, the constant complaint was that the mixture was too sweet. There were also soup or stew and jacket potatoes for those fit to eat them, and, popular with all, a brew that went by the name of tea. The black bread was most unpopular and was wasted; there was a great demand for white bread, but little to be had.

Typhus, in the presence of a known epidemic, we diagnosed by the high fever and violent headache often leading to delirium; tinnitus often followed by deafness, which continued during the weak, apathetic and sometimes mentally deranged condition known as the post-typhus state. The spleen was sometimes palpable. The appearance, speech and gait were best described as drunken. About the fifth day of the fever the typhus rash appeared on the trunk, inside of the legs or arms. This was paler than a measles rash and in dirty, flea-bitten patients not always easy to distinguish. The dehydrated state and dirty mouth often led to violent parotitis. There were fatal chest complications and some dry gangrene of the extremities. I have heard it said that in typhus the hair falls out and after convalescence grows again, but we did not observe this happen here. For the headache we gave aspirin and for the rest could only give the vitamin glucose mixture. The parotitis mostly cleared up but sometimes required drainage. The deafness often persisted. The mortality rate was estimated at between 10–20% at the age of 20 but was said to be almost 100% at 50. A comparatively large number of R.A.M.C. personnel (30 or 40) contracted the disease and also half a dozen students (none from St. Mary's). All of these had been inoculated against typhus, although some of the students only an extremely short time before. There were no deaths among the inoculated and the disease was said to be of about 25% the severity seen in the non-inoculated.

I did not hear of any proved cases of bacillary, dysentery. The diarrhoea was due to the weakened gastro-intestinal condition and the unaccustomed food and was very difficult to influence. We used a German drug, "Tannalbin," but were quite ignorant of suitable dosage. Eventually Tabs. 3 every 2 hours to a total of 12 seemed to have the desired effect in some cases, also a chalk and opium mixture appeared which helped.

Constantly the fit were being evacuated to Camp III. The Belsen standard of fitness was "an individual capable of collecting his own food and maintaining himself," and naturally many of these fell sick in Camp III and had to be transferred to the Hospital Area – Camp II. But all the time the numbers in the huts in Camp I were decreasing and it became possible to space out the patients more conveniently and attempt a certain standard of cleanliness in the huts. In this, as with the feeding, we were assisted by labour, provided by the Hungarian Army, which for the most part required constant supervision. The hospital accommodation was as follows : Camp II, 7,300 beds to be taken over by the 29th General Hospital, 4,000 beds under 9th General Hospital. In this way a hospital area was formed in the women's part of the Camp, in clean huts with patients treated by a Mobile Bath Unit before admission. This area was controlled by a group of students, largely U.C.H., and good internee nurses and was a great credit to them. Col. Johnston reported, "In my opinion, a higher standard of care and treatment is being achieved here than in any other hospital area, the reason being of course, the adequacy in numbers of staff employed there." The patients of this area were evacuated to the Round House, where they were treated by the same team.

By the middle of May, thanks to D.D.T. the typhus epidemic was on the wane, and the sick were being evacuated to the hospitals in Camp II and to a nearby German military hospital. This hospital was soon renamed the Glynn Hughes Hospital after Brig. Hughes D.D.M.S., 2nd Army, who was our most cheering and inspiring guest in the mess. Work was now started on burning the empty huts, although the camp was not yet completely evacuated. The enthusiasm of the firebugs with flame-throwing tanks and bulldozers was so great that it was with difficulty that Col. Bird, the Garrison Commander, in his trusty jeep followed by a fire engine managed to keep the conflagration within decent limits. On May 21st, with suitable ceremony and thanks, the last hut was destroyed and those who were not already there went to work in the various hospitals.

Here it was possible to give more individual medical attention to patients and with the arrival of fresh R.A.M.C. units and equipment Belsen standards were gradually forgotten. Tuberculosis was raging and was being diagnosed by physical signs in 20% of patients, who were then segregated. Serum and plasma were poured into the starvation cases, with varying results. Some blew up more than ever and paracentesis abdominis was frequently performed. The surgery was rarely aseptic and hardly needed to be; it was, at any rate, good to see the pus flowing freely after its long imprisonment. But with the 29th General Hospital we welcomed, a goodly contingent of nursing sisters; discipline was re-established; we learnt our place – it was almost time for us to go. Before we left we held a very enjoyable dance and were pleased to have with us those who were replacing us. In some respects it was nearly as good as a Mary's dance, in fact there were some who could hardly be expected to make the distinction. Also before we left some of us revisited the remains of Camp I. Here was the very abomination of desolation; destruction and dirt and still the smell of burning filth offended the senses. In the distance, at the South end of the Camp, was the crematorium furnace with its tall smoke stack and nearby were the mounds of the common graves containing the bodies of scores of thousands of all the nations of Europe. We also thought of the thousands of survivors, many maimed and ruined in mind and body; we thought of the tales they had to tell of this and other camps, and the pathetic photographs of happy family groups, now with a sole survivor. We had little time to think of these things before, but we will remember the terrible end of a wrong political idea.

The St. Mary's team consisted of the following students: R. Armitage, T.C. Brown, J. Hankinson, T.D. Hawkins, P.O.C. Jackson, G.W. Korn, A.B. Matthews, J. McLuskie, A.V. Price, G.C. Thick, R.W. Watson, J.L.C. Whitcombe.

(It is still difficult so many years later to even imagine the colossal, brutal and inhumane treatment of so many thousands by the German nation of the time. These acts of barbarism alone would have justified World War II, and lest we forget of what man is capable, let us reflect on the continuing cruelty executed since then in many more local conflicts, by various nations.)

(John Hankinson qualified in 1946 and obtained his F.R.C.S. in 1950. He was Surgical Registrar in the Neurosurgical Department of St George's Hospital and then Consultant Neurosurgeon to the Newcastle General Hospital, Newcastle-upon-Tyne. He was the author of numerous medical papers.

Thomas Colin Brown qualified in 1947. He obtained the Diploma in Public Health in 1957 and the Diploma in Industrial Health in the same year and for a time was a Squadron Leader in the Royal Air Force Medical Branch.

Thomas Desmond Hawkins qualified in 1946, obtained his Fellowship of the Faculty of Radiologists in 1959 and the F.R.C.R. in 1975. In 1979 he was elected F.R.C.P. He was Consultant Radiologist at Addenbrooke's Hospital Cambridge, and elected Dean of the Medical School in Cambridge. He was elected President of the British Society of Neuroradiologists and in retirement became President of Hughes Hall Cambridge. He wrote many articles and a book of scholarship entitled *The Drainage of Wilbraham, Fulbourn and Feversham Fens*.

Gerald Woolf Korn qualified in 1946. He obtained his M.R.C.O.G. in 1954. He was appointed to the staff of the University Hospital, Saskatoon.

Andrew Edward Matthews qualified in 1947 and obtained his M.R.C.O.G. in 1957. He served some time in the Royal Air Force Medical Branch.

John McLuskie qualified in 1947 and obtained his Diploma in Child Health in 1950.

Gordon Caton Thick qualified in 1947. He obtained his F.F.A.R.C.S. in 1953 and was Consultant to the Hertford Group of Hospitals.

Roger William Woodcroft Watson qualified in 1946 and resided in Christchurch, New Zealand.

John Leslie Clarence Whitcombe qualified in 1947. He obtained his Diploma in Tropical Medicine and Health in 1950 and his Diploma in Industrial Health in 1962. He was Consultant to the Anglo-American Corp. of South Africa and late Chief Medical Officer, Wankie Colliery Co., South Rhodesia.)

CHAPTER 30

After Arnhem

The following script of a talk broadcast to South Africa by Major Lipmann Kessel, M.B.E., M.C., R.A.M.C., is reproduced by kind permission of the British Broadcasting Corporation.

In the winter of 1936 I went to Amsterdam as a member of the Rugby football team of South African Medical students from London. During the four days we spent there I made some very good friends, but I certainly had no idea at that time that my next visit to Holland would be with the British Army. I left Holland in 1936 by an ordinary cross-Channel steamer and returned in September, 1944, by parachute ... You can understand that I had a very personal interest in this journey. It was very painful to hear of the way that the Nazis were treating the Dutch people, and I got very excited at the prospect when my Commanding Officer told us that we were booked to go to Holland, to help kick the Germans out. As soon as we knew where we were going, all my brother officers asked me to teach them a few phrases of Dutch, and when we dropped near Arnhem and had arrived at the hospital in which we were going to work I went along with my Commanding Officer to act as his interpreter. Our first meeting with the Director of the Hospital nearly ended in disaster, because after I'd spoken to him for several minutes he remained very unfriendly towards us. I was puzzled and said in English: "What the devil's the matter with you, I wonder?" Immediately his face beamed with a smile. "Potverdikkie!" he said, "You are English. I thought you were German!" So much for my attempt to speak Dutch! You see, it is nearly eight years since I left South Africa, and I had forgotten most of my Afrikaans and was speaking to him in a mixture of bad Afrikaans and bad German, which certainly did not sound anything like Dutch!

I worked in the hospital in Arnhem for about four weeks looking after our men who had been wounded in the fight for the town. Then the Germans took us to a prisoner-of-war transit camp on the Dutch-German border. We decided that it was better to get away while the going was good rather than wait until they'd got us into a real camp in Germany.

So I escaped from this camp as soon as possible. I left with three other chaps by crawling through the barbed wire on a very dark, rainy night. A few days later we contacted some underground workers. A month after this I tried with some friends to get across the Rhine to our own troops again, but we were caught on the way by a German patrol. There was a lot of noise from shouting and shooting and I managed to slip away from the scene of the trouble with two others. We walked the whole night in a northerly direction, away from the front line, taking our direction from the stars. We were so tired and hungry after some hours that we decided to ask for help at the first house which we came across. We felt pretty sure that it would be safe to ask for help at any house if there were no German soldiers actually billeted in the house itself. When dawn broke we lay down in the bushes about fifty yards from a farmhouse, where we could not be seen although we ourselves could watch the house. Soon a young woman came out of the back door and we could see her busy with the morning work in the yard and kitchen. I was a little afraid to approach her because I looked a pretty terrible sight with my filthy wet clothes and a three days' growth on my face. I didn't want to frighten her – that would be a bad introduction. However, there was nothing else for it, so I walked up to her and said straight out: "I am an Englishman, can you help me?" . . . The young woman looked straight back at me without blinking an eyelid, "Come in," she said, "we are all right here." Nothing else. I called up my two pals and in no time we were sitting in the kitchen, enjoying a plateful of good hot porridge. We rested there for the day and went on our journey when the sun set. When we met our friends from the underground again two days later, they told us that there were many Germans living in the area of the farm where that young woman had helped us at risk of certain death if she was caught. And all so simply – no fuss at all – just "Come in. We are all right here." How can I ever forget those words?

After this episode I spent a further three months in Holland: most of the time I was bitterly cold and we could never have survived without the help which the people gave us. Nothing was too much trouble for them. They did everything possible to look after us and help us to get back to our own lines again. They made us feel how closely they were in the fight together and that whatever they did was dictated not so much by their compassion for us as by the sole aim of speeding the day when the hated Fascists would be driven from their farms and homes and village streets. I finally found myself, after much touring about, in Sliedrecht, the river town which is famous for the skilled river-dredgers and watermen who come from there. Here I met a local lad called Jan who was born and brought up on the rivers and canals near his home town. He knew every little nook and crevice of the water system at the mouth of the Maas-Waal Rivers and the language of the tides and winds came to him as second nature. We set out in a canoe one night to cross to the British lines. It was a journey of about five miles, and after we had paddled for about twenty minutes we came to a lock at the place where a canal ran into the river. Jan went out to find the keeper of the lock, and after he'd climbed back into the canoe, the gates swung open and we went into and through the lock. The keeper would accept nothing from me, in spite of the fact that we'd hauled him out of bed at one o'clock in the morning to do a very dangerous job – to open the gates for a single little canoe. He was just a Dutchman doing his job.

Unfortunately our canoe began to take in water, and half-way on our journey the canoe filled and capsized and we had a very unpleasant ducking in the icy water. So there we were in the middle of the German positions with a leaky canoe, very cold and very wet. It wasn't so good! However, my luck held and we managed to sneak through the lines along the banks of the canal, and after two very hungry and cold days we arrived back in Sliedrecht from where we'd started. After a week's rest we did the trip again – this time in a good canoe – and got to the British lines after four hours' hard paddling without much incident. By the way, I went on a very good six weeks' leave to London after that, but not for Jan: he paddled back to Sliedrecht again to carry on with the good work.

(So many brave acts such as those of the young woman and Jan occurred during World War II and have gone unrewarded – they go some way to redeem the brutality inflicted by others.)

V.E. DAY

On the day before the great day, a certain general restlessness could be sensed in and around the hospital and medical school. A total disregard for private property, particularly in the matter of wireless sets, was noticed, especially after the afternoon bulletins. Almost hourly for the rest of that day at least one hard-worked houseman had his room invaded, his last chair sat in and his wireless turned on. After the announcement that the morrow was the day, various small scouting parties were observed departing westwards, and on their return they reported good prospects for the next night.

Tuesday started quietly and everyone was waiting for the Prime Minister's speech, which, thanks to some kind person's foresight, was relayed in the Hall, where an almost Christmas-like scene was enacted with considerable numbers of nurses, staff and students gathered to listen.

In the evening we listened to the King, which for us was a double privilege, as in the preceding situations we had the honour of having one of our nurses speak on behalf of the women of the Auxiliary and Nursing Services. After this we automatically repaired to the West End and shouted, cheered, walked, waved flags and walked even more; judging from my own feet, the next few days must have been a chiropodist's paradise.

The day after was still a holiday but was spent by most in rest and recuperation. In the evening, they tell me, there was a bonfire!! Need I say more? – except to thank two Sisters, one of whom lost her curtains and the other a large part of her garden with such good grace.

W.B.W.

Barbed Wire and Beri-Beri

A lot, possibly enough, has been written in the last six months about conditions in Japanese P.O.W. and Internment Camps. It is only because I think that the Military Internment Camp, Hongkong, was an average sample, neither relatively good like the camps in Manila and Shanghai, nor indescribably horrible like some of the camps in the interior of Java and Sumatra, that I venture on a very brief description of one aspect of life in it, an aspect which occupied an increasingly large proportion of our consciousness as time went on.

To judge my mortality figures, Stanley Camp must have been one of the most fortunate in the whole of the Far East. Out of a population of 2,500 to have had under 150 deaths, including 14 by bombing and seven by execution, in three years and eight months was more than just lucky. It is attributable to the fact that we were never visited by a major epidemic, though why the camp was spared will always be something of a mystery for cholera and smallpox were rife in the city of Hongkong, and diphtheria took a very heavy toll in the Sham Shui Po and Argyll Street camps, on the other side of the harbour. There were enough cases of typhoid and typhus in the camp to give rise to the gloomiest prognostications, and dysentery and malaria were always with us, but somehow they never spread as we were always afraid they would, and from first to last shortage of food and nutritional diseases remained our most serious problem and constituted the most serious and sustained threat to health and life.

There must be many thousand people in Great Britain now to whom the rice shortage occasions no concern. The basis of the camp ration was, as it was in all camps in the Far East, rice. The amount varied from time to time but the average ration was 12 ounces per person per day. The other fairly constant rations were: pea-nut oil, one quarter to one half ounce a day; salt, one-third ounce daily; sugar, one ounce for 10 days. Vegetables were also provided throughout, their quality and quantity varying with the season, and apparently also with the temper of the Japanese, from sweet potatoes, yams and taro-root to spinach stalks, turnip tops and chrysanthemum leaves. Meat, in the form of water buffalo beef was supplied fairly regularly in 1942, but in very small quantity. This was followed in 1943 by dried and salted fish, but throughout 1944 and till August, 1945 meat and fish were not seen. The basic ration was supplemented, irregularly, in various ways, of which the most valuable were consignments of soya beans and rice polishings sent into camp at intervals during the latter two years by the local international Red Cross representative. Red Cross parcels were received on three occasions: November, 1942; September, 1944, and March, 1945, and, while they lasted, had a tremendous effect on the physical well-being and also on the morale of internees. Lastly there was a black market, and at times considerable amounts of food came into the camp by devious underground routes from Chinese friends and through trading with the Formosan guards. It is impossible to assess the quantity of food that came in this way, but its effect in raising the general nutritional level was not very great for it was by no means evenly distributed over the population, only those relatively few people benefiting who had been lucky enough to get into camp with their personal valuables to trade with the guards. There cannot have been more than half-a-dozen wedding rings left in the camp by the time we were released.

The rations provided an average of about 1,600 calories per day, with 30–45 grammes of protein, 15–30 of fat and the rest carbohydrate in the form of white highly-milled rice, mostly deteriorated by long storage. The minimum monthly average was just over 1,000 calories in February, 1942, and the intake was raised to a peak of 2,300 by the international Red Cross parcels in November of the same year. The diet was seriously deficient in all other nutrient factors except Vitamin C and iron, especially so in B complex factors, the average intake being less than ½ mg. each of Bl and riboflavine.

One thousand six hundred daily calories is theoretically only sufficient to provide for basic metabolic needs, but the range of adaptability of the human body was clearly shown in the high level of physical work which was maintained throughout. Quite apart from the labour demanded by the Japanese, which consisted mostly of agriculture and digging "fox holes" and occupied 300 or 400 men most days, much manual labour was necessary for the maintenance of a camp in which no facilities were provided: splitting and chopping logs for cooking fuel, trench-digging for refuse disposal and latrines, rice grinding on hand stones, cooking, sanitation, anti-malarial work and many other necessary activities demanded at least two hours heavy work of all able-bodied people daily.

Inadequacy of total fuel value of the diet manifested itself most measurably in loss of weight, which was rapid at first and settled to a slow steady rate of fall only interrupted by the arrival of the international Red Cross parcels. The average loss of weight among all men at the end of captivity was about 45 lbs., or rather over 25% of their normal weight, though falls of over 100 lbs. and/or 50 per cent, of pre-war weight were not uncommon in men formerly very fat.

Hypotension (average B.P. 95/65 among 50 men in May, 1942), and bradycardia were observed in the early days but tended to return towards normal after about two years. The contribution of hypo-proteinaemia to these phenomena could not be estimated as biochemical investigations were, of course, out of the question, but many cases of "famine oedema" were seen in the first summer but not afterwards. Subjective manifestations were faintness, giddiness, "black-outs" on change of posture, undue fatigability and general muscular weakness, especially of the ciliary and extrinsic ocular muscles, which latter gave rise to diplopia and blurring after very short periods of reading.

Avitaminosis of all kinds except scurvy, were seen in large numbers, 85 per cent, of the population exhibiting signs of some avitaminosis during the period of internment. "Wet" or oedematous beri-beri was the first to appear, the first case occurring after just two months of captivity. Of this condition little need be said for the 760 cases were entirely "text book" except that, happily, cardiac involvement was uncommon and consequently deaths few. The incidence was brought dramatically to zero by the general administration of a daily dose of 1 mg. of thiamine and remained negligible while supplies of this preparation lasted – which unfortunately, was not for very long. The neuropathies formerly known as "dry" beri-beri did not appear for several months but, in the whole three and a half years, 840 cases were recorded. Contrary to previous experience among the Chinese, the typical flaccid diplegia of the text books was by no means the commonest syndrome. Pain and intolerable paraesthesiae often related to temperature sensation were outstanding features and gave the condition its popular name of "burning" or "electric" feet. The incidence of this condition did not seem to bear any relationship to the Bl non-fat calories ratio of the diet, as did "wet" beri-beri, nor was pure vitamin Bl particularly effective in treatment, not more than 20 per cent, of cases being cured, and they the mildest and a further 25 percent somewhat improved by doses of Bl as high as 200 mg. daily. The almost certain exclusion of any extrinsic toxin as an aetiological factor and the satisfactory response of most of these cases to such dietary supplements as soya beans, peanuts and rice-polishings, when these were available, as well as other evidence whose description would be too lengthy for this brief and superficial note, indicate to me, at any rate, a clear answer to Peter Meiklejohn's question of 1943: "Is thiamine the anti-neuritic vitamin?" and that so called "dry" beri-beri is caused, probably, by deficiency in two or more factors of the B complex of which thiamine is one but not necessarily even the most important.

Other B complex deficiencies were common, pellagra and ariboflavinosis, usually superimposed upon one another, being the commonest of all deficiency syndromes. The only deviation of the clinical picture from the description of numerous writers was that not a single corneal lesion was ever seen in a case of ariboflavinosis even when the other lesions were far advanced. A home-brewed yeast was reasonably effective in the treatment of these patients. Two other conditions connected in some way with the B complex presented very serious problems.

Tropical macrocytic anaemia, in the absence of all good concentrated sources of B complex and in the extreme scarcity of liver preparations, carried a mortality of over 20 per cent. We were fortunate that there were only some 50 cases. In a way the most distressing of all was nutritional retrobulbar neuritis, or, as I am told it is now officially called "captivity amblyopia." Neither we, nor, I believe, any observers in any of the other camps, were able to prove the aetiology of the condition, but many indications pointed to some member or members of the B complex as the causative deficiency. The syndrome was clear-cut, its main features being diminution of visual acuity, central or paracentral scotoma, disorders of perception such as flickering or shimmering of images, and headaches or retrobulbar pain. Examination of mild or early cases showed no retinal changes, but as the disease progressed temporal pallor of the disc appeared and in severe long-standing cases optic atrophy was apparent with degenerative colour changes at the macula. A constant finding was diminution of the visual field for colour discrimination. This is possibly the earliest detectable sign for it was present in a number of people examined in the course of routine who were symptom-free. Considerable constriction of the peripheral fields was present in a proportion of cases but was probably due to coexisting avitaminosis A, as, in such cases, it was associated with hyperkeratosis and other skin lesions and with prolonged dark adaptation, and, with them, responded to treatment with shark's liver oil; whereas the state of cone vision was unaffected. Visual acuity was not always a true indication of severity of the condition, for many patients learnt to improve their vision by looking "off-centre" and dodging their small central scotoma.

It cannot be said that any of these cases, of whom there were 360, were cured during internment. There was no response to Thiamine, nicotinic acid, or vitamin A, which were the only single vitamins we ever had: a series of patients showed improvement on high dosage of multivitamin capsules rich in B complex, when we received some in the international Red Cross supplies and many were kept more or less stationary when their diet could be supplemented with B complex foods such as beans and peanuts. Even since release response of the more severe cases to all kinds of therapy has been most disappointing and it is to be feared that when the changes have progressed far enough for disc pallor to be discerned, they are largely irreversible. As may be imagined, treatment of all these conditions was sketchy in the extreme, as with all medical treatment in the camp. Although most doctors, pharmacists and nurses took in a few medicines with them, they were first "concentrated," and this meagre supply was occasionally replenished from Red Cross sources, the dispensary cupboard was often bare and prayer and fasting the order of the day. There were some ingenious improvisations mostly on the surgical side, but some on the medical side, too. For instance: small packet of china clay found on the hillside yielded a good "Mist. Kaolin," and a suspension of the powdered asbestos lagging of an old boiler also provided a useful intestinal absorbent; while lye, made from wood ash, was not only indispensible for washing clothes but served as an alkali when taken internally and was a good anti-pruritic lotion applied externally. The Japanese were not helpful. A favourite response to any appeal for drugs or medicines was: "Any fool can cure people with medicines – you are a doctor – you should be able to cure them without medicines" – to which I did not know the answer.

D.A.S.

(This was certainly not the worst of Japanese camps but from the figures given an enormous percentage of the internees suffered serious ill health and many were blinded from retrobulbar neuritis and optic atrophy. The seven executions were also unforgivable.

The psychological trauma was unmeasurable and continued after the war ended. It is an incredibly naive sentence that 'The Japanese were not helpful'. The Japanese had a total disregard for the dignity and welfare of their prisoners of war and inflicted unbelievable horrors on prisoners beyond the boundaries of humane acceptance.)

The Late John Diver

We have received the following appreciation from Capt. A.W. Frankland R.A.M.C.

I should like to write a few words of appreciation of John Diver as a friend and contemporary after he had come down from Cambridge, and as a fellow medical officer at St. Mary's Hospital, and who was taken prisoner with me at the fall of Singapore.

My first contact with him during the war was at Millbank in 1941, when we were doing a tropical medical course there. I learnt – though not from him – that he had previously done an extremely good job of work in the evacuation of Dunkirk. I heard a rather similar account from his own men very soon after the fall of Singapore, although until that time I did not know that we were even prisoners together.

In 1942 besides his duty as a reception medical officer in one of the areas of Changi Camp, he was acting as liason officer between the British and the Dutch, and I know most Dutch medical officers used him as a sort of father confessor for all their problems. During this time his leisure hours were employed in exercising his voice in a male voice choir.

Later, while medical officer of a working party in Singapore, medical officers in Changi Hospital will particularly remember him for his kindness in bringing to us on his monthly visits such unheard of luxuries such as bread and occasional tins of jam and fish which he was able to buy in the town. Although I was never to see him again after he went up to Thailand I heard a lot more of him. The men who came back particularly mentioned his name, for his untiring energy under the very adverse conditions and for the way he stood up to the Japanese with the consequent beatings up on more than one occasion. He returned to Singapore at the end of 1943 in a poor state of health, but after convalescence, because of his reputation gained originally in Changi and later in Thailand, he was asked by the commanding officer of the ill-fated Normanton Camp, Singapore, to go as their medical officer. It was here under truly terrible conditions with almost no drugs and dressings and what was always a very low and ultimately starvation diet, that he showed not only his skill as a medical officer but also his untiring efforts on behalf of all the men and officers in the camp. Dreadful wrecks of humanity used to be allowed to be evacuated to Changi or Kranji hospitals occasionally from this camp some of whom I saw after the end of the war in Kranji Hospital. I believe many thought if he had allowed himself to be evacuated sooner to slightly more congenial surroundings he would have lived, but his sense of duty would not allow him to leave the camp until he was too weak from beri-beri and starvation to carry on. His death at Changi Hospital a few days later and so short a time before our release was a great shock to all who heard of it. There is no doubt that in the words of the men at Normanton Camp, "he martyred himself in their cause." I should like to associate myself, together with all those who knew him and worked with him, in expressing my sympathy to his parents in the death of this very gallant officer.

(Here is yet another man worthy of the highest decoration, and truly a credit to St Mary's Hospital Medical School and the medical profession.)

Nagasaki

We have received the following description from a correspondent:

While on our tour from Tokyo to Hong Kong with a draft of returning age and service groups we were allowed to proceed to Nagasaki for a few hours to inspect the damage caused by the atomic bomb. As I believe I am the first Mary's man to have witnessed it so far the following description may be of interest to readers of the "Gazette."

The town and its environs may be likened to a section of a wheel, the hub representing the harbour area and the spokes being valleys in which the town is built. It was in one of these valleys that the bomb was dropped. The docks had already been very badly damaged by ordinary high explosive, but very little had been dropped higher up the valley.

As we left the dock area an appreciable change came over the type of devastation, until we breasted a slight rise and the whole appalling scene appeared before us. For a distance of about three miles down the length of the valley and two miles across there were standing the shells of not more than a dozen buildings, and all these were either modern ferro-concrete structures or factories mainly made of steel girders. The Mitsubishi torpedo factory was pushed over to an angle of 45 degrees. The Nagasaki Hospital and Medical School, extremely modern buildings, were standing but completely gutted by the tremendous fires that raged afterwards. A building which one might have imagined to be able to withstand the blast was the prison, but this was situated near the centre of the explosion and was just a heap of rubble. The great majority of the buildings which were presumably the usual Japanese wooden houses were just charred ashes, and amongst these I was able to identify, to the gruesome interest of my companions, skeletal remains of their quondam inhabitants. The Japanese A.R.P. regulations were such that workers were not to take cover during a raid unless there were more than six planes overhead, and in this case there were but two, the plane that dropped the bomb and a reconnaissance machine. I am not at liberty to disclose any of the details of the bomb, such as they are that I know, but will conclude this sketchy description of the scene by the somewhat Chestertonian remark that it is indescribable, and that any gentleman who is in future desirous of making war should pay a visit to Nagasaki to ensue his recognition of the horror that may be loosed.

Pacific Letter

St. Mary's warriors in the Pacific thanks to an excellent mail organisation, are fully close up on the great events there on the occasion of the Centenary. Although the other representatives are separated from me by varying distances of ocean, I am presuming to represent them in sending our congratulations and our best wishes for the future.

My spies have kept me fully informed of all the fun and games, and I have received a more sober account in a copy of the "Times" that came to-day. I felt a telegram would be appropriate and I accordingly searched through the phrases of the E.F.M. telegram service, but could find nothing to cover centenaries though the Passover, Mothers Day, Thanksgiving, and

"Happy Occasions" were well catered for. "Anniversary" was the nearest I could get and as such it was sent.

What with "VE" Day and the Centenary we have obviously missed a big occasion, but what I regret missing most was the symbolic burning of those monstrous obstructions in Norfolk Place, whether in honour of "VE Day" or the Centenary my "reliable sources" do not inform me. Whichever it was, my two shins, both supraorbital processes, and my nose, recalling their almost nightly trauma of three years ago, wish to associate themselves fully with the cry that must have gone forth – "To the Barricades."

To us a welcome sign that the future is being well catered for was the receipt of the circular requesting our views on post-war post-graduate instruction. We are all looking forward to the day when we receive our "bowler hats" and we welcome this evidence of personal interest in our future which would be so much more valuable than any refresher course from the Government in power.

Destroyer life is not what it was. The modern vessels are built to stay at sea for too long and if the big ships choose to mill around the ocean indefinitely, the destroyers will follow them round – and like it. Those old Destroyer gatherings in the Wardroom which were so good for one's morale and bad for one's health, are things of the past, for we only seem to see our colleagues when we come alongside to transfer mail or "beef-and-spuds" or the big ships paper work. As far as the war itself is concerned it is a rather comfortable one for us as the Japanese Fleet has ceased to exist and the "Kamikaze" ("Divine Wind" – a delicious expression) Air Force are keener to splay out their Honourable brain on bigger game than us. We have seen a few of these gentlemen on the job and it is difficult to believe that there is a human being in that machine that speeds on towards its target, though often a ball of flame long before it is anywhere near. The resultant explosion is spectacular to a degree although the damage inflicted has been so far negligible. A Medical Officer in one ship which was the object of a suicide attack has a perfectly preserved Japanese eyeball as a momento and it should make an interesting addition to his Hospital museum.

We have been lucky in having Australia as a playground for our rest periods. This is no place to describe all the details of what constitutes a "rest period" but suffice it to say that no less than five of our ship's company have found that they are now married. I have been most hospitably entertained by the medical fraternity of Sydney who in spite of a very full day, have always found time to show me hospitals or entertain me in less technical ways.

"And here is a news flash" – which puts most of what I have already said into the limb of the unimportant. We gather the Japanese are prepared to accept the terms of the Potsdam announcement. I think a pause is indicated there while we listen for more . . .

There should be some printer's sign there to indicate the passage of time for I am finishing off this verbal ramble in times of peace. My ship is relegated with the job of "Tokyo express" and we are speeding with mail and general cargo to that city. Before I finish I must tell you of the Mary's people out here. Indeed the whole purpose of writing was to bring the Pacific to you in Paddington.

Surgeon Commander Spero ashore in Sydney is the same charming host he was when in "Renown." Charm is also lent to the R.N. Hospital by the presence of Jill Hippisley. I had a quiet celebration of Victory with Michael Walker a day or two back. He is now Acting Senior Medical Officer of his very large Aircraft Repair Ship. Dooley Muller is almost the Senior Member of the Wardroom of his very hospitable cruiser and he and I have an occasional liaison through binoculars when our ships come close to each other, and somewhat closer liaisons when in harbour.

Frazer is in a Minesweeper but I am afraid I discovered his presence too late to contact him.

The Centenary Gazette has just arrived and makes most exciting reading. The history of the hospital is thoroughly well done and makes me feel ashamed how little one knew of its earlier struggles and of the personalities of those Victorian giants many of whose names are, medically, household words.

Peace brings a hope of an early return to civilization for us and rapid progress with these great plans for our Hospital. We all look forward to the day when we can don a white coat and act like human beings again, pushing into the background the memory of these, for most of us, completely wasted and sterile years.

Best Wishes and congratulations to the Gazette on its continued existence.

R.P.M. Miles, H.M.S. Quality, B.P.F.
H.M.H.S. Tjitjalengka, c/o G.P.O., London.

30th September, 1945.
To the Editor St. Mary's Hospital Gazette.
Dear Sir,
You will be glad to hear that the hospital was represented at the surrender ceremony in Toyko Bay, for the Missouri was only about a quarter of a mile away from us. We had arrived two days previously and shortly afterwards Roger Miles in Quality, and John Price, in Troutbridge, joined us. I met both of them, but unfortunately we were never actually all together at the same time.

On September 4th, this ship moved in to the harbour at Yokohama to take on ex-prisoners of war. We acted as a base hospital for about a fortnight, and found that quite a number of men recovered sufficiently in two or three days to undertake the journey by air. We eventually left on September 16th with about 400 sick on board. Both Miles and Price very kindly came in several days to help to deal with the rush of patients and we were very grateful for their assistance. Troutbridge escorted us as far as Manus and then went on to Sydney.

I was able to get into Tokyo one morning, driving the 16 odd miles from Yokohama in a truck. This used to be a great industrial area, but the destruction is so great that hardly a building is left standing, let alone undamaged, along the whole length of the road. The two big cities, too, show very few areas which have escaped. I believe a lot of the damage was caused by fire, but it certainly destroyed what there was there. Little corrugated iron shacks every few yards serve as dwelling houses for what Japs there are left in the area.

Medically, the work on the ex-prisoners has been very interesting. Very many of them have beri–beri, and one suddenly developed acute cardiac failure after six days in hospital on strict rest. The disease in many cases is responding only very slowly on treatment, and I have had to put several back to bed with recurrence of oedema and tachycardia. There is a lot of pulmonary T.B., amoebic dysentery and ascaris infection. Chronic amoebiasis is a great bugbear in this area, and most of us now tend to suspect all cases of P.U.O. of having amoebic hepatitis until it is proved otherwise.

Yours sincerely,

Geoffrey Cutts.

Editorial

December 1945

For the first time for six years we are celebrating a peace-time Christmas, and although there are still many clouds on the horizon and on occasions the outlook may appear more formidable and foreboding than even during the war, we have much with which to bless ourselves. Immediate dangers have passed, many families have been reunited, and there are even some things in the shops which we have not seen for many years. Crackers in the West End, and lights in the streets begin to give the right Christmas atmosphere and are a portent for the future which is very welcome. Let us for a brief period enjoy the present without contemplation of the future, and by creating a spirit of cheerfulness and comradeship out of the good things which are available, store up a supply of hopefulness and courage which will carry us far into the New Year. Do not let future planning overwhelm present enjoyment; sufficient unto the day is the good thereof, is a better motto than its more familiar counterpart. Laugh and be merry for who knows what pleasures the morrow may bring. The only people we are really sorry for are those whose morrow brings an examination. A particularly pleasing gift from the various bodies to both the examiners and examinees would be some modification of dates so that examinations did not occur just around the Christmas time. Even to them and to all other of our readers, may we wish a happy Christmas.

(Alexander William Lipmann Kessel was awarded the M.B.E. and then the M.C. He qualified in 1937 and obtained his F.R.C.S. in 1947. He became a Consultant Orthopaedic Surgeon to the Fulham and Kensington Group of Hospitals. He wrote many papers on orthopaedic subjects.

Alfred William (Bill) Frankland qualified in 1938, gaining his B.M., B.Ch. and his M.A. in 1940. He obtained his D.M. in 1950 and his F.R.C.P. Hon. in 1995. He was Physician in charge for Allergic Disorders and Director of the Allergy Department of the Wright Fleming Institute. He was the author of many papers and has an international reputation and lectures widely throughout the world.)

Addendum

These letters from World War II are few in comparison to those from World War I, and the reasons for this have been covered in Chapter 26.

For those of us who were peripheral to the struggle of World War II, perhaps it is right that we do not forget the horrors of that war, which we have read about in other publications and perhaps seen also on film. These letters do not give the message that this war was the most enormous and monstrous conflict mankind has ever known.

The New Penguin Encyclopaedia gives the following facts:

In World War II, the most destructive war in history, three million Russians were killed in action, three million died as prisoners of war, eight million people died in occupied Russia.

Britain and the Commonwealth lost 600,000 men, the United States of America over 300,000: Germany lost 3¼ million military and six million total casualties, with also a loss of one million prisoners of war. France suffered ½ million dead, Japan lost two million military casualties with over ¼ million civilian deaths.

Four million Jews were murdered in extermination and labour camps and two million more in mass murders in Eastern Europe. The infamy of the German wish to exterminate the Jewish race beggars belief and this infamy was added to by the atrocious and unforgivably barbarous treatment with which the Japanese treated their prisoners of war. There was cruelty beyond comprehension, repeated and witnessed by survivors over the many years of the conflict. These facts must never be forgotten as they are a testament to how base and vile such human beings can be.

Unlike in World War I the civilian casualties in World War II and the destruction of major cities throughout Europe was on an unprecedented scale.

A new phase of warfare was entered when the Allies dropped the Atomic bombs on Japan, and the devastating results ended the hostilities of World War II.

Roll of Honour

1899–1902 South Africa

A.B. Douglas
R.H.E.G. Holt

G.W.G. Jones
G.U. Jameson

G.C. Parsons
R.P. Fort

1914–1918

C.W. Bond
A.E. Bullock
P.D.M. Campbell
H. Chell
H.N. Dale-Richards
W.H. Edmunds
S. Field
H.E.B. Finlaison
O.A.M Gibson
E.F. Gillet
W.A.S. Graham
J.A. Hawkridge
W.F. Higginson
D.R.N.O'N
   Humphry-Davy

J.W. Jackson
J.E.L. Johnson
F.C. Lambert
J.T. Leon
R. Lewitt
F.F. Lobb
W.F. Macalevey
N. Manders
G.C. Matheson
J.H. Meers
R.H. Menereau
H.C. Mulkern
E.J. Nangle
J.F. O'Connell
P. Oliver

A.U. Parkhurst
R. Pedder
F.W. Quirk
J.B. Rawlins
G. Ryley
F.M. Smith
V.R. Stewart
E.P. Stratford
H.H. Tanner
H.H. Taylor
H.J.A. Tootal
A.W. Venables
A.G. Whitehorne-Cole
E.O. Wright
R.J. Wooster

1939–1945

F.J.D. Armstrong
T.L. Butler
R. Clarke
W. Darby
C.V.R. Davies
C.H. Dent
J. Diver

D.W. Fell
H. Gimpleson
I.G. Hepburn
I.S. Jacklin
C.C. Kirby
I.L.B. Macfarlane
P.M. McRae

A. Moir
J.E.T. Munn
T.P. Myles
W.L. Patton
D.V. Phillips
S.K. Squires
G.L. Tapsall

Epilogue

The letters in this book take the reader on a journey through the nineteenth and twentieth centuries. They contain a history of the social climate that changed from the late 1800s to 1945. The status of master and servant was to change, and along with that came a greater willingness to question authority. This change has strengthened since 1945. The written and spoken word also changed: such remarks used by Handfield Jones as 'we passed through a topping forest', and 'these soldier types are fine fellows when you get to know them', would not be used now.

Punctuation changed, the comma was frequently used as were the colon and semi-colon; less so today. Indeed the art of letter-writing was to decline at the time of World War II but even more so since.

There appears at the present time to be less patriotism among the general population; at the time of the Boer War there was pride in fighting for one's country and even dying for one's country. The loss of the British Empire since World War II is perhaps reflected in the loss of pride in the general population. Indeed it is doubtful if the average civilian feels the same pride in being British, which he or she once believed was a God given blessing. Along with that past pride there was an element of arrogance, but its loss is more the pity. Today there is more criticism of our past history, but there is so much of which to be proud and there was more good in the Empire than there was ill. Much of our past pride and patriotism is reflected in these letters.

The letters have all been written by St Mary's Hospital doctors, and a few by St Mary's nurses. They have running through them a comradeship and a pride fostered in the Medical School which they regarded as special, as did other doctors regarding their own medical schools.

Dr Charles Wilson was appointed Dean of St Mary's Hospital Medical School in 1920. He was an extraordinary man, later Lord Moran, President of the Royal College of Physicians and physician to that greatest Englishman, Sir Winston Churchill. Lord Moran remained Dean until he retired in 1945. When he was first appointed the Medical School was small and badly housed. He decided it must have a brighter future. He believed that the students should be special and to achieve this he concluded that personal choice of students was better than choice by competitive examination. He travelled the country and chose the students himself. He looked for men of character and courage, capable of working in a team and gentlemanly in behaviour. He found these qualities in the best public schools, shown also in sporting ability, especially on the rugby field. St Mary's could boast of many rugby caps and many played also for the Barbarians. Four St Mary's men captained England and one captained Wales. There has been criticism of his philosophy, but the critics should examine the academic achievements of the School which includes a large number of F.R.S. awards, Presidencies of many Royal Colleges and of numerous medical and surgical societies, major advances in the fields of renal disease and hypertension, vascular and transplant surgery, immunology and the development of the anti-typhoid vaccine and the discovery of penicillin, both world-shattering in importance, and the award of two Nobel prizes, Fleming and Porter.

Much has changed since the days of Lord Moran but there is still a strong emphasis on choosing students with wide interests in addition to academic ability: there is also now a female to male ratio of about 60 to 40 per cent.

The letters in this book display the pride each doctor holds for his alma mater and the courage of many as demonstrated by Jacklin and McRae, among others, in their enormous sacrifices for their fellow man.

St Mary's Hospital Medical School is now united with Charing Cross and Westminster in Imperial College School of Medicine. Hopefully that spirit found in St. Mary's will continue to be fostered in Imperial, and long may it do so.

Index